BODIES in FORMATION

EXPERIMENTAL FUTURES:

Technological Lives, Scientific Arts, Anthropological Voices

A series edited by Michael M. J. Fischer and Joseph Dumit

BODIES in FORMATION

An Ethnography of Anatomy

and Surgery Education

RACHEL PRENTICE

DUKE UNIVERSITY PRESS

DURHAM AND LONDON 2013

© 2013 Duke University Press

All rights reserved

Printed in the United States of America on acid-free paper ∞

Designed by Heather Hensley

Typeset in Minion Pro by Keystone Typesetting, Inc.

Library of Congress Cataloging-in-Publication Data appear on the last printed page of this book.

Duke University Press gratefully acknowledges the support of the Hull Memorial Publication Fund of Cornell University, which provided funds toward the publication of this book.

TO the extraordinary
physicians, anatomists,
designers, researchers, and
engineers who took time to
teach me about their worlds.
Medicine is better
because of your skills
and dedication.

CONTENTS

ACKNOWLEDGMENTS

Looking back over the years that this project has existed in one form or another, I am awed and humbled by the generosity and support—intellectual, personal, and financial—that I have received from informants, mentors, peers, colleagues, and institutions. It is a reminder that academic work is at its best and most rewarding when it is done within the context of a community. We spend days, months, years even, alone in front of our computers, but we forget at our peril all the people who made those days and years of writing possible. Many academic communities have contributed to this book, and I count myself fortunate indeed to have worked with such extraordinary people. Any mistakes or omissions here are mine.

"These people you're writing about must be geniuses," a friend of mine said after reading an early chapter of this book. I had not put it in so many words, but openness to exploring and implementing new ideas gave the people I worked with in the field insights and achievements that one could easily call genius. The first and deepest debt of gratitude I owe is to the people whom I worked with in four academic medical centers in North America. In particular, the doctors, engineers, educators, and others I worked with in the medical school that I call Coastal University provided me with an intellectual home and an extraordinary education in matters medical and technological. Their generosity, openness, support, and good cheer were literally life changing. They accepted me as a colleague and, over time, as a friend. Every page of this book either directly or indirectly reveals their influence. The group's director gave me a home in the laboratory and showed me engineering at its broad-ranging best. The surgeons in the group taught me a tremendous amount about medicine and, as important, taught me how deeply caring physicians can be. If there is nuance in my portrayal of physicians' work, it is because of them. The anatomists, educators, computer experts, and students at Coastal all provided insights, support, and friendship.

The surgeons, anatomists, and researchers at Urban University in Canada furthered my education in medical practice over two summers. They allowed me to observe surgeries ranging from gall bladder removals to organ implantations. Allowing a stranger to observe while one does the intense and difficult work of surgery requires tremendous trust. I hope that I have honored that trust appropriately. These surgeons, too, provided insights that inform every page of this book. The anatomists at Cedar University and one anatomy professor in the Boston area all helped me understand that field's terminologies and spatial relations, as well as its history and controversies. Names of universities and names of most actors in this book are pseudonyms.

Professors Sherry Turkle, Joe Dumit, Hugh Gusterson, and Evelynn Hammonds, my dissertation committee while at MIT, provided the core of an excellent education. I often find myself sharing their insights with my own students and thinking about their brilliant work as I pursue my own. Sherry stood by me through thick and thin and provided support as my dissertation advisor. Susan Silbee came to MIT not long before I finished, bringing energy, dedication, and tremendous ethnographic skill to many graduate students, myself included. Dave Kaiser modeled everything a great academic should be (I hope I paid attention). Lucy Suchman introduced herself to me at a conference in Boston and has been an important colleague ever since. The work and the support of this extraordinary group of scholars have meant a great deal to me.

My work has had the good fortune to be read and shared by many peers in writing workshops, beginning with a student workshop at MIT and continuing with my faculty peers at Cornell. I am especially indebted to readings by Meg Hiesinger, Natasha Myers, Rebecca Slayton, and Kaushik Sunder Rajan. Each of them pushed me in ways that mattered immensely. At Cornell, various incarnations of a faculty writing group have kept me going. Anindita Banerjee, Durba Ghosh, T. J. Hinrichs, and Marina Welker all provided smart, careful feedback and lots of good cheer. Maria Fernandez, Sherry Martin, Sara Pritchard, and Kathleen Vogel provided amazing readings, often under urgent deadlines, and pushed me to be as clear as possible.

Tim Choy and Stacey Langwick read a very early version of the manuscript. I have referred to my notes of that conversation often.

My thanks to Ken Wissoker at Duke University Press and to Lawrence Cohen and an anonymous reviewer for supporting this project and for providing several excellent and constructive critiques. My thanks also to Dr. Claire Wendland, who read the manuscript and provided superb comments. Many thanks go to my colleagues in Cornell's Science & Technology Studies Department, who provided intellectual engagement and support for my thinking and writing. Mike Lynch provided excellent advice at a number of critical junctures.

This project has received tremendous institutional support, beginning with an Ida M. Green Fellowship in my first year at MIT and continuing with a U.S. Department of Education Jacob K. Javits Fellowship, which supported most of my graduate education. A Hugh Hampton Young Fellowship funded a final year of writing. At Cornell, I received support from the Institute for the Social Sciences and the CU-ADVANCE program, which supports female faculty. A year at the Cornell Society for the Humanities under Brett de Bary's extraordinary leadership gave me time to write and introduced me to marvelous scholars and thinkers from across the humanities. I am particularly grateful to Denise Riley for encouraging me to take hold of Maurice Merleau-Ponty's work and not let go. I am putting the final touches on this manuscript in the wonderful academic haven that is the Center for Advanced Studies in the Behavioral Sciences at Stanford University. I cannot imagine a better place to finish a project or start a new one.

Some of the empirical material for chapter 4 first appeared in "Drilling Surgeons: The Social Lessons of Embodied Surgical Learning," *Science, Technology & Human Values* 32(5) (September 2007): 534–53. An earlier version of portions of chapters 6 and 7 first appeared in "The Anatomy of a Surgical Simulation," *Social Studies of Science* 35(6) (2005): 837–66.

Last but not least, I would like to acknowledge the contributions of a number of feline companions, who tucked themselves into file drawers and onto piles of paper for long naps while I worked. Jasper, Cora, and the late Sushi made long hours in front of a monitor warmer and happier.

Two moments reveal the complex relations of bodies and technologies in the increasingly mediated world of biomedicine.

A surgical fellow delicately and painstakingly works to excise a tumor located deep in a patient's liver. He has spent several cautious hours opening the man's abdomen, peeling away layers of muscle, and retracting ribs to expose the cancerous organ. The fellow, whom I will call Dr. Marcos Alexander, is by all accounts an excellent surgeon.[1] Dr. Nick Perrotta, the staff surgeon supervising the operation, uses ultrasound to visualize the tumor and then, while watching the ultrasound monitor, uses a cautery to sear a line on the liver's surface. Marcos uses this line to guide his deep dissection of the tumor. At one point, his knife accidentally strays perilously close to one of three hepatic arteries, which supply blood to the liver. Nick, who has watched Marcos work for much of the tumor dissection, guides him past the artery, verbally helping him navigate between artery and tumor. Had Marcos severed the artery, the patient could have died. After the narrow miss, Nick jokes about the effect the accident could have had on Marcos's career: "[Marcos] would have some time, do some fishing." No one in the operating room laughs, but the joke told Marcos what was at stake.

I am eating lunch with two surgeons, Dr. Harry Beauregard and Dr. Ramesh Chanda, as I have done most days for several months. Harry and Ramesh have been working together to build a virtual-reality simulator for teaching minimally invasive pelvic surgeries. To perform minimally invasive or "keyhole" surgeries, the surgeon threads a camera and instruments into several small holes in the patient's body and then watches the surgical action that is taking place inside the patient's body on an overhead monitor. Putting surgery on a screen provided the inspiration for the construction of simulators for teaching. As a first step toward construction of the simulator, Harry made a graphic model of a woman's reproductive organs by using photographs of cross sections from a dead donor's pelvis. Ramesh used the same photographs to model the woman's bones and muscles. A computer expert embedded the models into the simulator. As Harry slices his apple with a surgeon's precision, I ask them a question that has nagged me for weeks: "Is it OK to let your students kill the virtual patient?" Harry and Ramesh look uncertain. While casting around for an answer, Ramesh spots Dr. Anna Wilson, another surgeon, who happens to be standing at a nearby printer. "Hey, Anna," he says. "Is it OK to let your students kill the virtual patient?" Anna does not hesitate. "Of course," she says. "They're going to do it anyway." Harry and Ramesh remain unconvinced. They say they are responsible for teaching proper surgical behavior. Avoiding harm is paramount. They might look the other way if a student intentionally killed the virtual patient, but they would never condone or encourage it. Their uncertainty stems from their role as teachers working with a virtual surrogate for a living patient. The stakes of failure differ from teaching in the clinic, but these two instructors remain unclear about their roles in this new regime of practice.

These two examples of medical training at the beginning of the twenty-first century depict a near-fatal slip of the knife and an ethical quandary. Marcos's slip is an opportunity for a lesson, couched in the form of a joke, about the medical and professional stakes of surgical practice. The moment reveals the intensity of relations among practitioners, trainees, and patients in the operating room, the high-stakes clinical setting of traditional surgical teaching. The ethical quandary emerges from the differences between treating a live patient and practicing on a virtual one. It shows how surgeons view their ethical responsibilities as instructors and how new training technologies may challenge this responsibility. During a typical medical residency, trainees work with human patients under the supervision of senior physicians. Skills are learned on the job. In contrast, advocates for medical education reform want to move some skills training out of the clinic and into spaces where medical trainees can work on virtual patients. The ethnographic action of this book takes place in these moments of practice, instruction, and change. In the first situation, a fatal slip is not an option. In the second, "death" is an opportunity to reset and try again.

Biomedical education at the start of the new millennium remains among the most grueling and demanding professional training regimes anywhere. Medical education reworks the trainee's body and being. Over the years, trainees become professionals who are prepared to bear the profound responsibility for treating others. Two questions guide this book: How do physicians become prepared technically, ethically, and emotionally to cut open a human body to examine or repair it? And how do changing technologies and practices for learning and working with bodies alter their meaning?

Medical school in North America typically involves four years of course work followed by a clinical residency that lasts from three to seven years and may be followed by a year or two doing a fellowship in a subspecialty. A majority of medical schools require students to take an anatomy course in their first year. Many include cadaver dissection as part of that training. One medical education expert said dissection is one of very few laboratory experiences remaining for most medical students. Cadaver dissection has long been a significant rite of passage for medical students. Yet time for anatomy lectures and dissections has been reduced from a full year in the 1950s to as little as six weeks today. Cuts in anatomy teaching have occurred in part because the field has declined as a research science and because medical schools have devoted increasing hours in their curricula to the biological and molecular sciences. As gross anatomy has declined as a research science, the number of qualified anatomists also has dropped, leaving many medical schools desperate for trained instructors. Yet anatomical language remains biomedicine's lingua franca, a foundation of biomedical epistemology and communication.

Following medical school, hospital residencies have been the foundation of clinical education in North America for more than a century. Medical trainees have learned their craft by working as apprentices to many masters, cultivating medical techniques, values, and wisdom within the culture of biomedicine. Medical residency involves "trading labor for training" in the words of one young surgeon. This formulation is literally true, but it collapses the technical, affective, and moral totality of residency into the abstract word "training." Those who elect surgery as a career spend years developing their craft, moving from fumbling attempts to perform rudimentary tasks, such as tying sutures, to embodied abilities to improvise from general principles and to judge when an operation might benefit a patient and when it is best to avoid surgical intervention.

Since the mid-twentieth century, balancing clinical care, research, and medical training has become a constant challenge for academic medical centers. Since the 1980s, three clinical trends that have been dictated primarily by finances have affected residency education negatively: shorter patient stays in the hospital, pressure to push more patients through the system, and the movement of many services once provided by hospitals to ambulatory care and other outpatient facilities (Ludmerer 1999). Shorter patient stays prevent residents from seeing the life course of a disease. Pushing more patients through the system curtails time for contact with patients and teaching by clinicians. Moving many types of treatment to outpatient facilities means residents spend less time with patients suffering from minor conditions and devote more time to contact with very ill patients, giving trainees less experience with more common ailments and preventing them from witnessing the course of many treatments. The redistribution of services and new modes of providing medical services have led to new challenges for residency education. Further, concerns about preventable errors have led hospitals and managed care organizations to seek new metrics for quality of care, fostering the bureaucratization of medical training (Kohn et al. 2000; Stevens 1999, xxv).

Institutional pressures on medical schools and teaching hospitals, as well as the increasing sophistication of computing and visualization technologies, have led technology designers to construct new tools for biomedical training and practice. These have included minimally invasive surgical tools and simulators designed to teach students anatomy and give them opportunities to practice surgical skills. These technologies have changed the ways that surgeons operate and are beginning to change the ways that trainees learn. They have challenged supporters of traditional teaching—for example those who support cadaver dissection for anatomy teaching—to rethink and to justify the pedagogical value of long-standing teaching practices.

As these historical trends have changed medical training, biomedical practice itself has become increasingly complex. Contemporary biomedicine in North America contains many regimes of practice, interrelated techniques of perceiving and acting that shape the physician's mode of intervening in bodies and that produce particular kinds of relations between practitioners and patients. Analyzing the professional development of medical trainees requires interrogating how trainees incorporate vast amounts of medical knowledge and how they become technically and morally qualified to intervene in human bodies. This book examines anatomy and surgery, two among many areas of medicine in which long-standing practices face challenges from technological innovators.

Anatomy and surgery, as they are taught and practiced in North America at the turn of the millennium, reveal how bodily relations in biomedicine contribute to the formation of medical professionals. Anatomists and surgeons use dissection to open bodies. These techniques of the body (in the two senses of techniques learned by bodies and techniques for working on bodies) build from the fundamental biomedical assumption that disease is located in the biological body. Both fields hew closely to the mechanical model of the human body that makes biomedicine unique among the world's medical systems (Kuriyama 2002). Opening bodies for investigation or repair is a major clinical technique. Because anatomical and surgical techniques involve direct action upon bodies, the relation between action and learning can be observed directly. Anatomy and surgery training combines development of technical skills with procedural knowledges, which accumulate and lead to the development of such higher-level abilities as intuition and judgment. Anatomy and surgery educators teach medical craft skills, often while pursuing research that promises to transform their fields through technology, especially computational visualization, modeling, and simulation. And both require emotional and ethical negotiation of strong taboos against invading another's body (Rabinow 1996; Richardson 1987). Finally, these related disciplines train practitioners in unique forms of perception that change with the introduction of new technologies.

Although both anatomy and surgery involve dissections of the human body, they cannot be treated as identical. Anatomists and surgeons have developed unique methods for opening, manipulating, and altering bodies. Anatomists dissect bodies to see and identify parts for either pedagogical or research purposes. Most North American medical students take an anatomy course in their first year that combines cramming names and locations of tissues, organs, and structures with cadaver dissection, which teaches them to open the body and locate structures in a complex, three-dimensional space. Developers of anatomical teaching tools hope to supplement or reduce expensive traditional means of teaching, particularly cadaver dissection. Further, they are working to build digital anatomical objects, such as graphic models, that can be incorporated into other technologies, such as simulators for teaching surgical skills.

Surgery, on the other hand, remains one of biomedicine's most distinctive and technologically intensive means of treating bodies. Surgeons dissect bodies as a necessary step in clinical intervention. Surgeons can require nearly a decade of training after medical school to master their craft and become qualified to intervene in patients' bodies. Surgical simulator development includes research into technologies that could speed up surgical learning and further digitally assisted modes of practice, such as minimally invasive surgery and robotic surgery. Both anatomy and surgery involve intense relations between bodies, relations that raise the question of what trainees embody when they dissect. These different purposes shape the practices and meanings of both kinds of dissection. This book examines the complex process of medical embodiment within the context of anatomical learning and surgical training.

Embodiment in Surgical Learning

Charles Bosk quotes a surgeon who said, "Surgery is a body-contact sport, there is no question about it. You can't be a good armchair surgeon" (1979, 13). The phrase "body-contact sport" reflects surgery's action orientation, particularly the ways that a resident becomes a surgeon by doing surgery. Approaching learning as it occurs from the outside in—in practice—reveals how practitioners come to embody biomedical knowledges and values. I argue that medical embodiment goes beyond the acquisition of skills to include the development of perceptions, affects, judgments, and ethics that occurs through bodily practice in a clinical milieu. The term "embodiment" calls attention to ways that human activity makes the subject. This approach reveals how human actions and interactions produce affects, knowledges, and judgments. By examining bodies as they act in the world and the persons that emerge from these actions, I show how physicians, especially surgeons, are made.

Studying the relations of bodies to objects and other bodies in surgical practice moves the focus of observation away from the visual and cognitive models that are ubiquitous in medical and social science accounts of medical learning and practice toward what happens when bodies interact with the world (Mol 2002). The role of physical interaction in the development of medical knowing remains underexplored. By focusing on practice, I treat training as a fully embodied activity, one based on the intertwining of learning and treatment, action and response, thought and feeling. This intertwining is complex. Medical education requires the accumulation of many abilities over time. Thus, the cultivation of a physician's body requires the emergence of higher-level abilities as lower-level information and skills become subsumed within them as trainees engage in meaningful practice.

My examination of bodies as they come into being through interactions—with instruments and other bodies in the hospital—builds on recent works in anthropology and science studies that demonstrate how practices produce subjects and objects. Science studies researchers have used practice as an analytic lens to focus on difficult questions about the ontological nature of scientific subjects, objects, and practices that arise when social constructivism gets taken seriously (Despret 2004a; Keller 1984; Knorr Cetina 2000; Mol 2002). Annemarie Mol (2002), for example, shows how, in practice, atherosclerosis is ontologically different in different sites of practice: it is a thickened arterial wall when a pathologist looks in a microscope, and it is pain during walking for a patient. Mol wants to show the extraordinary multiplicity of medical objects and ways of knowing them and coordinating them in medical practice.

Science studies scholarship on apparatuses, practices, and phenomena closely scrutinizes relations of subjects, instruments, and objects. Laboratory and clinical ethnographies reveal the power of opening up apparatuses, watching scientists as they use their hands and bodies to make things, and examining precisely the sorts of objects and ways of knowing that emerge from these actions (Knorr Cetina 2000; Latour and Woolgar 1979; Mol 2002; Myers 2007). Apparatuses in this view have their own agencies and indeterminacies that go beyond the intentions of their builders. Taking material agencies seriously means insisting "on the constitutive intertwining and reciprocal interdefinition of human and material agency" (Pickering 1995, 27). While humans exert themselves on objects, objects also have agency. This reciprocal agency helps explain how science and scientists are made (Keller 1984; Knorr Cetina 2000; Turkle 1995). The agency of persons and objects in medicine can help explain the formation of physicians, but medical practice also often builds around intense "moral dramas" (Good 1994, 85). In addition to specific techniques and knowledges, medical professionals must learn ways to grapple with issues that challenge their emotions, ethics, and judgment. Medical training often includes tacit and explicit lessons about these aspects of medical care. As such, affects, ethics, and judgments merit investigation, not as interior constructs inaccessible to social analysis, but as constituted by medical training and practice. Good doctors are made, not born.

If we take the approach promulgated by some anthropologists that how such things as affects, ethics, and judgments get constructed within a milieu is precisely what is at stake in the analysis of subject formation, then these seemingly interior constructs become products of sociotechnical interactions. Saba Mahmood draws on Aristotelian, Foucauldian, and anthropological works on practice to argue for a powerful role for practice in the affective and ethical formation of subjects. She writes, "*Habitus* in this older Aristotelian tradition is understood to be an acquired excellence at either a moral or a practical craft, learned through repeated practice until that practice leaves a permanent mark on the character of the person" (2005, 136). Practice, according to this view, makes ethical behavior a technique of the body.

Drawing from the strengths of both science studies and anthropological approaches, medical embodiment becomes an analytic frame that brings together the careful specificity of laboratory studies with the analytics of subject formation from anthropology. Using this approach, I treat perceptions, affects, judgments, and ethics as embodied through situated practice. Medical training embodies medical skills and medical subjectivity through specific practices. Technology developers and promoters have opened many long-standing medical practices to new scrutiny, making them more accessible to actors and analysts alike.

The narrative of this book tacks back and forth between close examination of traditional medical training and analyses of technological challenges to medical practices. This allows me to focus on the material practices of medical training. I show biomedical work as uniquely embodied. Like trainees in many professions and crafts, medical trainees come to embody distinct ways of knowing, acting, and being through lived social and material arrangements, relations, and actions; they become physicians by acting and interacting with colleagues and patients, technologies and pathologies, bodies and persons. Advanced medical training, especially training within particular specialties, leads physicians to develop unique regimes of practice, culturally distinct styles of interacting with persons, bodies, and pathologies. The development of new technologies for teaching and treatment brings practices from other fields, such as engineering and computer science, into medicine, fostering the development of new techniques for working with patient bodies, such as diagnostic work done across large distances using telemedicine technologies. Three themes related to the technical, ethical, and affective formation of physicians run throughout this book: the relation of practice to the formation of medical subjects, the ways in which a focus on embodiment can correct a visual and cognitive bias that runs through academic and practitioner discussions of biomedicine, and a separation of the formation of medical objects from the often pejorative concept of objectification.

Practices and Subject Formation

A medical trainee embodies the technical, ethical, and emotional lessons of biomedical work over time, gradually incorporating techniques of the body, becoming a physician by practicing medicine. Theories of practice provide a powerful means of analyzing the formation of physicians, especially within the context of clinical work. Practices as they contribute to subject formation have received much anthropological attention, particularly in relation to three decades of scholarly focus on bodies (Lock and Farquhar 2007; Mahmood 2005). Margaret Lock and Judith Farquhar argue that, since the 1970s, "lived bodies have begun to be comprehended as assemblages of practices, discourses, images, institutional arrangements, and specific places and projects" (2007, 1). The significance of this statement lies in its refusal to treat bodies as automata controlled by minds or by societies. Instead, this approach puts bodies into active relation with the world. The Deleuzian word "assemblage" suggests that the arrangements and relations that compose bodies contain multiple elements that can be disassembled and reassembled, implying possibilities for change over time. To analyze medical education and practice in a moment when technologies are changing rapidly, I show how medical embodiment develops and changes as trainees and physicians learn and work, revealing the power and durability of ways of sensing, feeling, and acting in medicine that develop with accumulated practice, as well as continuity and change in relations among bodies that occur with technological change.

Physicians' affective and ethical responses to patients emerge as trainees develop technical skills within the situated milieu of a teaching hospital. Anthropological literatures on practices as they make and remake subjects often begin with Marcel Mauss's observation that bodily techniques, everything from swimming strokes to walking styles, vary widely across cultures and histories. Mauss argued that these "techniques of the body" are trained, involving imitation of techniques accomplished by someone with authority or prestige. Mauss's approach finds social meaning in the techniques themselves, in what social actors do with their bodies. Glossing Durkheim, Mauss argues that techniques of the body meld physiological, sociological, and psychological into the "total man" (2007, 53). His focus on the interplay of bodies, societies, and psyches represents one reason to return to this early twentieth-century theorist.

Many scholars have cited Mauss's ideas about culturally unique techniques of the body. Less often cited is Mauss's observation, contained in an apparent aside about how swimmers diving with their eyes open are bolder in the water than those who dive with eyes closed, that techniques of the body also produce affect (2007). By treating affect as a product of training, I show how medical educators inform trainees' affective responses and learning. For example, within the world of biomedical training, some anatomy programs promote emotional learning by encouraging medical students to participate in such activities as memorial services for cadaver donors and their families, reminding students that the cadavers they dissect are the bodies of former persons and deserve respectful treatment. These anatomy instructors work from the assumption that students who learn to treat their cadavers with respect will extend that respect to their patients.

Another reason to return to Mauss is methodological. Mauss's focus on what bodies do when they perform techniques calls for a specificity that can be productively adapted for studies of anatomical and surgical learning. I show how simple acts can contain different meanings for surgeons at various points in their education and careers. The first incision in a body, for example, may represent a highly charged event for a new medical student doing a dissection, an interlude on the way to more interesting work for a chief surgery resident, or an opportunity to teach surgical landmarks for a staff surgeon. Yet a fundamental biomedical commitment to limiting harm done to patients and a largely uninterrogated belief in the power of biomedical treatments to heal underlie these differences. By focusing on specific techniques as they develop and change over time or with the introduction of new technology, these meanings can be opened to analysis.

Medical students must become not only technically qualified but also ethically qualified to practice. Ethics in biomedicine often are discussed in abstraction: as principles and dilemmas in ethics courses, as prescriptions by professional ethicists, and in philosophical discussions about the Hippocratic Oath. "First do no harm" is adapted from Hippocrates' *Epidemics* and is a moral imperative that physicians are reminded of constantly.[2] But the ethics of doing no harm are only occasionally invoked explicitly. Instead, they are constantly reinforced within the context of day-to-day medical training. Focusing on practice shows how trainees and instructors in medical schools engage in practices and commentary that keep the principle present even while teaching technical skills. These institutional and pedagogical practices instill technical, affective, and ethical dispositions for relating to patients. Although the technical aspects of these abilities often are made explicit, their affective and ethical components typically are not. Affect and ethics in this analysis are neither natural internal states nor consciously adopted positions. Rather, they are embodied through action in the clinic. This makes them durable, part of the becoming body of a physician. This also makes them resilient and resistant in the face of rapid change.

Surgery requires the development of bodily techniques that cumulatively lead to a powerful "feel" for bodies, pathologies, procedures, and instruments known variously as intuition, judgment, and, ideally, wisdom. A surgeon I know uses a sports metaphor for medical embodiment, saying that after about a thousand procedures, surgeons get "in the zone," reaching a level at which they have experienced most things that could go wrong and have learned solutions to most problems. Surgeons use many metaphors to sports, to war, and occasionally, to other activities that are highly physical and highly skilled, such as dance. Sports metaphors for surgical work reflect the traditions of macho behavior among surgeons (Cassell 1991, 1998). They also reflect surgery's connection to areas of human endeavor, such as sports and dance, that combine intense physical training with strategy, choreography, improvisation, and, often, coordination with a group.

The notion of embodied dispositions that guide actions resists models of learning that assume that the learner masters a set of rules or plans (see Suchman 1987 for a discussion of rules-based learning). Yet rationalizing forces in biomedicine, including the development of treatment protocols, evidence-based medicine, and procedural checklists, increasingly encourage physicians to follow strict procedures that dictate their actions (Berg 1997; Gawande 2009; Timmermans 2003). As scholars have shown, the move toward rationalized medical practice has had mixed results: checklists can help reduce procedural errors (Kohn et al. 2000), but rules-based decision making can lead to rule-bound thinking that limits practitioners' abilities to reason through unusual or unusually complex cases (Groopman 2008). Supporters of more bureaucratized means of ensuring performance often are also supporters of technologies, such as training simulators, that can provide trainees with opportunities to practice outside clinical settings and can chart their progress using clear-cut, precise, and mechanized means of assessment. These technologies would allow medical educators to control the content and assessment of medical skills more than they can in clinical settings, where clinical care (with all the contingencies and needs of a patient population at any given moment) is a primary goal. Thus, new training technologies often are accompanied by more bureaucratic methods of assessing achievement. These new technologies and practices can lead to new techniques of the body and new modes of medical subjectivity.

Practice, Vision, and Cognition

Returning to the surgical scene that began this book, the surgical actions described involve several practitioners' bodies. Opening an abdomen, peeling aside layers of muscle, and retracting ribs is hard physical labor. Visualizing a deep tumor requires ultrasound machinery and the ability to read what it registers. Searing a line on the liver requires coordination of hands, eyes, and instruments, as well as the ability to fluidly translate between two and three dimensions. Dissection of a tumor that lies deep in the liver and close to a major artery requires skilled use of the knife and simple bodily techniques that steady the surgeon's hands. Making a corrective joke requires timing and a sense for how to balance the seriousness of a possible mistake without rattling the fellow who nearly slipped. Surgery involves the whole person.

Yet medical educators often describe medical learning as the formation of mental models. The cognitivist notion of medical work has dominated clinical research into medical decision making since the 1970s (Berg 1997). The advance of computational tools for diagnosis and visualization has strengthened this cognitive focus, in part because cognitivism has pervaded the computational sciences, especially artificial intelligence. In the field of anatomy, tensions exist between dissection proponents, who assume that anatomy training develops bodily, affective, and ethical ways of knowing bodies, and technology designers (some of whom are also anatomists), who assume that learning entails the formation of mental models of anatomical language and structure. The cognitive approach to learning ignores the embodiment of technique, perception, and emotion in the development of a physician's craft. This cognitive focus has consequences for medical pedagogy and for medical technology development as designers replicate the cognitive approach in the tools they build.

The cognitive bias among medical practitioners and technology designers likely is the product of Euro-American traditions that split mind and body, as well as of the cognitive explosion in the biological sciences. I have heard simulator designers talk about their field as "applied cognitive science." Even surgeons, who are fully aware of the physical nature of their work, tend to talk about the "mental models" they want trainees to develop.[3] Eyes and minds are, of course, active in medical work, but examining what physicians do with their bodies as they act and interact reveals the significance of other senses, instruments, and actors in medical learning and practice.

The cognitive focus is accompanied by a related bias toward the visual, a bias reflected in the focus on the visual in Euro-American thinking about the senses generally (Geurts 2003). This bias creates several problems for the analyst. First, emphasis on the visual neglects the connection between seeing and doing. Much of surgical action, for example, involves techniques intended to create the conditions needed for the surgeon to peer into the body, but these techniques are as much about making the body available to action as to vision. Second, a visual bias neglects other senses, including touch, proprioception (the sense of one's body in space), sound, and smell, which also play a role in biomedical practice. For example, surgeons must develop a feel for variations in toughness among different types of tissue and among different individuals. Third, as with the language of mental models, a focus on sight puts emphasis on the construction of a representation. For example, analysts have focused on the visual aspects of anatomical learning (Good 1994, 72) and on the construction of a surgical operative site that resembles an image in an anatomical atlas (Hirschauer 1991). Biomedicine is undeniably visual, as these ethnographers show, but focusing exclusively on how anatomical and surgical dissection constructs a visual representation misses both the pedagogical purpose of naming structures and locating them in three dimensions in anatomy training and the pragmatic purpose of effecting change in the patient's body during surgery.

Focusing on specific techniques and the *habitus*, the "acquired excellence at a moral or practical craft" (Mahmood 2005, 136), that develops as a trainee learns bodily techniques in a clinical setting allows me to move beyond a visual and cognitive bias that often is shared by medical practitioners and observers alike. By showing those practices that cultivate medical and surgical ways of acting, being, and believing, the analyst can see how much of the work of learning and practicing medicine emerges from bodily work that is not exclusively visual. Vision is a significant component of medical work, but its significance can be overstated. One anatomist, for example, said he gauges his progress in opening the spine more by sound than by sight. As he chisels through bone, he cannot see when he reaches the spinal column, but the sound changes as his work progresses. The auditory signal does not need to be converted into a visual image to provide him with the information he requires.

The concept of mental models also misses the indeterminacy of what can lie inside a practitioner's mind. Oliver Sacks, in an article on mental "imagery," describes wide variations in states of internal representation among people who went blind as adults. These range from absolute darkness and an accompanying atrophy of visual concepts, such as "in front of," to powerful mental images augmented either by rich imaginings or by cautious checking against real-world referents. Even among those with unimpaired sight, how the world outside is "seen" varies internally from precise, three-dimensional visual images to complete darkness. Sacks (2003) describes at one extreme his mother, a surgeon and comparative anatomist, who once studied a lizard skeleton for just a moment, then drew a series of lizard skeletons, each rotated 30 degrees from the last, without glancing at it again. He contrasts her extraordinary visualization abilities to those of a vascular surgeon who said he was unable to visualize anything in his mind's eye (he said this mental blindness ran in his family). He could not have operated without having embodied some understanding of human structure, but it was not visual knowledge, that is, he did not "see" human structure in his "mind's eye."

Sacks suggests that the mind may have its own language, one that is not visual or linguistic or auditory or tactile, but is all these things and then some. His tales of variations in visual imagining suggest that knowledge defined as mental imagery is misleading, neglecting the rest of the body's role in knowing. The consequences of a visual or cognitive bias are significant. The purely cognitive model of medical learning erases two bodies: the patient's or cadaver's body becomes a model, and the practitioner's body becomes a mind. The practices and affects related to dissection and other forms of medical learning disappear and the problem becomes the ancient and insoluble philosophical problem of the correspondence between a reality in the world with a model in the mind (Bergson 1998; Mol 2002; Plato 2007). Treating medicine as largely a visual or a cognitive undertaking creates a philosophical aporia, a gap between representation and reality that is impossible to bridge. Beyond philosophy, the representational bias in medicine creates two problems. First, it focuses pedagogical and technological research on whether new techniques and technologies produce an accurate mental model of an external reality rather than on the pragmatics of what the trainee or practitioner can do. Second, the language of mental models erases bodily, social, and relational ways of knowing that have little to do with mental constructs.

Examining medical embodiment as the construction of a sociotechnical assemblage of the sort that Farquhar and Lock describe reveals much greater depth and complexity of bodily relations in biomedicine. One surgeon I worked with said that she tells her residents to become part of a shoulder (or other body part) when they operate. The act of opening a shoulder to find pathology is itself an invasion of the body; residents must become aware that they and their instruments are constructing a body that has been invaded by instruments and opened to vision and action at the operative site. The residents and their actions form part of this body during surgery. The surgeon indicates to her residents that they cannot extract themselves from the bodies of their patients: they are deeply implicated in what happens in the operative site. In this sense, the surgeon resembles animal experimenters as described by Vinciane Despret: "The experimenter . . . involves himself: he involves his body, he involves his knowledge, his responsibility and his future. The practice of knowing has become a practice of caring" (2004a, 130). Despret shows how experimenters often try to extract their presence by removing all traces of the effects they have on an experimental system. She also shows that this is impossible. Care, in Despret's sense of the word, reflects a deep affective engagement with the subjects of one's research, an investment in bringing one's knowledge, one's body, and one's being to bear upon the work of understanding. Surgeons, like experimenters, are never outside the reality they make with their patients.

Surgeons make the surgical body. By wielding particular kinds of instruments in the operating room, surgeons create a body that is mechanical, a body that can be fixed by opening up, patching, replacing, and rerouting its pieces. The process of learning surgery is a process of mutual articulation: surgeons learn the surgical body by creating the surgical body as they work in the clinic. Surgeon-body and patient-body come into being together. This process of becoming is not the construction of a representation. Treating surgical work as mutual articulation leads us out of the aporetic gap between representation and reality. The surgeon does not have to make the operative site correspond to an anatomical representation or to any "natural" body that could exist without the surgeon. Instead, the surgeon has to create a body that is available to surgical intervention. Yet availability to intervention must be constrained by the necessity of keeping the patient alive and able to be returned to something closer to its preintervention state. While there are conventions of practice that facilitate vision, these are simultaneously practices of intervening and of representing (see Hacking 1983).

Objects and Objectification

Biomedical modes of explanation and perception locate pathology in anatomy. This structural conception of disease and illness has ancient roots (Kuriyama 2002), but also provides the epistemological foundation for surgical practice. For example, one day in the operating room, a hand surgeon opened up a knuckle to reveal the arthritis inside. She pointed out that the joint's surface was pinkish, like chicken bone, and said the discoloration was a sign of degraded cartilage. I was uncertain about whether I had seen the arthritis. "Arthritis" was a linguistic object but not yet a material object for me. Later, however, the surgeon opened up another patient's knuckle to reveal its pearly-white, healthy surface. I could see the difference and began to have some understanding of what arthritis looks like to the naked eye. Arthritis had become a material object for me. In this moment in which arthritis became a material object, the first patient's personhood was present in a brief discussion of how her injury and a subsequent infection may have caused the arthritis without her awareness. Arthritis-as-object and woman-as-patient remained ontologically distinct during this interaction.

Much of the social science literature on biomedicine describes how practitioners objectify their patients, reducing them to bodies or pathologies, treating their conditions as material-biological phenomena divorced from related social and historical circumstances that may be pathogenic (Clarke et al. 2003; Hahn 1983; Scheper-Hughes and Lock 1987). The biomedical reduction of patients to clusters of symptoms can be dehumanizing (Young 1997). Some patients argue that many physicians fail to see them as persons. Objectification often is considered pejoratively, as an unfortunate function of modernity that "connotes a lack of agency and even motion, a distancing from the world, a lack of self-recognition, an abuse of others" (Keane 2007, 10). The social and political stakes become who or what gets to count as person or thing (Johnson 2010; Langwick 2011). Objectification becomes problematic when it leads physicians to ignore sociohistorical pathogenic factors or to give patients too little agency in processes of understanding and dealing with pathology.

One can, however, construct objects without objectification in the pejorative sense, such as when the surgeon taught me how to see arthritis. The same hand surgeon tells nervous patients that she plans to "borrow" their arm for a while, but that they should not be concerned: she plans to "give it back." Clearly this move alienates patients' arms from their personhood. But examining the process reveals that this objectification is temporary. By asking to borrow a patient's arm, the surgeon temporarily separates it from the patient's personhood, creating psychological distance between the patient and surgical actions upon the arm. This objectification makes the surgery affectively easier to grapple with for patient and surgeon. Patients can use objectification of their own bodies to distance themselves from painful procedures or poor outcomes, a phenomenon Charis Thompson calls "ontological choreography." Thompson (2005) documents how some patients in fertility clinics will describe their infertility as a problem of ovaries or hormones, rather than a problem of self. Similarly, anatomy students and surgeons often objectify bodies to create distance, to appeal to the patient's agency, or to show respect and compassion. That is, patients and practitioners regularly separate body part from person to make pathology or treatment possible or acceptable. Objectification in biomedicine can contain nuanced behaviors that trouble assumptions that objectification always is alienating or dehumanizing.

Further, the argument that socially informed perception constructs the objects of perception can lead to a slippage between objectification and object formation. Object formation, such as the visual apprehension of arthritis, is a function of medical perception that is broader than the more explicitly ideological concept of objectification. By separating the processes of object formation from objectification in biomedicine, one can disaggregate the effects of medical perception from the loss of patient personhood. The objects of our perception, as Merleau-Ponty describes them, begin with the visual apprehension of a field and then the mental discernment of figure (object) and ground (2002, 78). What gets to count as figure and what gets to count as ground can be socially or psychologically conditioned. Thomas Csordas makes Merleau-Ponty's observations more obviously sociocultural by showing how perceptions are always already socially shaped, before they end in conscious apprehension of an object (Csordas 1990, 1993, 1995). Thus, the perception of arthritis as roughened cartilage reflects a long-standing biomedical tradition of seeking anatomical sources for pain or affliction. The identification of potentially pathological objects clearly is part of biomedical training, which teaches physicians to use sight, hearing, smell, and touch to discern an enormous number of objects—roughened cartilage, gurgling lungs, a perforated bowel, a lump—that may indicate disease or abnormality. Much as geologists learn to read the landscape for cues about its formation, its structure, and its disasters, physicians learn to use their senses to read bodies to understand their variations and their pathologies. Physicians develop a perceptual syntax that begins from the assumption that pathology has its basis in biology and allows them to use their senses to diagnose pathology and to extend those senses into diagnostic technologies.[4] Thus, medical training brings many objects into the trainees' world.

Surgeons learn to see and feel differences among tissues and pathologies through years of opening and comparing bodies in the operating room (see Foucault 1973 for an anatomical comparison). Surgical perception brings together human perceptual capacities that are partly situated in our material beings as humans with our particular biology (see Haraway 1990; Merleau-Ponty 2002), with historically and culturally situated training of perception (see Deleuze 1988; Foucault 1986, 2005; Rajchman 1988), and with the specific practices of physicians (Howell 1995; Mol 2002). Historical circumstances, social formations, and material-discursive structures shape how things are "*made* visible, how things [are] *given* to be seen" (Rajchman 1988, 69). The specific socially and historically situated practices of medical education play a profound role in creating and shaping biomedical perception. This entails the bringing into being of vast numbers of medical objects, many of them parts of human bodies and their pathologies. Throughout this book, I show many processes by which physicians come to recognize objects and some processes by which they learn to objectify patients. By separating object formation from objectification, I hope to show that the construction of objects in biomedicine is a foundational practice, rooted in the anatomical search for disease. When the malady becomes conflated with the patient, then object formation becomes objectification.

Technological Change

Residency programs have struggled to ensure high-quality clinical education in light of structural changes, such as growing numbers of medical school faculty who devote their careers almost exclusively to research and the financial squeeze put on academic medical centers as a result of managed care. Efforts to reduce errors in hospitals also have played a role in attempts to retool medical education (Kohn et al. 2000). Physicians who are redesigning medical education want to move some teaching out of clinical settings and make trainee practice more systematically organized and more thoroughly assessed (Fried and Feldman 2008; Satava 2008). Because of the catch-as-catch-can nature of residency training on hospital wards, however, many of these efforts cannot be achieved without providing objects for trainees to practice upon whenever they want and as often as they need. Further, educators must attempt to anticipate the kinds of technical skills physicians will require in the future. Biomedical trainees and practitioners increasingly interact with advanced technologies for learning, imaging, and practicing medicine. Many of these technologies, such as the specially designed cameras and tools used for minimally invasive surgery, require extensive training to use properly.

Technology designers have worked for more than three decades to build digital technologies, such as virtual bodies, which have moved some physician training out of anatomy laboratories and operating rooms. Explicitly and implicitly, physicians and designers who are bringing new technologies and new ideas about practice into medicine challenge the methods of medical teaching that prevailed during much of the twentieth century. Some argue that the current system of medical learning requires overhaul (Fried and Feldman 2008; Satava 2006). Others defend traditional curricula but say that requiring trainees to develop some skills before they work on living patients would make operating-room teaching safer and would ease crushing time demands on surgeons in teaching hospitals. When I finished fieldwork in 2006, some residency programs had introduced simulators to teach rudimentary surgical skills, such as manipulating the camera for a minimally invasive surgery. Exactly how these technologies would combine with other recent changes in medical training, such as mandated cuts in residents' hours, remained unclear. But debates about the merits of traditional methods versus new technologies for medical teaching offer practitioners, designers, and social scientists opportunities to question current pedagogy.

To build medical teaching technologies, designers—who include physicians, engineers, and computer scientists—are disassembling physicians' habits, customs, and ways of thinking and acting. Similarly, patients' bodies are being made digital, reduced to pixels that can be reconstructed as graphic models. Both patients' bodies and practitioners' bodies are being articulated graphically and mathematically, so they can be reassembled in virtual worlds and made manipulable. This reworking of bodies and actions is not neutral: technology designers build their own assumptions about bodies, actions, and practices into their machines, assumptions that are changing medical practice (see Forsythe 2001). Not least, the concept of "practice" shifts from learning to work as a professional within the situated milieu of the hospital, with all the social lessons such practice entails, toward a greater emphasis on repetitive drills undertaken outside the clinic and on formal assessment of skills acquisition. This may affect physicians' abilities to communicate and interact effectively with patients, or it may simply bring practitioners into the clinic with a stronger set of skills.

The rationalizing logics moving into medicine from technical fields dedicated to quantification, precision, and "efficiency" have three features. First, they make bodies into informatic "body objects," digital and mathematical constructs that can be redistributed, technologized, and capitalized. Second, they are allowing medical knowledges to be distributed among more technologies and practitioners. And third, they are mathematizing embodied practices that become naturalized with training and practice, such as a physician's ability to detect cancerous changes with touch, so that they can be recomposed in computers and other instruments. While rationalizing drives in medical education remain partial and fragmentary, many proponents of simulation and formal assessment seek a thorough technological and bureaucratic restructuring of medical training, especially surgical training, as it has been practiced since the early twentieth century. This book explores some ways that the introduction of new technologies and rationalizing logics has begun to reshape medical education and practice. Keeping practitioner embodiment firmly in view allows me to show how new technologies and practices encourage subtle shifts in medical perception.

Finding the Body in Biomedicine

This project began more than a decade ago in a fluorescent-lit computer room in the basement of a building at MIT. Assigned by a pair of professors to write about a "computational object," I considered writing about virtual frog dissection, but the programs I found contained crude and uninteresting photographs and line drawings of specimens. I found myself drawn instead to the extraordinary and disturbing images of a male and a female cadaver created from the image databases of the U.S. National Library of Medicine's Visible Human Project. The decontextualized and strangely colored images of two naked cadavers with closed eyes and bodies flattened in death begged for analysis. The National Library of Medicine had contracted with researchers at the University of Colorado to create image databases of two cadavers, each as anatomically normal and pathology-free as they could find. Researchers procured the bodies of a thirty-nine-year-old man and a fifty-nine-year-old woman. They imaged the bodies using computed tomography (CT) and magnetic resonance imaging (MRI) technologies, then froze the two bodies and ground away cross sections, taking photographs as they revealed each new section (Spitzer 1996). They made the resulting databases easily available to researchers for medical and computer modeling projects. The project gained notoriety because the male body was that of a death row inmate, Joseph Paul Jernigan, who was executed by the state of Texas. The choice of a prisoner's body for the project received wide media attention (see also Cartwright 1997, 1998; Csordas 2001).[5]

By imaging entire bodies, the library hoped to create complete anatomical image databases that would provide the foundation for anatomical modeling and other medical research applications. Project directors argued that computational anatomy could supplement or even substitute for cadaver dissection. I wondered about the sensory aspects of such a shift. What would anatomy students experience if they undertook cadaver dissection on a virtual cadaver? Would the loss of touch or smell or sound leave them lacking some fundamental aspect of the experience? As a pilot study, I asked a dozen people—with and without medical training—to look at these images and tell me what they thought. Some had sensory questions similar to mine. Others asked how a doctor would become properly attuned to the person inside the body if training was limited to virtual bodies. These early questions structured some of my research, leading me to explore how biomedical practitioners and technology designers use virtual tools.

When I began this project, I planned to study the differences between virtual and actual dissection by attending anatomy courses. My first major surprise came when I visited a laboratory doing research into computer applications using graphic and anatomical models. I learned that few anatomists use Visible Human or other virtual bodies for much more than identifying structures in images of anatomical cross sections. The sophisticated and frequently beautiful models developed by the computer experts often gathered virtual dust in some digital cubbyhole. The models suffered from what one anatomist identified as a gap that left projects stranded between public funding for basic research and private funding for development. Yet researchers in laboratories around the world were using these digital images and others like them for research into medical teaching technologies. Though little used for training medical students, they had become standard bodies that computer experts could use to verify their algorithms and compare them to others' work.

Curious about how anatomists deployed images, models, and real bodies in their courses, I spent six weeks in the summer of 2001 taking an anatomy course designed for physical and occupational therapists. I learned some anatomy and began to explore the responses of some students, including myself, to dissected bodies. In the anatomy laboratory, I marveled at the depth of muscles in the back and the number of layers of muscles in the palm of the hand. Learning to read bodies in three dimensions is a critical aspect of anatomical learning. This begins with terms such as *medial* and *lateral* (toward and away from the body's centerline) and *superficial* and *deep*, which locate anatomical features in the body's space. Over time, most physicians develop a profound understanding of the body in three dimensions. In the anatomy laboratory, the senses also aid dissection: anatomists use the sounds and the feel of changes under their instruments to guide their hands. Although practices such as smelling or tasting a patient's urine to diagnose diabetes have either disappeared or are being replaced by numbers on a graph or readouts on a machine, sensory training remains a strong component of medical education.

The human body as depicted in the anatomy course I took is an extraordinary wonder of nature, and I marveled that bodies work as well as they do. Seeing the beauty of the dissected body is easy in an engraving by Vesalius or a print by Leonardo. But finding the beauty in a preserved cadaver in the laboratory often requires work to overcome the feelings and associations evoked by the cadaver. Many students I spoke with described taking some time to become accustomed to dissection. One researcher said the disturbing qualities of working with cadavers "just went away" over time, returning only occasionally when some aspect of the cadaver reminded participants that a specific person had once inhabited the body.

The same summer as the anatomy course, I visited several laboratories seeking one where I could reside as an ethnographer documenting the development and adoption of digital teaching tools for medicine. I first visited the laboratory that I call the Coastal Information and Medical Technologies Laboratory on a hot, dusty day in August 2001, winding my way past Coastal's hospital and several major laboratory buildings to find the unimposing brown stucco building that housed the technology development laboratory. Medical schools across North America have spent the past thirty years negotiating the tension between traditional teaching and the promise of digital tools to save time or reduce costs. Coastal remains at the more traditional end of the spectrum, using digital teaching tools primarily to strengthen and supplement existing lectures and laboratories. Simultaneously, the university also has been a leader in the development of digital technologies since the 1940s. On my first day at the laboratory, I spoke with surgeons, engineers, computer scientists, and education experts. I watched demonstrations of computer applications the group had developed. Laboratory researchers had extensive practice giving demos and presenting their devices and programs, all with a medical pedagogical purpose. I examined a program intended to teach embryology, which received scant attention in the school's curriculum. Researchers hoped that the embryology application and others like it would provide effective supplements to the standard curriculum. I also looked at the beginnings of a virtual emergency room, a blocky set of graphic corridors filled with oddly angular and awkward virtual people. The project, partly supported by a prominent video game development company, would simultaneously allow researchers to create the emergency room as a teaching technology and allow the developer to test their company's three-dimensional rendering software. This blending of medical, computational, and industry research is a common arrangement among laboratories in this field.

"I feel as though I'm missing something," I wrote in my notes while sweating in a train station after my visit. "Maybe it's the focus on the body as a human body." Initially, I worried that interest in the body was missing from the laboratory, but I later realized that the people I had spoken with that day were deeply immersed in building technologies designed to teach trainees how to work with specific body parts. Yet none of these researchers invoked "the body" as the kind of macro concept that has become ubiquitous in the social sciences and humanities, especially since the 1980s. The body as concept did not exist for these engineers, surgeons, and educators. Nor was "the human body" particularly important. Rather, what mattered to these researchers were parts of bodies with which one could do things.

The fragmentation of bodies is a hallmark of biomedicine, whose epistemic foundations rest upon the assumption that pathology is located within specific anatomy. When physicians seek pathology in organs, tissues, chemistries, regions, or systems, they assume that the whole body, including the person inhabiting the body, is largely irrelevant to the inquiry, except sometimes as a vehicle for symptoms (such as skin problems caused by food intolerances). Bodies are ubiquitous in this world, but seemingly contradictorily, "the body" is not a particularly useful object for medical practitioners. As Annemarie Mol (2002) has shown, medical bodies are multiple; a body may be different for different types of clinician and patients. Not only are bodies multiple for different actors, but body regions are multiple across medical specialties. The pelvis, for example, is a complex system of bones and joints for an orthopedist, a network of vessels for a vascular surgeon, and a cluster of reproductive organs for a gynecologist. Understanding biomedicine's reduction of bodies to parts, pathologies, and bodily phenomena is key to understanding object formation in biomedicine and the means of constructing technologies for teaching medicine.

I arrived for a longer stay at Coastal in November 2001, expecting to spend my time shuttling between the technology design laboratory and Coastal's anatomy laboratory. I had coffee with the anatomists many mornings and spent afternoons trying to understand what researchers did to build digital tools. The laboratory focused, among other areas of interest, on haptics, the study of the tactile and kinesthetic forces at work on the human hand. Surgical simulators with haptics might enable surgeons to get a feel for surgical tasks in a way that simulators without such feedback would not. After playing with the haptic devices in the laboratory, I realized that I would need to know much more about surgical work and the tactile and kinesthetic relations among bodies in surgery. As a result, I spent an afternoon dissecting a cadaver elbow with a surgeon and anatomist, which deepened my conviction that the use of senses other than vision is an understudied component of medical work. Whether because of the use of my hands or because of the emotions connected to dissecting (though this moment was less charged than others), I remember the lessons (how to cut, where to find the ulnar nerve) and the sensations of dissection more vividly than many other laboratory experiences.

I began spending the occasional Tuesday in the operating room watching one of the laboratory's surgeon-researchers do hand surgery. I observed about twenty procedures in operating rooms at Coastal, but I later realized that a genuine discussion of operating-room practice would require far more observation time. So I spent a summer watching surgeons and their trainees affiliated with the medical school at a school I call Urban University in Canada in 2006.[6] I chose Urban in part because surgeons there were researching new methods for teaching using simulation. Physician-researchers at Urban were developing a simulation center intended to bring together several types of simulated teaching. They also were creating new training and evaluation methods intended to take advantage of the user's ability to reset and retry simulated surgeries.

Observing surgeons expanded some of my inquiries, encouraging me to think further, for example, about the translation between two-dimensional imaging technologies and three-dimensional bodies. Surgery also raised its own emotional and ethical questions, such as the meaning of "do no harm" in a field in which treatment begins only after violence has been done to the body. Further, though I saw surgeons get angry or frustrated when things did not go well, I never saw the emotional toll that surgery takes. I watched an entire operating room groan with dismay upon opening a patient and discovering metastatic cancer. I wondered whether such experiences ever got discussed. For myself, I had to leave the operating room for several weeks after a nine-hour liver implantation that should have taken four hours. I had been standing on a stool overlooking the patient's abdomen while surgeons sewed and resewed blood vessels that kept springing leaks (evidently a function of the patient's physiology). I waited until the surgeons finished to retreat, but the tension, the heat under the lamps and layers of clothing, and the smell of blood left me drained and overwhelmed. The surgery left me with much greater respect for surgeons' fortitude and stamina. But I wondered then, and still wonder, how they cope with the peculiar combination of tension and concern for the patient that such an experience creates.

Overall, I spent eighteen months observing and interviewing trainees, physicians (mostly surgeons), technology builders, and educators. I was in residence in the laboratory at Coastal for ten months, then returned several times, as I continued to follow the laboratory's work. I spent three months at Urban. The ethnographic approach that I took entailed, in the words of anthropologist Rayna Rapp, "hands-on research that is open-ended, and locates the researcher as far into the experiences of the people whose lives are touched by the topic as she can figure out how to go" (1999, 2). My work included formal interviews, informal conversations, observations of surgeons performing operations, and observation of anatomical dissections done by surgeons, anatomists, and students. I went to two annual conferences in the field, Medicine Meets Virtual Reality and the American Telemedicine Association meeting. I sat in on dozens of hours of meetings related to anatomy and simulation projects being used to test a federal high-speed Internet system and on dozens more regarding a large server in development to store and make available physicians' image collections. My informants often opened exciting new avenues of inquiry during the least formal interactions. For example, a surgeon began an important critique of simulation that I hastily tried to write down as he and I hustled at his normal breakneck speed between the operating room and the lunchroom for a quick bite between surgeries.

Early on, I decided that the project would be about the formation of physicians and that patients would not be a significant focus of this project. Anthropologists and others have done important work comparing patients' perspectives to physician perspectives and have found surprising and sometimes tragic differences in understanding (Fadiman 1998; Mol 2002; Rapp 1999), but I chose instead to focus on differences in understandings within medicine and between physicians and technology builders. I organized a weekly coffee and discussion about medical topics for Coastal researchers. These typically focused on a news or academic article on a medical topic. Many long quotations from group sessions come from these meetings. During these sessions, physicians' hunger for conversation about their work became clear. It seemed as though the daily pressures of clinical work and technology research, as well as the discomfort of many nonphysicians with medical topics, left little time for these doctors and educators to reflect on the meanings and larger issues of their work.

Cumulatively, I gained a picture of medical training that is changing, but more slowly than technology builders and promoters might hope. Many of the computer technologies that saw the most rapid deployment in teaching were very specialized systems built by a specific faculty member for a particular course. Commercial development has continued, and some medical schools are pushing forward with simulators for training. But by and large, no revolution in medical training has occurred. Some of the technologies and practices I discuss in this book eventually will enter medical training and practice, and some will not. Regardless of the future of simulation for medical training, the technologies reflect rationalizing approaches and logics that already have led to changes in medical practice (see Berg 1997) and will continue to bring new logics, especially from engineering, into medicine. Movement among the spaces of medical teaching, surgical practice, and technology development became a necessary research method for this project. I had to establish what exists in typical medical training and practice before the changes that technologies might bring would make sense. Each of these spaces—anatomy laboratories, operating rooms, and design laboratories—informed the others. Technology designers have begun to open established medical practices to new kinds of analysis and new challenges. Questions technologies researchers raised about knowing and touch, for example, led me to spend more time focusing on surgeons' hands when I entered the operating room. The intertwining of existing practices and new technologies thus shapes the chapters of this book.

The Plan of the Book

The order of sections in this book is arranged by field site—anatomy laboratories, operating rooms, and technology design laboratories—because this roughly mirrors the historical development of these sites and is a common trajectory that practitioners tend to follow. But this movement should not be read as teleological: there is no inevitable movement from Vesalius to the virtual. Developments in one area fold back on others. Many projects that technology designers have worked on, such as developing a means of transmitting touch over a computer network, have led to scientific excavations of the role of such phenomena as touch in traditional medical teaching. Further, the promise of technological change has brought new urgency to preexisting pedagogical questions, such as the value of cadaver dissection.

The first section, on anatomy, considers anatomy laboratories as spaces where medical students begin to cultivate affective stances toward patients and as spaces where dissection as a pedagogical tool is increasingly contested. Chapter 1 looks at how medical schools implicitly teach students to objectify cadavers and, increasingly, to activate the person who once lived in the cadaver. Physicians and social scientists have long argued that dissection involves progressive detachment: students must learn to manage and temper emotional responses (see Fox 1988). This chapter seeks to nuance this narrative of detachment by reexamining cadaver dissection. It reveals that students' profound emotional and philosophical reflections on the cadaver's ontological status help prepare them for the complexities of treating patients' bodies and respecting their persons. A process of tactical objectification helps students manage the emotionally difficult work of practicing medicine, while also helping them to acknowledge their patient's humanity.

Chapter 2 opens up the controversy within anatomy teaching over whether to drastically curb or eliminate cadaver dissection. The chapter shows how reductions in anatomy teaching emerged from the rise of cellular and molecular biological sciences. It also shows how many who challenge dissection take a primarily cognitive view of anatomy education, arguing that students must learn names and structures of the body, eventually developing a "mental model" of human anatomy. Dissection proponents, on the other hand, argue that anatomy education introduces students not only to anatomical terms and structures but also to the ethical, social, and emotional demands of medicine. Anatomists' debates index a central concern of

North American biomedicine today: Should good healing engage a physician's mind, body, and emotions, or should physicians focus exclusively on marshaling and utilizing biomedicine's extraordinary accumulation of information and powerful tools for diagnosis and intervention?

The second section examines the technical, ethical, and perceptual lessons of surgical residency. Chapter 3 considers medicine's hidden curriculum—the informal lessons of teaching through clinical apprenticeship—and the ways medical learning becomes embodied. The chapter describes physicians' cultivation of affect and judgment as preparation for the care of others. These seemingly subjective aspects of a physician's professional persona begin with "prestigious imitation" of superiors (Mauss 2007, 54). Physician affect becomes structured in clinical interactions, where trainees have to manage their own feelings and, often, those of patients. Judgment, in this sense, becomes less the application of abstract rules to real-world situations than an affectively informed product of accumulated practice and observation in a structuring environment. Putting the trainee's body at the center of analysis brings the agency of the practitioner together with the effects of clinical interactions. This approach allows me to consider technological and institutional change in conversation with embodied learning and practice.

Chapter 4 shows the ways that technical training in surgery embodies lessons about surgical ethics. In particular, it reveals how surgeons teach control as a technical and ethical value in the operating room. Senior surgeons utilize verbal and nonverbal teaching methods in the operating room, ranging from almost subliminal guiding of a resident's hand, which shapes the action while giving the resident a sense of near-total autonomy, to jokes that convey deep lessons in more or less lighthearted ways (Goffman 1961b; Katz 1981). By examining how trainees simultaneously craft surgical sites and their own knowledge, I connect surgical socialization to embodied material practices. This chapter examines interactions of surgeons, trainees, patients, and technologies in several surgeries to consider the lessons a trainee incorporates while in the operating room. It reveals how surgical teaching that appears purely physical contains ethical lessons about the values of control in the operating room.

Chapter 5 examines minimally invasive surgery, revealing how doing surgery while looking at a monitor subtly shifts surgeons' perceptual relations to patients' bodies. This chapter explores the relationship between open surgery and minimally invasive surgery, a relatively recent addition to a surgeon's suite of tools. It shows how perceptual changes evolving from minimally invasive techniques result from the practice of open surgery and from the stance surgeons adopt in relation to the patient's body. The chapter counters literatures that find remote and digital technologies disembodying. Further, it reveals the ways new technological practices both emerge from existing practices and lead to genuinely new perceptual experiences.

The third section, on technology design laboratories, considers challenges to traditional medical ways of knowing coming with the introduction of new technologies and rationalizing logics into medicine. Technology design laboratories bring together researchers from diverse fields, including engineering and computer science, medicine, and education. Researchers with exceptionally different ways of knowing must negotiate and build medical technologies for teaching anatomy and surgery. Chapter 6 argues that virtual reality and other simulation technologies in medicine have become central to reformers' efforts to shift clinical apprenticeships toward a mode of learning that is more standardized and more bureaucratized. This evolution changes the mode of practice that occurs during residency from practicing within a profession to practicing to master a skill, a shift toward a disciplinary model of practice that resembles other kinds of skills training. This shift in the notion of practice represents one way that instrumental logics—logics that break down the actions of the human body and reorganize them with efficiency, optimization, or capitalization in mind—are moving more deeply into medical teaching and into the bodies of patients and practitioners.

Chapter 7 breaks down the elements of a virtual-reality simulator for teaching surgery to explore the ways simulator researchers have broken down the bodies and embodied relations of patient and practitioner. This chapter examines in depth the development of a simulator for teaching surgical skills to reveal the ways that technology builders have constructed relationships between user and simulation, that is, interactions between eyes and screen, hands and devices, virtual instruments and virtual bodies. Each of these interactions can be seen as a form of articulation, or bringing into being, of bodies, instruments, and relations.

The conclusion considers ways that the disassembly of bodies and actions taking place in medical technology design reveal how instrumental logics enter, challenge, and reconstruct bodies and practices in medicine.

Bodies are being rebuilt to meet the needs of computers. Practices are becoming decontextualized, partial, and removed from patients. But unexpected new relationships among bodies in medicine also are emerging. Technical logics can have depersonalizing effects, but technologically mediated medical practice remains the art of human healing.

one

"A FASCINATING OBJECT"

With some doctors, I get the feeling they're not seeing
the part of me that's not my body.
A PATIENT

Take my body. Use it well. Become a good doctor.
TAKEN FROM A NOTE WRITTEN BY A FUTURE CADAVER
DONOR TO MEDICAL STUDENTS

On the first day of a cadaver demonstration in an anatomy course I took, a student had to leave the laboratory because tufts of hair emerging from the cadaver's ears reminded her of her grandfather. In that moment, the cadaver became a former person, one who reminded the student of someone she loved. For her, the cadaver was no longer a scientific object. This phenomenon is common among medical students: some detail, such as ear hair or a tattoo, brings the cadaver's personhood to the fore, making dissection emotionally difficult. Students also often have strong emotional reactions when they dissect anatomical areas that evoke a cadaver's humanity and personhood, such as genitals, faces, and hands.

Cadavers are persons and things. This ontological duality cannot be resolved, but it can be managed through practices that encourage students to interact with cadavers as persons or as objects. Cadavers remain the most important objects-subjects in a formative rite of passage in North American medical schools: the anatomical dissection. Cadavers help students become physicians, in part by helping them shift from treating bodies as persons to treating bodies as the objects and the subjects of clinical inquiry. Although dissection as a pedagogical practice is in decline, most North American medical students still dissect cadavers in the anatomy courses they take in their first year. Defenders of dissection say the experience provides two benefits for medical students. First, dissection demonstrates a real, if not in vivo, example of the body's structures, and it helps students begin to develop a biomedical stance toward patient bodies. Second, it helps medical students to begin to craft their own bodies as practitioners while they craft others' bodies.

The cadaver often is a medical student's first exposure to medicalized human bodies, to bodily interiors, and to death. Students must grapple with the emotional intensity of destroying a human body. Dissection, whether it takes place in an anatomy laboratory or operating room, requires working against many ethical, legal, and religious traditions that prohibit doing damage to living and dead bodies. Several physicians I spoke with alluded to these taboos, saying what they do would be considered "psychopathic" in any other context. But medical and surgical education, as well as broader faith in biomedicine, makes dissection an important and accepted learning experience. In the past, students kept their feelings about dissection to themselves. Describing the anatomy course he took in the 1940s, Dr. Richard Hunt, a retired anatomist, said, "If you had weird feelings about the cadaver, you never dared tell anyone." Since the 1950s, however, anatomy programs have seen a steady rise in attention to students' affective socialization. Programs at the turn of the millennium do far more to give students opportunities to express their feelings and, in related ways, to engage in practices that summon the cadaver's personhood.

Biomedicine typically takes a "radically materialist" stance toward bodies, diseases, and treatments, approaching humans and their diseases as grounded almost exclusively in biology, excluding other explanatory frameworks (Scheper-Hughes and Lock 1987). Marilyn Strathern argues that biomedical physicians also seek, often in relatively impoverished ways, to "activate the person," who often gets erased amid biomedicine's objectifications of bodies and pathologies (2004, 8). In this chapter, I examine how anatomy training constructs cadavers as persons and as things.[1] I also explore how anatomy courses manage student emotions, how students respond, and how similar constructions of patient bodies as persons and things come into play in clinical settings. Finally, I draw upon anthropological literatures on embodiment and emotion to connect medical training to the cultivation of an affective stance toward patients and their bodies. Students in anatomy laboratories learn to treat bodies within a materialist paradigm, while also cultivating means of engaging the patient's personhood. In other words, students learn to put the cadaver's ontological duality at the heart of what I call "tactical objectification," the ability to objectify the body or call forth the person as needed.

Objectivity and Objectification in Biomedicine

By the early 2000s, many medical schools had cut their anatomy curriculum from a year or more (which was common in the 1950s) to a semester or even a few weeks. Medical school administrators argue that cutting anatomy teaching has enabled them to make room in the packed curriculum for more leading-edge sciences. They also chafe at the cost of running a willed-body donation program that provides medical schools with teaching cadavers. During eighteen months of fieldwork from 2001 to 2006, I interviewed anatomy instructors at four medical schools, took a summer anatomy course, and did participant observation of anatomy courses, dissections, and other activities in two laboratories. Even among programs that remained most committed to traditional anatomy teaching, anatomists and technology builders often discussed the reduction or elimination of dissection at other schools, debated the merits of dissection versus demonstration with previously dissected materials, and considered how they could use imaging and modeling technologies to replace or supplement dissection. The threat to dissection as a pedagogical practice raises questions about what lessons, beyond knowledge of anatomical structures, the dissection holds for students.

Many nonphysicians I spoke with worried that biomedical training alienates physicians from their patients' humanity and that virtual anatomy or virtual dissection might further distance physicians from their patients. They expressed concern that a physician's sense of touch, empathy, or morality might remain underdeveloped without the experience of dissection. Physicians expressed concerns about the effects on medical students of reducing the hours spent dissecting or of eliminating dissection altogether. They argued that trainees must prepare themselves for the emotional rigors of clinical work and acquaint themselves with death and dead bodies.

There is something paradoxical in the notion that future physicians should study dead bodies, however real, to understand their patients' humanity, but the history of medical and scientific objectification of bodies coexists with the "still present sense that the body and its parts are always more than things" (Rabinow 1996, 149; see also Richardson 1987). Laypeople and physicians alike find significant ontological differences between "former" persons and scientific models ("never" persons), differences related to a cadaver's ongoing personhood. They see engagement with the cadaver's personhood as vital to physicians' moral and emotional development. The cadaver is never just an object.

A growing literature in science studies shows that the construction of an object of inquiry often involves the simultaneous construction of the scientific self (Daston and Galison 2007; Knorr Cetina 2000; Turkle 1995). In contrast, the social science literature on dissection has focused primarily on the achievement of a practitioner's "objectivity," including students' attempts to detach their treatment of the clinical body from opinions and emotions, or on objectification of the patient's body, finding that medical education teaches practitioners to set aside the patient's personhood and treat only the body. Medical students in the 1950s learned the value of "detached concern," the belief that medical empathy requires professional distance (Fox 1988). One student, who performed his first autopsy in the 1950s, told the sociologist Renee Fox, "You have to overcome some of your emotion . . . and learn to look at things objectively and scientifically" (1988, 68, ellipsis in original). "Objectivity" in this usage becomes a synonym for emotional detachment. This is consistent with widespread faith in the values of science, objectivity, and the containment of emotion, which was stronger in the mid-twentieth century than it is at the beginning of the twenty-first century. These students' views of objectivity clearly fit within the construction of objectivity at a time when researchers considered detachment from self to be necessary for effective scientific or clinical discovery (Daston and Galison 2007).

Fox updated her study of medical students in the 1970s, arguing that, during the intervening decades, physicians had become much more concerned with developing the proper values and ethics in relation to patients. By the 1970s, physicians no longer valued the "omnipotent" physician or an attitude of "detached concern." Similarly, an objective stance would be viewed with some regret as interfering with "feeling with a patient" (Fox 1988, 100). Though Fox does not identify historical shifts that led to this change, she describes the trainees of the 1970s as far more concerned with issues of justice, equity, and resistance to the negative socializing effects of the medical "System" (96). Just a few years later, Donald Pollock (1996)

found that so many students described their struggle to retain their humanity and empathy, despite "the System," that this belief itself seemed to be a
hallmark of late twentieth-century medical education. He used physicians'
autobiographies to suggest that stories about bucking the system reflected a
concern with the rise of impersonal bureaucratizing and technologizing
forces in biomedicine. He argued that the concern with resistance represented an essentially conservative appeal to values of individualism and
moral responsibility, rather than a call for systemic reform (352). As Fox and
Pollock show, the value of detachment in medicine came under increasing
scrutiny in the latter half of the twentieth century as physicians sought to
distance themselves from a medical system perceived to be dehumanizing
and impersonal. The language of detachment remains ubiquitous in medical and social science depictions of medical training. Detachment does
occur, but I have observed more nuance than these depictions convey.

Anthropologists have documented biomedical practices that construct
the patient as an object (Good 1994; Hahn 1983; Scheper-Hughes and Lock
1987; Segal 1988; Young 1997). Scheper-Hughes and Lock (1987), for example, describe biomedical practitioners' pervasive separation of mind and
body, which leads to the uniquely biomedical construction of disease as
pathology contained in the patient's body, a construction that is not universally shared. They observe that the biomedical epistemology that objectifies
patients' bodies is simultaneously effective and alienating. Looking at anatomy laboratories, Byron Good describes medical students struggling to
alternate between seeing bodies as bodies in the anatomy laboratory and
seeing bodies as persons when they leave (1994, 73). These discussions describe objectification as an often unfortunate product of the biomedical
reductiveness that constructs ailments as discrete entities located in human
tissues—that is, as objects.

In most of these discussions of the development of objectivity and of the
objectification of bodies, the personhood of cadaver or patient, if mentioned
at all, is construed as a threat to detachment and emotional control. While
these authors' informants view empathy as desirable, they treat most emotions as negative or threatening states that training mitigates, either through
the socializing effects of instructors and peers or the rationalizing effects of
science itself. These views reflect European and North American cultural
traditions that treat emotions as internal forces of irrationality and disorder
that threaten reason and good judgment. "To be emotional is to fail to ra-

tionally process information and hence to undermine the possibilities for sensible, or intelligent action" (Lutz 1986, 291). This cultural bias shapes the view that emotional responses that go beyond compassion complicate good clinical practice, not least by clouding the practitioner's judgment.

The ontology of the body and the practitioner's emotional stance toward bodies and the persons who inhabit them clearly relate, but not in simple ways. Do patients or practitioners benefit from a practitioner's emotional detachment or from the objectification of a patient's body? Are the benefits of detachment or objectification clinical, emotional, or both? Answers to these questions are diverse: for every patient who wants an empathic physician, another wants clinical reserve. And for every physician who prizes his or her own detachment, another fears that too much distance may damage doctor-patient relations.

Charis Thompson (2005) studies patients in reproductive clinics to explore questions of agency and objectification of bodies. She finds that patients engage in complex practices of coordination of ontologies of their bodies as a means of managing the complex relations of technological fertilization to ideas of self, nature, and society. Thompson calls this use of objectification of one's body "ontological choreography." She says patients in in vitro fertilization clinics often objectify their own bodies. They say, for example, "My ovaries are not cooperating" when a procedure fails. Conversely, they may take ownership, saying, for example, "I am pregnant" when a procedure succeeds (189).[2] By extending Thompson's important finding to practitioners and training practices, I show how medical training promotes and strengthens practitioners' abilities to engage in similar forms of ontological choreography by teaching trainees to objectify bodies or to activate persons, as needed. Practitioners learn these responses to distance themselves or their patients from difficult or disturbing biomedical procedures or to appeal to their own or their patients' humanity or agency.

Thus, ontological choreography is a common psychological move to create distance through objectification or to create ownership through appeals to personhood. I argue that medical training teaches and reinforces the trainee's ability to objectify the body or activate the person as needed.

Persons and Things in the Laboratory

Many ethnographic discussions of laboratories show how they reconfigure natural phenomena by reconstructing them as scientific objects. Human bodies in the anatomy laboratory are no exception. I have visited anatomy laboratories in several schools, finding them tucked away, on dusty top floors or in dark basements, far from the prying eyes of curious visitors who might wander by. Objects in anatomy laboratories—rolling steel tables, blue body bags, scalpels, and skeletons—locate them as spaces for investigation of human biology, connecting them to clinical work and, in a broader sense, to scientific research. Laboratories are "enhanced environments," where objects are detached from their natural order and "upgraded" to become available on demand to researchers (Knorr Cetina 2000, 28). The cadaver is the primary object of inquiry in the anatomy laboratory and, although "upgrading" might not be the correct word for embalming, the process slows decomposition, changing the cadaver's relationship to time to allow deconstruction by students rather than digestion by microbes.

While I was doing research in the anatomy laboratory at Coastal University, I observed several anatomy classes, assisted with dissections, and spent an afternoon dissecting an elbow. The lab is new and technologically sophisticated, but otherwise typical. It occupies the basement of a steel-and-glass building housing biology laboratories and classrooms on upper floors. The laboratory space resembles an operating suite, where most work takes place within a restricted core surrounded by peripheral functions. This arrangement creates the effect of a progressive introduction to dissection. The basement houses a main anatomy laboratory, a receiving area for bodies that is closed to the public, an office that keeps its anatomical identity understated, and several faculty offices. When I was there, instructors, technicians, and other staff had coffee in the lunchroom every morning. The scene would have fit a corporate or office lunchroom, except that dusty Vesalius prints depicting cadavers in classical poses competed with the cat calendar on the wall. Dark humor, such as one technician's remark that, after spending the day preparing donated bodies, he was exhausted from "lifting dead weight all day," punctuated the quiet flow of business.

One enters the main laboratory area through double doors with signs restricting access to those authorized. At the time, three human skeletons held together with wires dangled from the wall and greeted visitors when they entered the antechamber. To the right of the skeletons was a trashcan lined with a red "biohazard" bag in front of a bank of heavy steel sinks stocked with gloves, scalpel blades, and soap. The anteroom led to an inner room holding the dissecting bays, each containing a small shelf for anatomical atlases and other books, a small chalkboard, cubbies for backpacks and coats, and a large steel dissecting table. Cadavers on the tables were shrouded in bright blue plastic bags when not in use. The colorful bags make the space look less sterile and forbidding, despite their contents. A powerful ventilation system sucks out most odors, but the laboratory retains a faint, pervasive odor of embalming fluids and cleaning materials underlain with a slight odor of organic tissues that other chemicals never quite erase. Generations of medical students have said the smell of embalmed tissue generates powerful memories of the anatomy laboratory that persist for decades (Fox 1988, 58).

At Coastal, teaching assistants and technicians often wore surgical scrubs in the laboratory. Instructors and most students wore street clothes, occasionally donning scrubs or white laboratory coats over the top to protect street wear from chemicals. Anyone who planned to touch a cadaver had to wear gloves, but clothing changes were optional. The laboratory thus began students' transition into clinical clothing and safety practices. This mix of medical and casual garb made the laboratory, like the medical school itself, a liminal zone between university and clinic.

Students learned correct laboratory behavior both from explicit lectures and from modeling by instructors and assistants (see also Fox 1988; Segal 1988). Mark Smith, a third-year medical student at Coastal, said his instructors and assistants made dissection ordinary:

> Something that helps is that you see other people interacting with cadavers, like it's an everyday known process, like it's easy to brush your teeth. If everyone was in there freaking out, I think you would have a really hard time overcoming anything. But everyone is so calm about it and they are open to listening to your thoughts about it, if you want to involve emotions. They are willing to talk about it and they take it very calmly and so it's easier for you to slip into that same network.

Instructors, assistants, and peers made the experience mundane by treating dissection as business as usual: emotional reactions can be contagious, but so can calm. Mark suggested that daily practice habituated students to dissecting dead humans, making dissection an ordinary part of their daily routine, like brushing their teeth. The availability and sensitivity of instructors and students in talking about emotional issues further eased student worries.

Standardizing procedures make cadavers resemble something closer to a model than a human being. Before embalming, cadavers are shaved, giving them a more uniform look. Embalming both preserves the cadavers and changes colors and textures. Vivid reds and whites become browns and grays. The degree of embalming seems to affect students' perceptions of personhood. Fox's informants in the 1950s described their cadavers as "mummified," whereas bodies dissected at autopsy, immediately after death, appeared much closer in time to living people, producing powerful emotional responses in students (Fox 1988, 57). Students now dissect cadavers that, to reduce chemical exposure, have undergone less embalming and look less mummified than in the past. And the anatomical dissection now provides some of the emotional lessons that the student autopsy, which has largely disappeared, once offered (Fox 1988). The degree to which a body resembles either a dead and desiccated object or a living person—that is, the body's apparent distance from life—affects students' emotional responses.

Many anatomical procedures, including embalming and shaving, have instrumental purposes, but they also strongly situate the cadaver within the realm of technoscience. A shaved and embalmed cadaver nestled in a blue bag atop a table amid a roomful of similarly laid out cadavers becomes homogenized, losing some of the distinctions of facial features, skin color, and hair color that typically identify persons. A look at Vesalius's sixteenth-century *De Humani Corporis Fabrica* or at eighteenth-century Florentine wax cadavers reveals how cadavers have been displayed differently (for images of these waxes, see Taschen 2001). Vesalius depicted cadavers in poses similar to those of classical statues, occasionally placing them amid ruins, sometimes holding their own flayed skin. The eighteenth-century wax models, painstakingly made from observations of hundreds of cadavers, show bodies posed on purple pillows with gold tassels. One female wax model has a pearl necklace, flowing tresses, and an abdomen open to view. Cadavers posed to evoke classical art or nobles at rest can be jarring to twenty-first-century eyes because they are removed from twentieth-century traditions that construct cadavers as scientific objects rather than as persons set in nature or displaying their social status.

Most anatomy programs provide students with little information about the people who donated their bodies for dissection. Many programs give students the cadaver's age and cause of death to help them make clinical correlations. Some programs tell students the cadaver's first name, while others maintain strict anonymity. If no name is given, students often name the cadavers. Richard, the retired surgeon and anatomist, named his cadaver "Ernest," so he could describe himself as "in dead Ernest." Students who name cadavers personify them, but in a limited way, less as autonomous persons than as objects, like dolls, which receive names because the people doing the naming have strong connections to them. Naming the cadaver gives students control over and responsibility for this object-that-is-not-an-object. In many historical and cultural traditions, naming locates the person socially (Mauss 1985). Anonymizing the cadaver removes it from the person's social world, disconnecting it from its previous life, family, and position. Renaming by students brings the cadaver into their social world—the laboratory. The cadaver becomes a privileged object, not a person, but a quasi subject with whom students develop a bond that encourages many to take particular care of the cadaver and to remember it long after their laboratory experience ends.

Anatomical language further reinforces anatomy's status as a science of medical objects. Even the name of the body itself changes. According to Wendell Park, a clinician turned social scientist:

> We didn't say "dead body." We called it a cadaver. Once you use this term, it seems to me you're not seeing the dead body. It's in a medical context.

Wendell said that medical language shifts the body into a medical context where dissecting a cadaver becomes something very different from cutting up a dead body. Medical language distances the student from a body's personhood—a personhood that might be more evident if a student were to use the words "dead body" or "corpse." The term "cadaver" identifies the body as a medical-scientific object, not a person who once was alive. Linguistic anthropologists have argued that no empirical means exist to separate language and culture (Martin 2000). Anatomical language begins the acculturation of medical students, separating them from the ordinary world and initiating them into the culture of biomedical practice, in which anatomical terms are the lingua franca. Fingers become phalanges. Arms and legs become upper and lower limbs. Each nerve, vein, and artery and each of their branches receives a clinical anatomical name, rapidly immersing the student in a unique language describing the body and in the utterly unique culture of biomedicine (see Good 1994).

Fundamental laboratory practice furthers the dead body's semiotic reconstruction as medical object. The basic setup of the dissection has changed little since medical education became standardized in the early twentieth century. Students typically work in groups of four students for each cadaver. They dissect and compare tissues to depictions in an atlas to identify, name, and fix those structures in their memories. The exposure and identification of tissues focus student attention on body parts and their names, the objects that compose the human body, rather than on whole bodies. By this biomedical logic, diseases are found in organs, tissues, and systems, rather than in the whole body or in phenomena located outside the body (Scheper-Hughes and Lock 1987). Histology, molecular biology, and biochemistry further reduce the body's functions and dysfunctions to its smallest structural underpinnings (Good 1994). At each level, the notion that persons, rather than bodies, get diseases becomes more abstract.

Despite the cadaver's strong contextualization as object, the fact that it is a former person remains inescapable. Instructors often cover faces and genitals until students dissect those areas. Students also begin by dissecting the cadaver's back, legs, or chest, areas considered less likely to be disturbing. Many students say the cadaver's personhood overtakes them when they dissect highly charged areas, such as hands, genitals, and faces. I argue that these body parts strongly evoke personhood among contemporary North American medical students for three reasons. Hands mark these bodies as human and often are tools for action and communication. Genitals mark gender, which is among the most powerful bearers of identity. Especially in North America, genitals also typically remain hidden to others in all but the most intimate settings. And faces mark bodies as belonging to individuals with inner lives, lives whose vicissitudes have been such an important part of Euro-American concepts of self and person.

Like body parts, marks on a body, such as a tattoo or a tan line from a wedding ring, give the cadaver a history and a social life. When I partially dissected a cadaver arm, the arm had a tattoo with the words "Vivien Leigh, 1944." The tattoo gave the cadaver a history and a social identity that I could speculate about. The arm no longer belonged to a generic body; it came from a person whose "specific embodiment" (Haraway 1990, 190) had come to the fore. I wondered what led the man who died to put Vivien Leigh's name on his arm.

In these emergences of personhood, the opposing category is significant. Laboratory practices strongly situate the body as an object. The cadaver becomes an example of human anatomy, similar to a model. The object-cadaver can be named, manipulated, cut into pieces, and, ultimately, destroyed. But the person-cadaver is the remains of an individual who, at one time, had control over his or her own body. The person was born, named, raised within a family and community, and was a person who enjoyed the rights typically given to persons. The bodies of persons retain some of their sacred associations, associations that neither an increasingly secular world nor faith in scientific materiality can dispel (Bynum 1992; Rabinow 1996; Richardson 1987). But concerns about personhood and sacredness decline as the distance of body parts to the person increases.

Activating the Person

In recent years, medical schools have instituted more practices that evoke the persons who originally inhabited their teaching cadavers. Richard, who took anatomy in the 1940s, said his generation of medical students had more experience dealing with death prior to medical school but also was more reticent about expressing feelings. He described a large shift in how anatomy instructors introduce students to cadavers now:

> In the old days, it was push them into the room with the cadaver and, if they have sensitivity about it, then they're probably in the wrong place. And that is certainly not the way it is now. As you know, we have all these memorial services for the cadavers. We have an introductory series talking about where these cadavers came from, and that they wanted this to happen. We read some things, letters from donors, and that sort of thing, and we used to have a [plaque]. . . . It was actually by a donor who said, "Take my body. Use it well. And become a good doctor." At first, us old folks [asked], why do you have all this sensitivity business and all that? . . . But I have become convinced that it is a place where you can show by example some levels of sensitivity towards human beings, one another, as well as the cadavers.

Richard said that a historical shift had taken place in the ways anatomy programs introduce students to the cadaver. Most significant, instructors now explicitly address emotional aspects of dissection and demonstrate more sensitivity both toward cadavers and toward fellow practitioners.

Richard mentioned that anatomy programs increasingly encourage students to think about cadavers as former persons by discussing the voluntary nature of donation, reading donor letters, and encouraging student reflections on their own feelings by writing or drawing pictures about their expectations, anxieties, and fears. Letters from donors are a means of post-death address, a last word from the person who gave his or her body. The act of writing a letter to one's future dissectors marks the donor as a person who sets the process in motion. Letters give the dead a voice, stressing donors' agency in choosing to have their bodies dissected, agency that students say eases their qualms about dissection. As with the donor's injunction to use his body well, a letter from a donor sets up an obligation for the student: it offers the student something precious—a body—with the expectation that the student will learn from that body. The gift is altruistic (the donor receives nothing in exchange), but it nevertheless sends the student a powerful message about the donor's expectations and hopes (see Lock 2002).

Since the 1980s, most North American medical schools have incorporated memorial services into anatomy laboratory courses in North America as part of their efforts to humanize the social relations of medical practice. They invite family members of donors to attend. During these services, students present their reflections on their anatomy experience and the meaning of the donation.

When I did research at Urban University, Cassie Brown, an anatomist and biologist, had run memorial services there for more than a decade. She made students write memorial remarks for Urban's service. She said they are testimonials to the profound development that students undergo during their anatomy training:

> I make them write what the experience of dissection has meant for them. What they turn out is so profound. They grow from a caterpillar to a butterfly in that short time. You would cry, it's so beautiful. . . . They've talked about the nail polish on the fingers of their person. They relate intimately with this person that they're dissecting. And a kind of respect and a compassion builds up. And [those descriptions are] my proof.

Families of donors often told Cassie that they felt better about the future of medical care after attending such services, largely because of the medical students' words. Cassie's statement about nail polish may seem odd in this description of student metamorphosis, but it resembles statements I heard often from anatomy students: details that defy the cadaver's standardization and its construction as model bring forth its personhood. Respect and compassion grow from reflections upon these details and from weeks or months of relating with a former person, who gave his or her body so students could learn.

A memorial service for anatomical cadavers can mark the end of a medical student's first major transition into medicine. As the name suggests, memorial services shift focus from the cadaver body to the place the body will hold in the memories of students and family members. The ceremony returns cadavers to their original status as deceased family members, as persons whose bodies were treated as objects in the laboratory, but who must now be symbolically returned to their previous social milieu. Lesley Sharp (2001) describes how physicians who procure organs for transplantation objectify and dehumanize brain-dead persons, largely as a means of distancing themselves from the gruesomeness of dissecting a brain-dead body, whereas organ donors' family members seek to memorialize the person whose body parts have gone to prolong others' lives (see also Hogle 1999). In contrast, medical-school memorial services bring donor families and students together, bridging the distance between families and practitioners as students come closer to the perspective of those who have lost a loved one. Memorial services also may prepare students for encounters with surviving family members later in their careers. Anatomists describe such practices as helping students stay focused on the cadaver's humanity. Only persons, members of a social group, receive memorial services.

Prior to the enactment of the Uniform Anatomical Gift Act in 1968, medical schools in the United States culled their cadavers from the unclaimed dead. Fox cites a student saying that the lack of family connections made the dissection more "impersonal" (1988, 60). Students from other countries where dissections of the unclaimed dead still occur told me they had similar feelings. Bodies with no family to mark the end of a life are the most abject of former persons. An aspect of the personhood at issue in cadaver dissection is the individual's embeddedness in a network of social relations. Unclaimed bodies have already suffered social death.[3] In an apparent contradiction, North American medical students now take comfort knowing that their cadavers are "gifts" from voluntary donors. Voluntary donors were persons who had authority and agency to donate their bodies. The contradiction rests on the distinction between thing and person: unclaimed bodies become identified as things, whereas voluntary donors become identified as persons who exercised their right to determine the fate of their bodies. Both situations clarify the cadaver's ontological indeterminacy in ways that make dissection more emotionally acceptable.

Within anatomy programs, the language of "gift" and "donation" is ubiquitous, resembling the language of organ donation, which often is described as the "gift of life."[4] As Margaret Lock has written, such altruistic gifts represent donation as a choice, one consonant with the North American ideology of "the right to dispose of one's property as one wishes" (2002, 318). The notion that our bodies are our property is deeply ingrained in North American values. In some traditions including those of ancient Rome and the antebellum southern United States, persons were legally distinguished from slaves because slaves did not own their own bodies (Kopytoff 1986; Mauss 1985). More recently, legal cases that deny patients rights to profits from inventions made with their tissues and bodily substances wrestle with conflicts between ownership and an ongoing sense that the material body, regardless of how fragmented or alienated, retains some essence of the person (Landecker 2000; Rabinow 1996).[5] Two aspects of donation language are significant: first, that the donation is an individual choice, which is strongly valued in North America; and, second, that a right of disposal is a right granted to legally recognized persons, who are deemed competent to make such a decision. The language of gift invokes a person who is capable of making such a gift. Anatomy programs use the words "gift," "donation," and "donor" to tactically call forth the cadaver's personhood as a legal entity capable of entering into a contractual relationship to give a medical school control over his or her body after death.[6] The voluntary nature of the gift underscores donors' desire to have their bodies used for medical research after their deaths. A person thus becomes someone who owns his or her body and can choose to give it away after death.

Emotional Preparation

While discussions of medical training within the social sciences tend to put boundaries around medical school and residency, most medical students have spent years preparing for medical school, and rites of passage occur throughout and beyond a resident's early years of clinical practice (Hahn 1983). In contrast to the science courses that dominate the early years of medical education, the anatomical dissection often is a medical student's first experience that bears some resemblance to clinical work. Most anatomy programs prepare students in various ways for their first day of dissection. Some anatomists I have talked with say they prefer to avoid "the touchy-feely stuff" of addressing students' emotions, but even these teachers talk with students about the significance of donating one's body to medical schools and the need for students to maintain respect for the cadaver.

The preparation done in the course I took at a Boston-area medical school in 2001 was typical of the anatomy programs I have observed. Dr. Jerry Kaplan, the instructor, stated in a lecture that the bodies were donated, and the donors knew what would happen to their bodies. Respect for cadavers was required, he said; medical schools would expel any student caught doing anything inappropriate to a cadaver (see also Hafferty 1988). As he spoke, Jerry displayed two slides of a cadaver, front and back, on the screen behind him. This marked the start of a process of progressive desensitization as the time of our encounter with the cadaver approached. One young woman left the room when these slides appeared on the screen. When she returned ten minutes later, the slides were still up, but she kept her gaze focused on the table. Jerry also gave students a video he had made. In the video, Jerry gave several lessons in musculo-skeletal anatomy using a previously dissected cadaver. I watched the video in my office and found it more disturbing than looking at the cadaver in the laboratory. Other students described similar feelings, perhaps because the video allowed us to look at a cadaver out of context, away from the privileged space of the laboratory, which is a space of enclosure where dissection is sanctioned.

During his lecture, Jerry addressed possible student concerns by making a series of jokes. He said preserved skin looks a lot like chicken and could put students off chicken. He turned to a student in the course who had done dissection; she confirmed that she had been unable to eat chicken for months. The exchange had a bantering quality that made it funny, as though a reluctance to eat chicken is absurd. He then said anatomy programs use fewer embalming fluids than in the past, but that anatomists live long lives because they already are "half pickled." Finally, he said students sometimes ask if they need to wear safety goggles or other special garb. He said that neither HIV nor hepatitis survives cadaver preservation. Prions can survive preservation, he said, but there would be no danger of infection from them unless one ate body parts. Following the solemnity of Jerry's comments about respect for cadavers and donors, the jokes mitigated the seriousness of the discussion. They also served several didactic purposes.

Jerry's jokes index potential student worries about the cadaver's dangers. Corpses are considered polluting in many cultural and religious traditions (Douglas 1966). Hugh Gusterson discusses how nuclear weapons scientists joke about the body's vulnerabilities and, ultimately, about scientists' control over both bodies and fears. He argues that jokes give weapons scientists a sense of mastery by diminishing the appearance of radiation's harmful potential (1996, 116–17). In medicine, as well, physicians say dark humor helps them cope with the pain and suffering they face daily (see Shem 2003 for a fictional example of this). Jerry's jokes about pickled anatomists, lingering prions, and cannibalism suggest that students need not worry about physical contamination from the cadaver so long as they stay within the bounds of scientific and cultural norms. The comment about avoiding chicken made light of potential responses, acknowledging and normalizing physiological responses to affective disturbance. The joke gives students permission to feel physically and emotionally upset. The possibility of contamination is easily contained by medical science, but affective responses are real, embodied, and allowable.

On the first day of actual laboratory demonstration, students met Jerry in the lobby of the medical school's affiliated hospital in a rundown section of Boston. After following him through a chutes-and-ladders maze of elevators and hallways, we arrived at a long corridor filled with gray metal lockers. Jerry stopped us outside a set of double doors containing warning signs offering admittance only to those authorized to enter. Jerry said:

> You are all going into a caring profession. Or, if you're not, then the fact that you're in this class indicates that you care. If this bothers you, that's OK. I would be worried if it didn't. If you find that you can't do this, then leave the room.

This speech addressed the affective and moral formation of medical professionals. Jerry expected those who go into a caring profession to be bothered by the cadaver, to respond emotionally to death and dissection. Caring professionals are not only allowed to feel bothered, they should be bothered. Jerry said dissection had occasionally upset him and told a story about having to leave the laboratory in the middle of a dissection that he did shortly after his grandfather died. Like the jokes, Jerry's story about his grandfather normalized another common response to cadavers: their ability to evoke memories of aging or deceased family members and loved ones.

The story, one I have heard several anatomists repeat in one form or another, also calls forth the cadaver's personhood, linking it with family members, loved ones, and other people with whom a dissector might have a connection.

When we entered the large laboratory, we received another brief lecture about safety requirements for working in the laboratory. Then Jerry led us into an inner room that held the cadaver. The small room held cabinets, a sink, and a bench covered with tools and models of bones. At the center was a stainless steel table with the cadaver on it, zipped into a blue body bag. The partially dissected body was face down inside the bag, which Jerry had unzipped just enough to show us the embalmed gray-brown back. This, too, was part of Jerry's stepwise, often interrupted, occasionally distracting introduction to the cadaver. Jerry plunked two boxes of gloves down on the table in front of him and ripped them open with some force. He said the gloves were required if we wanted to touch the cadaver, but we should not feel obligated to do so. Throughout these first few moments, Jerry seemed unusually agitated and dramatic. He later explained that he uses this manic behavior to distract first-time dissectors from what they are about to do, using his body to pull students away from their thoughts and from the body on the table. In contrast, I have seen other anatomy instructors modeling unruffled calm when introducing students to cadavers.

Most students took gloves before gathering around the table. Jerry described how cadavers are chosen for student dissection: they are typically from the bodies of older donors, largely because instructors assume that students would find dissecting the corpse of someone of a similar age more troubling.[7] Thus, anatomy programs work to make bodies appear like and unlike the students' own bodies, helping them create distance, but never allowing them to forget that the cadaver was once a human being.

Jerry continued to tell stories about student reactions, including one about a student who had religious objections to dissection but did not realize it until she saw the cadaver, which made her leave the room. This story provided students with another example of concerns the cadaver could raise. Later, he told a story about a female student whose evident glee in dissecting male genitalia disturbed him and other students in the laboratory. He said he finds this type of response far more difficult to handle than student terror. These stories again contain normative and moral lessons for dissectors: feeling disturbed is normal, feeling glee is not. Taken together,

Jerry's stories provided a rough typology of possible responses—religious, normal, and pathological—to interacting with dissected cadavers. His stories stand in contrast to the cadaver stories students tell, which are almost always apocryphal. In one such story, a student handed a toll-booth attendant a severed human arm. According to Hafferty (1988) these stories are displays of student bravado and unconcern about games played with body parts. Jerry's stories normalized possible responses in two ways, first by letting students know that emotional responses are common and acceptable and, second, more subtly, by channeling possibly inchoate affective responses in particular directions, in effect telling students how they might react and what types of responses would be acceptable. Like the anatomists cited above, Jerry equated properly conducted anatomical education to the development of the capacity to care for others sensitively and professionally.

Finally, without ceremony, Jerry unwrapped the body.

Wonder and Cadavers

Up to this point, I have focused on ways anatomy programs and instructors encourage students to focus on the cadaver-as-object, or cadaver-as-person, depending on the situation. Here, I turn to several student responses, including my own, to open up the affective and sensory experience of anatomy, beginning with a moment following an anatomy lecture that reveals how emotions can be a positive force in anatomy learning. A few weeks into the course, a small group of students stepped out of the anatomy classroom and walked to the bus stop, enjoying an unusually clear and dry summer's day. The lecture had covered the form and functions of the nerves as they enter and leave the spinal column, the conduit for all nerve signals our bodies send and receive. The symmetry, complexity, and coordinating abilities of the spinal nerves are extraordinary; they quite literally allow us to move, to feel, and to live. The group remained quiet, seeming lost in thought or just at a loss for words. Finally, a young man spoke, the first to acknowledge what I and perhaps others were thinking, "I don't know how anyone can study this stuff and not think about God."

The student questioned how scientists could examine the exquisite complexity and symmetry of the spinal column without imagining a unifying plan created by a supreme being. The student's statement resonates with histories of the search for divine purpose inside human bodies (Kuriyama 2002). Wonder at the body's design seems more personal and more sublime than the "gee whiz" response that many new technologies can evoke. Regardless of one's religion or lack thereof, the body's marvelous workings evoke wonder and philosophical reflections on sublime design, whether natural or supernatural. For Maurice Merleau-Ponty, wonder allows us to gain distance from our embeddedness in the world, making it a first move toward reflection, that is, toward discovery and toward philosophy (2002, xv). Idealization of scientific detachment has obscured the importance of scientists' emotions, but historians of science have shown that fascination and wonder often are integral to naturalistic inquiry (Daston and Park 1998; Fiege 2007). As discomfort begins to fade, fascination, wonder, even surprise, are among the first emotions medical trainees experience when studying and dissecting human bodies, but these sentiments too easily become submerged in medical student stories about churning through ever more information and social science narratives about clinical detachment. Dissection brings up many emotions for students, including fear, disgust, and concerns about death. But fascination and wonder can help students transcend the cadaver's disturbing humanness, revealing a world inside the body that is "strange and paradoxical" (Merleau-Ponty 2002, xv).

Students entering the anatomy laboratory for the first time rarely respond with wonder. In chapter 4, I show how emotionally charged aspects of surgical training defamiliarize trainees with their own bodies, creating an opening for the embodiment of new practices and new social ways of being. Here, I focus on the sensory experience of dissection and the ways these experiences form part of a profound emotional journey. I begin with a long excerpt from my field notes that retains much of the emotional and sensory immediateness of the experience. I choose to analyze my own field notes as I would any other informants' comments because they call for analysis.

Knowing my interest in anatomy, Jerry, the instructor, invited me to watch him dissect a cadaver's spine in preparation for a laboratory session. The procedure is called a laminectomy. Jerry showed me on a model spine how he planned to chisel open several vertebrae to reveal the spinal column and its associated nerves. This was the second time I had seen this cadaver, and I felt the same dread I had felt the first time. Jerry again hurried around the laboratory, frenetically finding gloves and putting blades on scalpels. I wrote the following notes when I returned to my office (they have been edited for length and to remove redundancies):

The procedure involves removing the dorsal parts of several vertebrae . . . to reveal the spinal cord beneath. It's a big, messy job. Dr. K. racked up a scalpel for me, but I couldn't cut. He began by gently removing some of the muscle on the back that hadn't already been removed. Cutting and peeling away flesh this gently was a little hard, but not impossible, to take. . . . He began to cut into the deep muscles of the back. He cut all the way down to bone, then had me run the scalpel through the cut to see how deep the muscle lies. In the lower back, the spinal column is inches deep, through about three inches of muscle, at least on this guy. As I ran the scalpel through the cut, I could feel it bumping over bone, which were the transverse processes. The transverse processes are very difficult to see (though you can see them as bumpy protrusions in the back). So that was the trick, revealing the transverse processes.

This description of the process is marked, first, by my decision not to pick up the scalpel. Some of this decision was squeamishness, and some of it was uncertainty about my role as an observer, not as a medical student. Many students told me that some members of their dissecting team were more reluctant to dissect than others. I was able to watch but did not find watching easy. The tone shifted as Jerry began to reach the deep parts of the spine. I became interested in the depth of muscle concealing most of the spine and the feel of the transverse processes under the scalpel, but my attention had begun to focus on details, on parts rather than wholes.

As the process got messier, my comments became more sensory:

The next step involved peeling away the muscle, and it was nasty. It basically involved hacking away large strips of muscle tissue and tossing them into the red bucket below. When he had cut down to bone, Dr. K. asked me to feel the depth of the muscle with my hand. It was really pretty incredible, but not fun. The dissection was a lot like butchery, except it was messier. I imagine that if you were doing this as a student, you would be more ginger [than the instructor] about cutting (I certainly still felt squeamish about touching the body). The next step involved chiseling away the spinous processes. This involved a hammer and a mallet. K. offered me the chisel, but I certainly wasn't ready to do that. He said, and I found this interesting, that he works both by feel (often not even looking at the body) and by sound. The sound of the chisel changes when he pushes through the bone into the underlying cavity. At that point, he began clipping away large chunks of bone. This was very messy. And I kept looking at the chunks of bone and muscle coming out of the back and getting set down next to the body for eventual deposit in the red bucket.

As I recalled how Jerry cut deeper into the cadaver's back, my comments became more visceral: peeling away muscle was "nasty," especially because he was "hacking away" at tissue. The feel of the depth of muscle was "incredible, but not fun." The combination of amazement and disgust marked the movement between interest, the move toward discovery, and aversion, shrinking away from uncomfortable knowledge. My revulsion at the messiness of the process continued, and I continued to decline invitations to participate, but when the discussion shifted to the sensory aspects of the process, I found myself fascinated by the relation of senses to knowing. This moment, when Jerry revealed his own sensory ways of knowing, broke into my disturbed feelings, not least by focusing me on the sounds of the work; it pulled me out of my gruesome associations and into what was actually happening at the moment. When Jerry described using sound to gauge progress, wonder and interest broke through the messiness.

As Jerry began to open up the spinal column, my tone shifted remarkably:

> K. removed one vertebra to reveal the spinal column below. At one point, he asked me to reach a finger into the cavity formed by the vertebrae to feel the cavity itself. All I felt at first was the sharp edges of cut bone, then I felt the cavity after he had opened the space a bit more. After snipping another six or eight inches away, he had opened up the spinal column to view. The spinal column was red, not white, as I had seen in books. This is because there's blood and lymphatic fluid running through it. It was also flat, not round as I imagined, but K. said that some of the flatness was due to loss of water after death. Then he snipped away the *dura mater*, a thin but tough membrane, which I actually felt. You could see the *cauda equina*, which looks much more like a horse's tail than any drawing I had seen. You could also see *dorsal root ganglia*, which were really cool. . . . After that, K. snipped a little further up to find the *conus medullaris*, the end of the spinal cord proper.

This paragraph began with the description of the feel of the cavity holding the spinal nerves, then discussed the visual differences between the cadaver's spinal column and my anatomy atlas's depiction of the spinal column. Although most of the paragraph is descriptive in tone, the underlying element of wonder (I looked inside a spine!) comes through in the description of touching the dura mater, the membrane covering the spinal nerves; the cauda equina, a bundle of nerve cells that emerge from the dura mater in the lower spine and resemble a horse's tail; and the "cool" dorsal root ganglia, small nodules on peripheral nerves that contain the cell body. The human body is composed of parts and anatomy students must learn to visually identify these parts, to name them, and to compare them to the images in an atlas to fix them in visual memory. Wonder helped fuel the inquiry.

Despite my thoughts that parts of the spine were "cool," some aspects of the dissection continually threatened to overwhelm my senses:

> At certain points in the dissection, the meaty smell rose up from the body enough that I had to step away. At other points, the view of the inside of the body was so fascinating that I wasn't at all aware of the fact that this was a dead human person. . . . Afterward, Dr. K. cleaned up and zipped the body back into the bag. I washed my hands, twice, but could still smell what seemed like the meat smell on my hands. Dr. K. and I went back to his office so I could interview him a bit, but truthfully, I was completely out of it. . . . I struggled through a few questions, then quit.

The cadaver's smell, an unforgettable combination of meat and chemicals, initially was the most intrusive sensory aspect of the experience, more than the tactile impressions, which were brief. Oddly, though, as years have passed, I remember the tactile feel of sharp bone and thick muscle more clearly than I remember the smells. Medical students often describe finding the smell of the anatomy laboratory overwhelming and indelibly etched in their memories. They also describe the same oscillation between being upset and being fascinated, a fascination that takes one away from the disturbing knowledge that one is cutting into a body. I struggled to focus after this first dissection experience, reflecting the profound turmoil that this experience—at once disturbing and fascinating—evoked in me.

Elements of the experience lingered after I left the laboratory:

Even after, I could still smell meat, though I'm certain it was my imagination. As I left, I realized that I really was pretty shaky. I got off the bus at MIT and walked across campus. I passed street construction and was looking at the archeological layers of cobblestones and other things under there when I noticed yellow-wrapped fiber-optic cables lying in the hole, looking like a spinal cord, as though Mass. Ave. had also had a laminectomy. A little further and I was passing the Stata Center construction site, and I saw a set of six or eight big pipes running from the base of a hole in the ground into its side. They reminded me of ribs. I thought this was funny, except that everything was reminding me of opened-up bodies. I had to wash my hands before I went to the Chinese food trucks, thinking that I needed to do it even before I touched the Styrofoam box. I went to the trucks thinking I was hungry. I ordered mango salad, which I thought was completely innocuous, except that the fried tofu on top looked like trabecular bone, which I had held in my hand so recently and, oddly, it seemed to taste like chemicalized meat. I couldn't eat much of it, and I certainly couldn't look at it. I also had to toss out the sweet pink lemonade.

After the dissection, my return to my office at MIT was plagued with sensory memories of the cadaver, including the smell lingering on my hands and, more unusual, the ways construction around campus provided visual reminders of the cadaver. Further, though the cadaver's flesh did not remind me of chicken, tofu reminded me of bone, and I was unable to eat it, even having a phantom taste of meat in my mouth.[8] The smell lingering on my hands kept me in psychological contact with the cadaver in a sense best captured by the word "incorporate," which, according to the *Oxford English Dictionary*, can mean "union" into one body or, more rarely, an "embodied realization." My series of embodied realizations kept me connected to the dissection, a passage through the body, to the point where the world around me revealed its spinal cords, ribs, and bone. In that passage through the world-as-body, I believe the body incorporated me, so I could later incorporate my knowledge of it.

I thought I had imagined the smell after I had removed my gloves and washed my hands, but I later learned that phenols from preservation chemicals leach through latex gloves and lodge in the esophagus. What I thought was an imaginary smell traveling with me probably was a real smell, a real incorporation of preservation chemicals that played a role in keeping the lab present after I left, possibly affecting even the taste of meat that I had while eating tofu. Throughout this description, the sensory aspects of the experience remain prominent: the feel of the spinal column, the sound of the chisel, the smell of meat. Late that night, I was reflecting on various theories of the medical gaze, while still remembering that I had run a scalpel across a dead man's spine. I wasn't finished being disturbed, but the next time I was in the laboratory, I found myself absorbing the anatomy and thinking critically about the experience, while also thinking about the man on the table. Writing field notes was a cathartic way of grappling with the intensity of the dissection. The sensations of touching the cadaver's insides have not left me, even years afterward.

As this passage reveals, the anatomy laboratory provides an introduction to the profoundly sensory nature of medical work. Sounds, smells, and tactile sensations not only indelibly mark the anatomy laboratory in memory, they also mark the beginnings of a sensory education. Richard, for example, recounted with fascination (and some disgusted glee) how physicians once tasted urine to diagnose diabetes (undigested sugars make it taste sweet, I am told). Another surgeon said she took delight in learning the music of the heart's rhythms and gurgles with a stethoscope and lamented that electrocardiographs and other equipment had rendered this acoustic knowledge largely obsolete.

Over the course of this passage, and despite my clear emotional struggling, a shift from disturbance to interest becomes evident. There is a movement from reluctance to participate, by not picking up the scalpel, for example, to emotional disturbance at the messiness of the process to fascination at the details of the body and the resemblance of body parts to their names, such as the cauda equina. The fascination eclipsed my awareness that this was the body of a dead person. Fifty years after his medical training, Richard said:

> I was scared, but I can't remember what the effect was of dealing with a human being in dissection because I got so intensely interested in the structure that the fact that it was a human being didn't seem to penetrate.

Fascination helps propel us away from our disturbing knowledge that the cadaver was once a person and into the details of the human body.

Doing Violence versus Inflicting Harm

Some anatomy students show a clear oscillation between objectifying and personifying the cadaver. In a newsletter for her peers, Allison Christie (2001), a first-year student at Tufts University School of Medicine, revealed several ways in which objectification can be tactical:

> This dissection is definitely something completely new. I don't feel at ease with it, but I am surprised by how easy it is to carry out. I am definitely enjoying learning about anatomy by taking apart an actual body, but I have been avoiding thinking about the cadaver as a former person. To me, this week, the cadaver on the table has been a fascinating object.

This is the first part of a much longer passage. Christie's language is embodied and emotional. She contrasts her discomfort, a bodily state, with surprise at her ease while dissecting. She enjoys taking apart the body. She says she avoids thinking about the cadaver as a person, though her statements indicate that some part of her can think of little else. She finds the cadaver a "fascinating object." In these statements, the student places herself within the long history of wonder at the workings of nature and the body. Surprise, pleasure in learning, and fascination stave off her unease at the knowledge that this is the body of a person.

She continues by objectifying her own body:

> I am sure that my brain is compartmentalizing the experience, because when I try to think about the person who inhabited this body, these thoughts are immediately pushed aside for as long as I am in lab. On the other hand, the numbness that surrounded my brain during the first few hours of dissection, protecting it from its own natural line of inquiry, seems to be slowly lifting. I hope that in a few more weeks those compartments will start to come back together, and I'll be able to handle a greater appreciation of what I'm doing.

By saying that her brain compartmentalizes the experience, relinquishing agency to her brain, rather than herself, Christie's description resembles the ontological choreography that in vitro fertilization patients engage in when they objectify their own bodies as protection against uncomfortable sensations or unpleasant news (Thompson 2005). In this case, she has objectified her brain to let it do the difficult work of sealing off the cadaver's personhood while dissecting. She further wraps her brain in a state of numbness, creating a second barrier between herself and the knowledge of the cadaver's person-hood. But her psychological anesthesia has begun to wear off.

Christie continues, considering the larger significance of what she is doing:

> I would like to be able to understand the cadaver simultaneously as a former person, as well as an object. I'm trying to work out why this is important to me. I think it has something to do with how I understand my purpose working in medicine.

She expresses a wish for psychological integration of the knowledge of the cadaver's ontological duality, its status as person and thing. I will return to her statement about her future, but here, she shifts registers from her brain and its numbness to herself and her desire to understand the cadaver's duality. Indeed, more than binary person and thing, the cadaver becomes multiple as the student elides several of its ontologically salient characteristics. Annemarie Mol (2002) describes how various practices brought to bear on a particular disease bring forth its many realities, making it ontologically multiple. By calling the cadaver "a former person," the student skips over the fact that the person is "former" because it—she never specifies gender—is dead. In this student's statement, the cadaver troubles the categorical distinctions we often make about bodies: person or thing, alive or dead, and, in this case, male or female.

Christie's next statement brings forth more of the bodily dimension of her ontological work:

> So, I need to be sensitive, but I can't be squeamish.

The student must maintain her sensitivity to patients, but she cannot let that become squeamishness about physical contact or invasive procedures. "Squeamish" appears often in student descriptions of their concerns about and responses to dissection. The word describes someone who is both easily nauseated, unable to swallow anything disagreeable, and, in older usages, unwilling or averse to doing something. The word perfectly captures students' emotional-physical responses: an embodied aversive reaction characterized by nausea. Christie wants to be "sensitive," to allow other bodies to affect her perceptions and her emotions, but sensitivity must not tip over into physical discomfort. She cannot let her bodily reactions overtake her.

Her emotions must be present enough to treat her patients as persons, but they cannot give way to physical discomfort.

She next brings out the destructive nature of dissection:

> I need to recognize that, although there is certainly violence in our dissection of this cadaver, there is no harm being done. I had to think about that for awhile, because it feels counterintuitive. It's all right to enjoy taking this body apart. It's all right to enjoy the process, as well as the information gained.

Here, she makes a distinction between violence and harm. She paraphrases, "First, do no harm," an oft-cited caution to physicians that hails from Hippocrates' *Epidemics*. Yet a student's training begins with violence done to a cadaver body. According to the *Oxford English Dictionary*, the Old English word "harm" means "evil (physical or otherwise) as done to or suffered by some person or thing." In contrast, the OED defines the Old French word "violence" as "the exercise of physical force so as to inflict injury on, or cause damage to, persons or property." The notion of harm begins with "evil," suggesting malicious intentions or a malicious deed. "Violence," on the other hand, can entail injury, with connotations of moral wrong, but "damage" does not always have decisive moral significance. She is doing violence—physical damage—to the cadaver, but she is not doing evil. Her intent is to learn anatomy, to learn how to work with bodies, and to learn to manage her own bodily responses during these encounters. And, though the body will be destroyed, according to the traditions of biomedical practice, she will not have done anything morally objectionable. She inflicts physical force on the cadaver, but she does not do harm. By making a distinction between "violence" and "harm," she clarifies her ethical position and gives herself permission to enjoy taking the body apart. Her ability to enjoy the process—to experience positive emotions related to discovery—hinges on this moral clarity.

Christie goes on:

> In the end, the gift of this experience will come around and be given back as I approach my living patients with knowledge and confidence. Eventually, I need to learn how intimate inspection, physical or emotional, can be done with respect and purpose.

Christie's use of the word "gift" and her notion of giving back through emotionally competent medical practice clearly speak to the ontological work that anatomy programs do to activate the person. Further, she fulfills her earlier promise to work out why the dissection is important to her future in medicine. She makes knowledge and confidence into a binary, a split of reason and emotion that is common in European and American belief systems but rarer elsewhere (Lutz 1986). Michelle Rosaldo argues that emotions are "*embodied* thoughts, thoughts steeped with the apprehension that 'I am involved'" (1984, 143). Christie is indeed involved with the dissection in profoundly embodied ways: it affects her entire being, mentally, physically, and emotionally. She is learning to manage her own embodied responses to dissection—squeamishness and pleasure—by structuring it with the intellectual distinction she makes between harm and violence. The clarifying effect of the linguistic-ethical distinction she makes eases her emotional responses; she can reason her way to emotional acceptance—even enjoyment—of dissection. She argues that her acceptance will be bound up with developing a positive emotional stance toward her patients.

Christie thinks about her future:

> This dissection is part of an important acculturation, by which my inhibitions will be broken down so that I can be responsible to my future patients. For this reason, I'm going to try in the next few months to confront my unease rather than ignore it, and to blend together my ideas about the cadaver as a specimen of anatomy and as a dead person.

Christie's acculturation will mean breaking down the internal restraints that could prevent respectful contact with patients. If we consider the compartments that Christie says she erected in her brain, this description becomes more embodied: she must break down the internal barriers that her "brain" has constructed and separate her knowledge of the human body's structure and workings from her emotional response to treating, and sometimes doing violence, to persons.

The culturing of a medical student, as Christie describes it, is a process of embodying a professional stance toward contact with patients: confronting her unease, learning to avoid squeamishness, while achieving sensitivity, respect, and confidence. In effect, she says she must embody the cadaver's ontological status as person *and* thing to become a responsible physician. Thus, the transition from medical student to physician entails making a set of sophisticated distinctions that affect her emotional, epistemological, and moral relationships with the cadaver: squeamishness versus sensitivity, unease versus enjoyment, harm versus violence. These distinctions rely in large part on the cadaver's dual ontological status as dead person and scientific object.

Though Christie's remarks are exceptionally eloquent, they are otherwise typical of the emotional and intellectual wrestling that medical students do when they dissect. Her comments could be analyzed in psychoanalytic terms by considering her dissociation and eventual integration of the cadaver's personhood, but she herself describes this process as "acculturation," and many medical students describe these kinds of responses, suggesting that they are cultivated in anatomy courses. Further, they speak very strongly to the ways anatomy programs engage students in practices that treat the cadaver as a scientific object and as a former person.

Person and Thing in the Operating Room

What's at stake in tactical objectification of the cadaver? First, the evocation of the cadaver-as-person stands in contrast to past practices in the anatomy and autopsy laboratories, where emotion stood in opposition to the desired goal of objectivity (Fox 1988). Students in the new millennium are encouraged to think about the cadaver as both person and thing and to think about their own emotions. Of course, not all medical students learn to manage this duality effectively. Many patients can give personal examples of medical objectification going wrong, typically when a physician does not seem to see or hear them. But, whether learned in the anatomy laboratory or elsewhere, I argue that good medical care often entails managing—not denying—the dual nature of body-as-person and body-as-thing. To examine this duality in practice, I recount two clinical examples that I observed in different hospitals. In both cases, tactical objectification does emotional work: for surgeons in the first case and for an entire surgical team in the second.

In the first case, Dr. Anna Wilson, a hand surgeon, planned to release a pinched nerve in a patient's elbow. The patient insisted that this be done under a local anesthetic, against the surgeon's wishes. She would have preferred to use a general anesthetic because the patient would be unconscious and it would allow her to maintain more control over the procedure. As the surgery began, the man complained loudly of pain and wiggled his arm. The surgeon and the resident stopped working. Anna told the patient that they would give him more anesthetic. He became very agitated. Not general anesthesia, he said. No, just more local, she replied. While the resident injected more anesthetic, Anna told the patient that moving his arm would be very dangerous. If his arm started to hurt again, he should tell her, and she would take care of it. "I am just borrowing your arm for a bit," she told him, "but don't worry, I'll give it back."

Patients often use the first person when discussing emotional pain, saying, for example, "I am in pain" or "I feel sad." Similarly, they also often use the third person when describing physical pain, saying, for example, "my foot hurts" (Lyon and Barbalet 1994, 57). This move splits the senses and the emotions in ways unfamiliar in many non-European traditions (see Geurts 2003). And it reveals that ontological choreography can be rooted in linguistic forms of objectification. Long before the surgery, pain and injury had probably already led Anna's patient to objectify his own arm, leading him to experience it as "not me." Anna further objectified the arm when she said she would "borrow it." The arm became alienated from the patient's body, first through its pain; second through the anesthetic, which dulled his arm; and third through Anna's statement that she wanted to borrow it, suggesting that it was property that he could temporarily give to her. Anna constructed the arm as an object that could be exchanged, an item that could be alienated from its owner and loaned to another. The request to "borrow" the arm invited the patient to exercise a different kind of agency: rather than agency to move the arm, he had agency to "lend" the arm to her, which was safer. For a short time, the arm was not his. But the loan was temporary. When the surgery ended, Anna would "return" the arm, and, after the patient healed, the arm could become again an unproblematic, mostly unnoticed, part of his body and life.

The arm's being, its ontology, shifted it from being a part of self to an object. And the choreography involved delicately making this move and then unmaking it. Only a person can donate his or her body or organ. Similarly, only a person can lend an arm. A temporal and ontological difference exists between a patient's arm and his entire body: a person can only promise to give his entire body after death, whereas an arm can be lent in real time. Further, the gift of an organ or body is irrevocable: some parts cannot be lent. By borrowing the arm, Anna addressed the whole person, the person capable of making the loan. By communicating with the patient directly and making him a participant in his own surgery, Anna demonstrated, in Strathern's words, "respect for the person as a subject rather than as an object" (2004, 8). Her activation of the person was especially important for this patient, whose fear of a general anesthetic suggested that he feared loss of agency or personhood or life that could result from loss of consciousness.

Through the rest of the procedure, Anna kept up a running monologue with him, telling him what she and the resident were doing, even noting that his pinched nerve likely was caused by an anatomically unusual tendon. The tendon ran across the elbow, rather than toward the shoulder (as it would in a more normal arm). This could have caused the pinched nerve. A tendon like his typically might be found only in birds, she told him. Her curiosity about the anomalous tendon echoed anatomy students' wonder at the human body. Anna's use of objectification was tactical, but it did not solely benefit the patient. She has talked about teaching the feel of various body parts by using analogies to food. Cartilage, she often tells trainees, feels like coconut. Or, similarly, she describes the nerves in the arm and hand as pasta that has been cooked al dente. The small ones are "spaghettini"; larger ones are linguine. She uses the Freudian term "displacement," which signifies the symbolic replacement of one emotionally charged object with a more or less charged object, to describe these linguistic objectifications. By likening a body part to food, she eases the psychological difficulties of cutting into a human body. This helps explain her comment likening the man's tendon to a bird tendon. For both patient and surgeon, the tendon becomes avian, not human, and it is taxonomically displaced from its problematic humanness before it is surgically displaced from its anatomically problematic location.

Objectifying the arm clearly eased the patient's distress. But what happens when the patient is unconscious? In another hospital at another medical school, I observed the removal of a liver tumor from an older man. After the attending surgeon and fellow removed the tumor, Dr. Jill English, the chief resident, removed the man's healthy gallbladder, a standard, uncomplicated part of this much larger surgery. As she finished, she told the team that the patient was "a funny guy," who looked at his CT scans and said he felt proud of his healthy gallbladder (so markedly different from his diseased liver). The operating team giggled at the thought of a man being proud of his own gallbladder, a humble and mostly unremarkable organ. The operation proceeded, but much of the tension that marked the difficult tumor removal had left the room.

The surgeons discussed the patient in the third person, even though he lay beneath their hands. Erving Goffman (1961b) has described the ways a surgeon might joke to relieve tension and to signal the end of the difficult portion of a procedure. But more was happening. The patient's remark seemed strange and amusing because most people do not admire their internal organs the way they might admire, say, their own eyes or their physique. Hidden deep inside the abdomen and disposable, a gallbladder cannot be a defining feature of the person. By talking about the patient's pleasure at the image of his gallbladder, the resident discursively connected the gallbladder to the person, even as she was disconnecting the gallbladder from his body. This marked the beginning of the return of this patient to consciousness, his return to a state where he would be addressed directly, in the first person, rather than the third person (see Young 1997). Removal of the gallbladder was the last step before starting the critical but relatively straightforward work of closing the abdomen. The hardest part was over. The amusing anecdote reminded everyone present, however, that there was a person connected to the body they were working on and that, even during the surgery's denouement, they had to exercise care for that person and body.

The Cultural Construction of Emotions

The formation of a physician requires the cultivation of medical techniques and the development of a medical stance toward patients. Medical trainees learn to manage their emotional responses to touching, invading, and sometimes doing violence to patients' bodies in the name of healing. As I have shown, cultivating the practitioner entails also engaging in practices that ontologically remake the patient's body. Focusing on the ways practices in the anatomy laboratory hone in on the object or activate the person shows how common distinctions among senses and emotions, thought and feeling, reason and morality begin to break down during dissection. Treating emotions as embodied through culturally and historically situated practices, rather than as individual internal states, allows me to connect students' anatomical practices to the emotional work they do.

Tactical objectification is a means of managing the emotional needs of patient and practitioner. A physician objectifies bodies as a survival tactic, but patients may find this tactic alienating. In the anatomy laboratory, for example, the medical student first separated herself from the knowledge of the cadaver's personhood by compartmentalizing her brain, that is, by objectifying and therefore distancing the part of herself that knew she was doing violence to another body. Objectification in this case was a defense of self against emotionally painful knowledge. Similarly, Anna objectified the patient's arm to distance herself and the patient from the violence she was doing to it. But the person cannot be allowed to disappear lest objectification itself become harmful. Thus, Christie reminded herself that she eventually would have to work both with a patient's personhood and with his body's thingness. Similarly, Anna activated the patient's personhood by making his arm something he could lend. Jill, the chief resident, activated the patient's personhood in the operating room as a warning to other residents: the patient was a person, and they would have to remain attentive to do no harm.

The fear that emotions might cloud clinical judgment fits with a long-standing equation of emotion with irrationality and lack of reason, but too little emotion or too much detachment is equated with coldness and disconnection (Lutz 1986, 290). Clinicians and social scientists alike have worried about the balance (or lack of it) between empathy and objectivity among doctors. Marcel Mauss makes "composure," or "resistance to emotional seizure," a result of the development of culturally specific "techniques of the body" that is "fundamental in social and mental life" (2007, 67). Mauss couches his statement in unfortunate early twentieth-century language of race evolution, reflecting a contemporary prejudice deeply rooted in European cultural traditions that emotions are wild and primitive and that they require containment by well-disciplined, rational thinkers. But his point that emotional restraint is culturally defined and developed provides a useful starting point for thinking about physicians' emotional training. Mauss provides an embodied perspective on emotional and cultural training that speaks to the prevailing North American view of biomedical physicians as composed and rational men and women of science who can grapple with the extremes of human suffering because they have mastered their emotions and developed a properly moral stance toward their patients and their work. Mauss's language of a culturally developed resistance to "emotional seizure" reflects a generally negative view of emotional expression as a force that threatens rational, civilized thought (see Lutz 1986). This view tends to privilege mind and rationality over body and emotion as the more "civilized" (and, not coincidentally, gendered male) half of these binaries (Lutz 1986; Martin 2000). Absent from this passage is the notion that positive emotions such as curiosity or wonder could motivate action and guide culturally defined "proper" behavior.

Later work in anthropology makes emotion a much more profoundly cultural phenomenon, showing that categories of what counts as emotion vary across cultures (Lutz 1986). Saba Mahmood (2005), like Mauss, draws on Aristotle's notion of *habitus* to argue that practices generate emotions and moral behavior. These practices eventually condense to become *habitus*, dispositions that generate emotion and moral behavior in largely unthought ways, becoming who someone is, rather than what someone does or believes (Mahmood 2005, 136–37). Although Mauss and Mahmood differ about the nature of emotion—it is part of humanity's primitive constitution for Mauss and is produced through culturally defined behaviors for Mahmood—both take the view that practices embody emotional configurations (i.e., actions make feelings). Anatomy programs expose students to experiences that locate the cadaver as an object or as a person. Laboratory practice constructs cadavers as objects. Memorial services resituate them as persons. Whether through specific instruction or by indirect means, many practitioners learn to tactically objectify the body or activate the person.

Conclusion

Building on the work of Mary Douglas, Julia Kristeva (1982) describes corpses as abject, uncanny objects that disturb the boundaries of person and thing, upsetting the categories that define our lives. Kristeva suggests that the corpse's abjection cannot be resolved in any simple sense. Its abjection is unthinkable, and it remains outside and constitutive of the categories that define our worlds. Twenty-first-century biomedical training demands that most trainees confront the abjection and uncanniness of a corpse, encouraging them to learn to tactically place it within one category or another—person or thing—to meet the demands initially of anatomical training and, later, of patient care. The corpse thus becomes a medical object—a cadaver—that is always multiple. But the cadaver's ontological multiplicity—and, by extension, the patient's—does not get resolved. Instead, practitioners learn to manage the body's duality to facilitate switching between treating the body-as-object and activating the whole person. This process does not always go well. But perhaps calls for reforming biomedicine might work from within this constitutive contradiction. Perhaps then the violence that often is part of biomedical treatment of the body will less often become harm to the person treated.

two

CUTTING DISSECTION

I think [dissection] will go because there isn't much evidence
that it makes much of a difference. It's going to go.
ANATOMY INSTRUCTOR

If you're dealing with a cadaver, you're dealing with a real human
being. That can translate later on when you're dealing with real
people. It helps you deal with human beings as human beings,
rather than as objects.
PHYSICIAN AND ANATOMY RESEARCHER

Dissection, long a rite of passage for North American medical students, has
faced drastic reduction or elimination in many medical schools. Anatomists
and medical educators have vigorously debated dissection's role in the medical curriculum since the 1970s, before computational tools became widely
available for teaching anatomy. Educators agree that anatomy is medicine's
lingua franca and that some mastery of the field's fifty thousand terms and
complex spatial relations is essential to good doctoring. They also agree that
medical students should begin to develop anatomical perception, the ability
to distinguish among types of tissues and to locate bodily structures in three
dimensions. The debate focuses on how anatomical knowledge should be
acquired, what tools best aid anatomical teaching, and what other lessons a
gross anatomy course can or should provide medical students. Profound
questions about the relationship between a doctor and a patient emerge
quickly when anatomists and educators squabble over resources and curriculum hours. When—during medical school or residency—does a trainee
develop a physician's stance toward patient bodies? How does a doctor come

to know—to examine, to speak about, and to practice upon—a patient's body without disregarding the patient's personhood? What kind of affective and cultural relations do physicians develop with their own bodies and with patient bodies in the anatomy laboratory?

This chapter examines dissection controversies. I explore structural, technological, and epistemological reasons that educators give to cut or to maintain programs. Gross anatomy's decline as a research science began in the late 1950s, as new anatomical findings became rare events and other biological sciences took off. The development since the early 1980s of digital tools for teaching anatomy provided promising alternatives to dissection, raising the stakes of the debate. Dissection's critics have argued that it is an expensive and inefficient means of teaching anatomical language and structure. In contrast, proponents defend aspects of anatomical understanding, such as dissection's role in introducing medical students to the reality of death, that cannot easily be technologized.[1] The debate also indexes a related tension in medical care between the canonical and the instantiated body—that is, between a body that is normal and generic and bodies that are unique and particular.

Stefan Hirschauer argues that surgeons acquire two bodies, their own as practitioners and the anatomical body of the patient (1991, 309). As I show, the two bodies are significantly linked: the assumptions about patients' bodies that accompany medical learning emerge from and are built into physician practices that start in the anatomy laboratory. Further, various practices for working with cadavers reflect different assumptions about bodies coming from diverse areas within medical work with unique methods that physicians use for investigating bodies. The debate reveals a tension between dissection, as an iconic cultural practice through which many of medicine's affective, relational, and physical lessons come into play, and anatomy learning, as the cognitive acquisition of names and the understanding of spatial relations.

Declining Sciences and New Technologies

As I discussed in the previous chapter, most ethnographies of anatomy education were written by sociologists who spent time in medical schools in the 1950s and again in the 1970s and 1980s (Becker et al. 1961; Fox 1988; Hafferty 1988, 1991; Segal 1988). These ethnographies typically consider the emotional socialization of medical students, focusing on uncertainty (Fox

1988), group work (Becker et al. 1961), and students' explorations of death (Hafferty 1991). In these works, the emotional work of dissection received more attention than the relation of technical practices to the process of cultivating medical students. The lessons embodied through touch, for example, have received scant attention. More recently, science studies scholars have explored relationships between the construction of scientific objects and the construction of scientists themselves (Gusterson 1996; Keller 1984; Knorr Cetina 2000; Turkle 1995). Dissection is an example of the mutual articulation of object and subject: students articulate anatomical structures so they can become articulate in the language of medicine.

The availability of digital teaching tools has not been the primary driver behind the decline in dissection. Other factors, such as anatomy's decline as a research science, the loss of qualified anatomy teachers, and the expense of maintaining body-donation programs, have been more significant. This resembles nuclear weapons design, another high-stakes research field that, during the same time period, also turned to virtual practice more for reasons of politics and economics than because digital tools offered pedagogical improvements (Gusterson 1996, 2001, 2005). After the Nuclear Test Ban Treaty of 1996, nuclear weapons designers working on the maintenance and management of existing weapons began using computer simulations to examine the effects of design changes to America's aging nuclear weapons. Weapons design research had already peaked, and it became increasingly incremental in the late 1950s. During the ensuing decades, the intense apprenticeships of young weapons designers gave way to formal programs involving more carefully structured and codified lessons. The field turned in on itself, becoming "involuted" (Gusterson 2005, 77). Anatomy has faced similar involution as new anatomical findings have become rare events and the field has moved more toward development of pedagogical techniques and supporting technologies.[2] Although the underlying rationales for the virtual turns in weapons design and anatomy teaching diverge, weapons designers and anatomists use similar arguments to defend traditional pedagogies, arguing that genuine learning is ensured only when trainees know the "real" objects they will work on, whether bombs or bodies. In medicine, this appeal to the real speaks to the ultimate aim of medical training: preparing students to treat individual patients.

Without material bombs and bodies to practice upon, weapons designers and anatomists alike worry that their trainees might lose their "feeling for the organism," a sense of intense relation with the object of inquiry that can foster intuitive and powerful insights (Keller 1984). The shift toward simulation as pedagogy demonstrates the complexity of motives for moving to digital training methods, including savings of time and money, the power of scientific and engineering logics, and the vast power of computational modeling. Further, researchers in both anatomy and weapons design use the "real" as a defense against the digital.[3] Despite similarities, the histories of the virtual turn in weapons design differs from that of anatomy in at least one crucial way: many anatomists defend dissection by appealing to the ways medical students in anatomy laboratories develop respect and compassion for their living patients in part by dissecting dead ones.

The digital turn in anatomy education is consistent with thirty years of research on medical decision making. Writing about medical decision-making tools, Marc Berg shows how competing models of physician decision making suggest that the "'scientific nature' of medical practice has become a *mental* category" (1997, 30, emphasis in original). According to Berg, the historical processes of modeling diagnostic decision making entailed recasting medical work as the cognitive work of individual physicians, rather than the social work of human groups. Noncognitive aspects of this work were treated as irrelevant. Defining medical decision making as cognitive work allowed designers of decision-support tools to draw from logics native to cognitive science and artificial intelligence to build digital tools and to design research protocols.

Berg argues for an examination of debates about rationalizing technologies by scrutinizing the distinct logics that frame them and the networks of relations, practices, and tools that lead to them (1997, 174). Showing the diverse logics in play in constructing computational tools removes the analyst from the difficulties inherent in adopting a normative position on a tool's effectiveness. Similarly, examining practices that develop around new technological systems allows the analyst to consider the technology and the milieu that shifts with its introduction. Lucy Suchman argues for a shift in designers' and analysts' thinking toward "recognition that systems development is not the creation of discrete, intrinsically meaningful objects, but the cultural production of new forms of material practice" (2002, 99). For example, physicians recognized the diagnostic potential of the X-ray very soon after Roentgen's 1895 discovery, but it took thirty years for institutional structures and material practices to develop enough that the X-ray could become a regularly used diagnostic tool. These included creation of institutional spaces and support, the rise of radiology as a profession, and the emergence of a new way of seeing bodies as envelopes surrounding skeletons (Howell 1995). This suggests that examining the practices that have materialized with cadaver dissection and digital anatomical study may be more fruitful than asking which method is most effective.

"A Dying Breed"

The word "anatomy" derives from Greek and simply means "cut up." It is synonymous with "dissection" and, in some uses, "analysis." Human gross anatomy is the study of human structure from organs and tissues, its largest components, down to a fuzzy border with histology, where tissues become cells. Anatomical terminology originated with animal dissections performed by Aristotle and Galen (for a discussion of Greek anatomy, see Kuriyama 2002). In 1543, Vesalius first codified anatomical terminology in *De Humani Corporis Fabrica*. Since the early twentieth century, two international organizations have worked to standardize and update anatomical terms, attempting to make anatomical language a universal language for biomedicine. They have collected their findings in a compendium currently known as *Terminologia Anatomica*. Anatomical terminology is one means of describing the body, of spatially locating densely packed tissues and their functions. Many anatomical terms describe structures by location and function. For example, the *flexor digitorum superficialis* is a set of tendons in the wrist that connect to the fingers (*digitorum* means "of the digits"), allowing fingers to flex (*flexor*). This set of tendons is more superficial—closer to the skin—than another set of flexor tendons that lie deeper in the wrist (*profundis*). Anatomical terminology is one way the discipline of gross anatomy cuts up (dissects, anatomizes) the human body, constructing it as a linguistic object in three-dimensional space.

Anatomy forms the foundation of biomedical epistemology, which builds upon the assumptions that disease can be isolated and located exclusively within the body's tissues. Anatomical language also forms a platform for medical communication: doctors can rapidly describe the location of pathology by using terms more or less common to all medical disciplines.[4] But language—the articulable knowledge of the human body—is not the only way to cut up the human body. Medical students also are expected to understand the spatial relations of organs and tissues. Though related to the logic of anatomical terminology, this understanding is visual and spatial. These two interlocking knowledges—language and three-dimensional structure—form the uncontested core of anatomical training.

In the 1950s, medical students in North America and much of Europe spent a year or more studying gross anatomy in lectures and in laboratories (Becker et al. 1961, 61). Laboratories typically have organized students into a group of two to eight students per cadaver. Students typically take turns dissecting and identifying structures using atlases and other guides. This group exercise has been considered an introduction to medical teamwork. Since the 1980s, medical schools in North America have adopted widely disparate approaches to anatomy, ranging from a year of lectures and laboratory to six to twelve weeks as a separate course or as embedded within a broad introductory course to human structure and function. Some schools have abandoned dissection in favor of using teaching models made from body parts, or previously dissected specimens (called "prosections"), and from medical images. Regardless of the particular solutions adopted, most medical schools in North America, Australia, and the United Kingdom have reduced the overall curricular time devoted to gross anatomy. Recent numbers for North America are elusive, but some estimate that anatomy instruction has been cut by as much as 80 percent since the 1950s (Zuger 2004). One study of Scottish medical schools showed declines of 60 percent to 85 percent in anatomy teaching contact hours. At the University of Edinburgh, anatomy contact hours dropped from 445 hours in 1983 to 67 hours (which includes 50 hours of laboratory time) in 2003–2004. Medical students at Edinburgh do not dissect cadavers. At St. Andrews, one of two Scottish medical schools where students still do whole-body dissections, laboratory time remained at 82 hours, a 32 percent decline from what it had been in 1983–1984 (Pryde and Black 2006, 18–19). In many poorer nations, medical schools have continued to teach using a traditional mix of lectures and dissections.

The decline in anatomy teaching parallels anatomy's decline as a research science. Human anatomy research began to wane after World War II as the medical sciences became increasingly cellular and molecular (Ludmerer 1999, 149). Researchers continue to make discoveries in human structural anatomy, especially in neuroanatomy, but most anatomists agree that the map of the human body at the level of tissues and organs is largely complete. Since the late 1950s, anatomy departments have become increasingly submerged within cell and molecular biology departments, sometimes renamed as "structural biology" departments. Faculty hired to pursue leading-edge biology research programs often ended up teaching gross anatomy, though many lacked expertise. In the 1970s, medical research became more of a full-time occupation and medical faculties hired fewer researchers willing to teach anatomy, creating shortages of qualified teachers (Ludmerer 1999, 292–93).

Dissection as an educational experience for medical students became controversial as a gap emerged between research programs and teaching needs. Anatomy instructors like to refer to themselves as "a dying breed."[5] Many departments now look worldwide to find qualified anatomists to teach their courses, relying on an aging population of North American anatomists, a few retired surgeons, and anatomists trained in countries with more traditionally structured medical education programs. One anatomy teacher at Urban University, who maintains a research program in the biological sciences, said anatomy teachers are

> in total demand everywhere. Universities all over the world ask, "Please come teach us gross anatomy. We have no gross anatomy teachers any-where left." And, in fact, that is true. No PhD program is spinning off teachers of gross anatomy at all, at all, at all.

With reductions in anatomy research and the accompanying shortage of qualified teachers, proponents of digital anatomy have stepped up their research efforts to develop pedagogical tools for anatomy teaching. By 2006, when I finished doing fieldwork, digital anatomy programs had become commercially available, and some digital tools were used to supplement traditional teaching (often to provide materials not covered by anatomy lectures). But traditional anatomy training through lectures and laboratories remained strong.

Digitizing Anatomy

As early as the 1950s, anatomists began to experiment with three-dimensional viewers and other technologies intended to help students understand the body's complex spatial relations, especially how three-dimensional structures correlate to two-dimensional radiological images. Dr. Richard Hunt, a retired surgeon and anatomist, described a chance encounter with stereoscopic photographs early in his medical training. Looking at three-dimensional images of the rib cage, he said he understood for the first time that ribs encircle the thorax at a downward and curving angle from the spine: the ribs are not perfectly horizontal. Richard contends that the understandings of spatial relations that such experiences provide can be especially important for beginning medical students. Though still a strong proponent of dissection, Richard has worked for decades to develop technologies that facilitate three-dimensional viewing of the body.

More recently, anatomists and educational publishers have worked to harness computing power to teach anatomy. These efforts range from relatively unsophisticated programs that help students identify and name body parts (an approach one anatomist I interviewed denigrated as "one click–one fact") to much more advanced computational and modeling efforts, such as the National Library of Medicine's Visible Human Project and plastination, the replacement of fluids in the body with polymers to create long-lasting models from real tissues.[6] Though all these technologies have limitations, many more teaching tools that compete with dissection have appeared in recent years. In this section, I detail one example of an anatomy education and research effort that reveals how researchers are adapting gross anatomy to a computational medium.

In the prestigious medical school that I call Cedar University, a small group of physicians, medical students, and computation experts is tucked into tight quarters filled with computers, anatomical texts and models, drawings, and graphic renderings of human anatomy. The group has worked for years to render the taxonomy of anatomical terms accessible to computer logic. Since Aristotle and Galen, anatomical terminology has accumulated slowly, punctuated by efforts at systematization, such as Vesalius's *De humana corporis fabrica* in the sixteenth century and the *Terminologia Anatomica* today. The investigators at Cedar want to make the anatomical lexicon not only searchable by computer but also available for use by expert systems, which would require that the terms be placed in a relational database describing hierarchical relationships among anatomical structures. Group members estimated that they eventually would have close to ninety thousand anatomical terms in their database. If the effort succeeds, this new anatomical taxonomy could be incorporated into future digital anatomy programs, eventually allowing computer applications to more easily correlate anatomical terms with graphically depicted structures.

The terms in Cedar's database would build on and modify classical anatomical taxonomies. Existing anatomical taxonomies contain ambiguities about relations among structures, many of which are clinically unimportant. An anatomist at Cedar explained to me, for example, that there are two types of skin, hairy and hairless. Anatomical taxonomies are vague on whether one type of skin is a subset of the other or whether both are a subset of "skin." The distinction is clinically irrelevant, but computational systems require ambiguities among relationships to be resolved. When ambiguities have arisen, the anatomists have consulted many sources and occasionally have simply decided on a relationship. Similarly, if an area of the body lacked a name, they invented one. Although human minds and clinical needs allow some relationships to be unclear or some parts to be unnamed, the computer's logic structures require precision. The resulting taxonomy will be a hybrid of standard anatomy and anatomy created for the database.

For years, Ernan Tomaso, an anatomist at Cedar, has collaborated with computer experts on this project. He argued that anatomists and computer scientists approach the same material very differently:

> The anatomists think about the way they view the body and the way they think about relationships. The cs [computer science] people think in terms of what is the best way to represent this. What system is best to represent this? To an anatomist, this is classification. To a cs person, it's how can you represent this in your application? . . . cs forces you to make it more explicit. It forces us to be consistent, logical, and explicit.

The effort to codify anatomical taxonomies according to the highly structured logic of computers requires the incorporation of some anatomical distinctions and terms that are not clinically significant. Although Ernan argues for the structuring effects of digital representation, he also recognizes that some anatomical relations would be unnecessary without a digital space to fill: clinical logic does not require as much specificity as digital anatomical taxonomy.

The reconstruction of anatomical taxonomies as digital representations is one of many efforts to make anatomical knowledge accessible to interactive computational systems. Cedar's effort reveals how anatomical and digital logics are being brought together in a platform that creates a more precise anatomical taxonomy, a taxonomy that adds terms and relations that did not exist prior to the digitization effort. This digital anatomy project reveals one way that computational representation is remaking the anatomical canon.

Open-Ended Exploration versus Instrumental Engagement

Specific arguments about dissection, which I detail in the next sections, focus on the role of open-ended exploration versus constant practice, acculturation versus abstract symbolic reasoning, and the meaning of mistakes, anatomical variations, and complex spatial reasoning. Many research-oriented medical schools have gravitated to teaching exclusively with lectures because laboratory-based courses require more faculty time (Ludmerer 1999, 309). Dissection proponents, including physicians, engineers, and medical educators, argue that anatomy is the last remaining laboratory experience medical students undergo. Proponents argue for the educational value of open-ended exploration, sometimes making an explicit analogy to bench science. As Dr. Anna Wilson, a hand surgeon sitting in on a discussion about anatomy's future, said:

> The human body is somewhat of a black box, and you have to explore it hands-on to get a sense of the context. If someone shows it to you, or it's on the computer screen, it's already packaged for you. You don't get to do that kind of exploration yourself.

Anna argued that exploring cadavers helps students contextualize anatomical structures and encourages them to organize material on their own instead of relying on lessons that are constructed by others (see also Becker et al. 1961, 110).

Dissection's skeptics argue, in contrast, that hours for anatomy education, including dissection, already have been so reduced that students must race through dissection, potentially eliminating the benefit of exploration. They often cite the high cost of maintaining a willed-body donation program. This reflects a curiously circular logic that justifies cuts in dissection due to the expense of maintaining a willed-body donation program that no longer makes sense given the short time students have to dissect. Dr. Gabriel Meier, an anatomist at Cedar, said he supports dissection, but he has begun to question its expense and its efficacy given how little time students have to study anatomy. He said:

> It's kind of become a sacred cow in anatomy, dissection. I am not saying that dissection is not important. It has its place. But it's the sort of a sacred cow that you mustn't cut back on it and you mustn't eliminate it.

But what must you do for a class of 120 to 130 students? You must generate at least twenty-five or thirty cadavers for a class of 100. And you have to have a body donation program that operates statewide that educates the public that it is a good thing to do. And then you've got to screen them. You've got to prepare them. You've got to embalm them. You've got to have a whole big setup here to deal with these bodies. And so it's a big, big expense. And then what has happened is the amount of time that is allowed to students to dissect has been cut back and cut back. So what they do is literally tear through, not having even enough time to really get the best out of it because they don't know what they are doing. They are trying to learn anatomy by doing dissection. And they destroy most of what they are trying to dissect because they don't know it. . . . If I sit down and dissect a hand of a cadaver, I do a very fine job and, even though I know it all, I always learn something new. But if a student is given a hand to dissect, before they know the hand, they're going to ruin 80 percent of the stuff you could ruin. What they have learned, they could have learned without dissecting the hand.

Gabriel worried that, by treating dissection as untouchable, anatomists were failing to recognize that students no longer have time to properly dissect, greatly diminishing dissection's effectiveness as a learning experience. He argued that dissection ought to be done with enough time and care that students learn from it. Gabriel also pointed to a difficulty inherent in the object itself: the body resists understanding. He described the human body as an immensely complex entity. He said that, even though he had been dissecting bodies for fifty years, he did not know every nuance of human anatomy. Individual variations, both anatomical and pathological, also are infinite. First-year medical students lack the skill to open a cadaver and properly illuminate its insides, he said, arguing that students should earn the right to dissect by demonstrating some anatomical knowledge.

The anatomical knowledge that Anna and Gabriel have far exceeds what first-year medical students are expected to learn. Anna, a surgeon who regularly reviews the anatomy of regions in which she operates, and Gabriel, an anatomist who learns something new every time he dissects, agree more than they disagree. Both Anna and Gabriel are anatomy experts who have learned the canonical body and many of its variations in depth. When Anna reviews anatomy before a surgery or when Gabriel dissects, they are reviewing and learning the finer points of anatomical structures. Both see the educational value of open-ended, unstructured dissection, but Gabriel would like to require that students learn some anatomy beforehand. By arguing for the value of structured exploration, as occurs in the laboratory, Anna and others acknowledge that clinical work contains many uncertainties and that trainees must develop an approach to problem solving and organizing information that later will help them confront these uncertainties. Dissection thus becomes, in part, a preparation for clinical problem solving.

In contrast, some anatomy teachers argue that anatomy courses should prepare students for board exams and early clinical training, not future medical work. During my first visit to Coastal University in 2001, I sat in on a meeting during which laboratory members, including engineers and anatomists, discussed the value of dissection. The meeting was about computer technologies that could supplement or replace dissection, but the discussion focused more on dissection. Dr. Graeme Fetters, a medical educator visiting Coastal from Australia, said that his program primarily teaches anatomical terms and visualization of structures by using photographs, models, a few cadaver demonstrations with predissected materials, and plastinated specimens. He said students in his program do some dissection in their first year, but he thinks the practice will be discontinued. "I think [dissection] will go because there isn't much evidence that it makes much of a difference," Graeme said. His program focuses on preparing students for their internships rather than for actual clinical practice and he sees little evidence that dissection contributes to student success during internships. Graeme's view may reflect the reality of medical school training for many students. In a 1961 study of medical education, Becker and others described how students in their first year of medical school rapidly realized that they had to set priorities about what to study, especially in "big courses," such as gross anatomy, that require mastery of massive amounts of information (Becker et al. 1961, 110). The students had two choices: they could study what they expected to be on the exams, or they could study what they deemed to be clinically relevant. Most students, even those who initially preferred the clinical view, eventually began studying for the exams.

Although many researchers, anatomists, and clinicians agreed that open-ended exploration can be an ideal means of learning, some argued that such exploration requires time that medical students do not have and resources that medical schools struggle to find. At stake in arguments for exploration or for a more limited use of dissection are the ends of anatomy instruction. If anatomy learning serves exclusively to prepare students for their board exams and their first weeks of clinical work, then a stripped-down program of demonstration and prepackaged learning modules may be the most efficient use of students' time. If anatomy education instead helps prepare students either for open-ended research or for the uncertainties and contingencies of clinical work, then an open-ended dissection might better suit this broader purpose.

The pedagogical effectiveness of exploration is difficult to measure, not least because the criteria to be measured remain somewhat unclear: How, for example, might instructors measure a trainee's ability to grapple with uncertainty or with unexpected findings? One intriguing study suggests that physical action itself has pedagogical value. The neuroscientist Francisco Varela argues that perception is most effectively trained as a product of exploration and action. He cites a 1958 study demonstrating that kittens allowed to freely explore their worlds developed more quickly than kittens experiencing identical phenomena as passive observers (1992, 331–32). Varela argues that perception begins with perceptually guided action (exploration) and that cognition emerges from repetition of perceptually guided action. His work raises important questions for anatomy instructors: What counts as action? Can taking a quiz to show memorization of names count as action, or does action, as in the kitten experiment, imply embodied exploration? Further, what do instructors measure when they give anatomy exams? Most written exams test the acquisition of anatomical names and locations. But can these exams also measure anatomical perception, the complex spatial and perceptual skills associated with dissection? Exams structure both course content and student learning, so exams come to define pedagogical significance for students.

Researchers building anatomy programs could inject more interactivity and exploration into their programs. They are limited not by the computational medium, but by the curricular priorities set by potential purchasers and users. As medical schools push to limit the time that students spend learning anatomy, designers likely will feel compelled to build applications that teach canonical anatomy as rapidly as possible. Designers could find ways to build exploration and anatomical perception into their teaching systems if medical schools defined them as values. The most important question is whether anatomy represents a ritualized introduction to medical culture or whether it is a more abstract exercise in learning language and spatial structures.

Acculturation versus Mental Model Formation

Challenges to dissection have made anatomists examine the lessons of gross anatomy and dissection in new ways, making anatomy's supporters step back to observe their own field much as an ethnographer might. A discussion about anatomy's future that I organized at Coastal indexes many of the issues related to anatomy controversies. Medical students take anatomy and anatomy laboratory during their first year, following a method of anatomy teaching that focuses more on the identification and names of structures than it does on clinical correlations. Most anatomists there supported continuing this method. Dr. Allan Smith, an anatomy professor, and Dr. Richard Hunt, a retired surgeon and anatomist, were strong proponents of the traditional anatomy program. Stephanie Porter, an educational technologies expert, played devil's advocate:

> ALLAN: And that is another reason why anatomy comes under attack because it can't say that new knowledge is being generated on a weekly basis. I mean, that's true.
>
> RICHARD: But neither is it in the French language, and yet if you go to France, it would be awfully nice to know how to speak French.
>
> ALLAN: I think we have to base our argument on exactly that. We don't try to compete with genetics or biochemistry in terms of the explosion of knowledge. We say, look, it's a language. It's an acculturation process, becoming a member of the medical community. And it applies to more of what lies in their futures, perhaps, than some of the other courses do because it's a fundamental language of description, of function, of nouns and verbs.
>
> STEPHANIE: And you can't replace it with a computer because . . . ?
>
> RICHARD: That you can talk to students about, and you'll find that the transition from undergraduate school to medical school is a very important period. And students time and time again will say, You know, I finally recognized I was in medical school when I walked in the room and here were cadavers, and we were doing something human, with human beings. And it's very important that they experience that, I think. They

learn a lot about death and dying. They learn a lot about family relationships because we spend a little time telling about where cadavers come from, poems by the donors and things like that.

The Coastal anatomists described gross anatomy as an initiation into medicine in several important ways. The discipline no longer is a productive research science, but it is medicine's language, the basis of medical cultures and communications (see Collins and Given 1994, 288). But the argument that anatomy is medicine's most fundamental language could support several types of curricula.

Language courses have moved toward a pedagogical model that emphasizes immersion (or some combination of immersion and memorization) over rote memorization. Dissection clearly gives students an immersive experience, one that can focus on identification of structures or on anatomical correlations to clinical problems. Many medical schools have attempted to immerse students by introducing them to clinical reasoning much earlier, an approach known as "problem-based learning." This approach allows instructors to build dissection around specific clinical cases or problems. Medical school instructors have hotly debated the merits of problem-based learning, focusing especially on the benefits of situated learning in the clinic versus the more thorough and systematic approach offered by traditional lectures. The debate focuses on the completeness of a highly structured approach versus the clinical relevance of a problem-based approach.

Proponents of traditional anatomy courses argue that problem-based learning is good in theory, but it leaves gaps because students are not exposed to the entire body during their clinical work. They advocate for an anatomy program that gives students a base to work from prior to making them learn in clinical settings. Many instructors have added more clinical correlations and clinical problems to their teaching, but others insist that learning to name and identify structures should remain a primary goal. Several anatomists told me that hospital staffs with active residency programs complain that interns and beginning residents often have insufficient preparation in anatomy. Allan and Richard argued that medical students must receive the best possible anatomical preparation for residency. Thus, anatomists argue about whether immersion ought to be immersion in terms and structures, immersion in clinical problems, or immersion in human cadavers.

Stephanie asked whether medical language could be taught using computers. Richard replied that medical students begin their acculturation into the medical profession with this investigation into human bodies, an investigation that can be highly charged and that includes lessons about death, dying, and the family relations within which most people are embedded. Anatomy is a confrontation, for many students their first, with death. Richard described gross anatomy as a transition from undergraduate school to medical school that includes learning a new language and new practices for working with the human body. Richard's description resembles an initiation as described by Van Gennep (1908), who documents three phases: separation from the original group, a liminal period of transition, and a final incorporation (*aggregation*) into the new order. First-year medical students leave behind their previous lives and begin their acculturation as physicians in the ritual space of the anatomy laboratory. Several physicians told me that, after the grueling hours of difficult studies required to get into medical school, the anatomy laboratory was the first experience that felt like clinical work.

The technical and sometimes gruesome nature of early medical education, as well as the sheer amount of time students must spend studying, isolates them from people outside their cohort (Becker et al. 1961, 88). Students enter a phase in which their relationship to the bodies of others bears little resemblance to previous experience. For example, some students struggle to separate their perceptions of the bodies they encounter in the anatomy laboratory from the bodies of people they see on the street (Good 1994, 73). During this phase, students begin to learn the norms and behaviors of the medical profession, their new group (Turner 1967; Van Gennep 1908). The memorial ceremony that many anatomy programs hold to commemorate the donation of cadavers also marks students' transition into the next phase of medical school. Dissection of a human cadaver remains, in most medical schools, the first, most important rite of passage into medical knowing.

Dissection proponents argue that the acculturation of medical students that occurs in the laboratory includes becoming accustomed to working with real bodies. Dr. Cassie Brown, an anatomist at Urban University, described how students become initiated into medicine during the first day of dissection:

> There's a medically sealed bag, and they have to cut it open. And I say, "Open it like a book. In other words, top, middle, and just flip it over like

this. Cut the bag first, you see." They're going to start getting familiar with their tools, but with the bag first. So you've got the green shroud flipped over but no face, no head or neck [is visible]. And then I show them what to do with the skin. I say, "First of all, you've got to find your bony landmarks: clavicle, sternum, and the low end of the rib cage." And they can all palpate that. So you do that. And OK, now they've touched. So they're getting used to it a little bit here. Because they've touched. And then they mark it [the body] if they have a felt pen. And I say, "Mark along here." And they do, so we're getting familiar now. And I say, "Now take your scalpel blade and just sort of sear the surface of the skin. Just score it." And OK, so that feels funny. They do that on both sides. Oh, and we're getting more used to it now. And I say, "Now cut a little bit deeper." And I show them that this is a layer of fat underneath. "And try, as you pick up one edge of the skin, try and separate it. Keep the fat with it and then, as you go down deep, you're going to see brown substance, and that's the first layer of the muscle." And they all do that. And so by the time I get through that first hour, they're pretty handy with knowing where it's going. That first lab, that's literally all they do. They get the skin open, like a book, in the same fashion that they cut the plastic bag. And then that's it. See, we're looking at muscle now. We're looking at *pectoralis major*. You can feel, you can see that bone was a clavicle and the other one was a sternum. And then we have a first rib. And they're seeing these bones now. Not through the skin, but they're seeing them. And then that's about it for that first day.

Cassie described the first dissection as an initiation both to working with the cadaver and to opening the body in layers. The first day begins with objectification of the cadaver as a distancing tactic. Students become familiar with their tools by cutting the bag open "like a book," then finding landmarks on the body, and cutting open the skin the same way they opened the bag, "like a book." Cassie's analogy is interesting: both cadavers and books open in layers. But books are much more familiar, creating a sense of the mundane for students. Students identify bony landmarks and use the landmarks to guide dissection. This requires them to match words to objects, initiating them into medical language and structure. Finding landmarks also requires students to touch the cadaver.

Cassie's statement that touching the cadaver helps the student become "used to it a little bit here" contains a complex, seemingly counterintuitive observation about the relationship between touch and self. Merleau-Ponty says that touch cannot be theorized in the same way as vision because we cannot describe what we touch without using terms that describe properties of the object itself. Tactile experience connects us very directly to the thing being touched. When we touch, we become aware of the tactile properties of the thing being touched. Touch encourages us to abandon what we imagine the object to be—a corpse—and to begin to grapple with the qualities that the object presents to our hands. Touch brings us into relation with the object, not allowing us to maintain distance by imagining what we think the cadaver is, but encouraging us to relate to the qualities that it presents to us—bony landmarks protruding from softer tissues, landmarks that become exposed bones over the course of the session. According to Merleau-Ponty, this relationship is not quite one of objectification. Rather, it is "a certain way of linking up with the phenomenon and communicating with it" (2002, 370). Touch grounds the connection between student and cadaver in the material sensations that the cadaver presents to students: leathery skin, greasy fat, hard bone. Though metaphysical concerns certainly creep in, the physical connection and the need to do the work of dissection and identification of parts holds the students' imaginations at bay.

Cassie said that the medical students she teaches have few emotional difficulties with dissection:

> When you start them gently like that, there's no problem. . . . They love it. It's not a matter of, Oh, we've got to dissect. It's exactly the reverse. Heart and lungs, they can relate to that. Everybody breathes. Everybody can feel their heart. Wow, I've got that in me. Is that what that looks like in me? So it's this intimate relationship with their own bodies that drives them.

When students touch cadavers and begin to identify structures, they forge a link to the body that leads to identification as the students discover the elements that all bodies, including their own, have. Cassie's interpretation of dissection fits my experiences in the anatomy classroom, where I periodically became aware of my own body, becoming conscious, for example, of my spine while the professor lectured about the spine's complex functions. In the previous chapter, I discussed the wonder that the body's marvelous workings can inspire. Cassie's comments suggest that some part of this wonder may result from connections students make between the anatomy that is exposed through dissection and their own anatomy.

On the other hand, Gabriel, the anatomist at Cedar, argued that the emotional preparation that dissection provides is minimal relative to the demands of clinical work. He argued that anatomists must help students deal with the emotional lessons of dissection but that such lessons go only so far in preparing students for the emotional rigors of clinical work:

> Medicine is a very emotionally intense profession. And people have to learn to deal with their emotions to become effective professionals. Seeing a bad wound is much more emotionally taxing than seeing a cadaver. I do think it is a major challenge for students coming in to deal with and one needs to consciously work around it and help them to positively and explicitly make it a learning experience and not just brush it under the table. So yes. But again, to my view, that alone, by itself, is not enough of a justification to expose students to cadavers. The biggest reason to expose students to a cadaver is because of the kind of mental image they are going to form for themselves of the way the human body is put together. If experiencing the cadaver enhances that mental image in some way, then there should be exposure to cadavers. But if it can be done other ways, cheaper ways, then we should not brush that under the rug.

Gabriel argued that anatomists must help students manage their emotional responses to dissection, but he separated this from mental model formation, which he viewed as the primary reason to dissect and the primary reason to seek less costly, possibly more effective, teaching tools. He separated emotion, which must be addressed as part of the learning experience, from cognition, which he maintained was gross anatomy's primary purpose. Gabriel presented a view of anatomical learning very different from Cassie's. Cassie described dissection as an embodied experience for medical students: touch initiates learning, and identification and fascination fuel student inquiry. In contrast, Gabriel argued that anatomy students must acquire abstract mental formations, language, and structure. Other considerations, such as students' emotional responses, must be acknowledged but should remain separate and subordinate.

Gabriel, who has worked since the 1970s on computational visual and linguistic models of anatomy, defined the most important aspect of anatomy learning as the acquisition of language and structure, allowing him to describe anatomy pedagogy in terms familiar to computational researchers:

> I thought that in order to be able to reason anatomically as a physician, because that's what you have to do when you are examining a patient or when you interpret any kind of medical data, for that you needed two things. You had to have a mental image, a mental model of what was underneath the skin, and you also had to have a kind of a more abstract symbolic model of the knowledge, of what were the relations, what was the kind of information that related to certain kinds of things. That sort of dual modeling problem has been a part of our big anatomy research. The research now is concerned with modeling, creating graphical models of the human body . . . but parallel to that, to make sense, to give meaning to that graphical model that is represented by pictures or 3D graphics or whatever, you have to have a mental model, and I call that a symbolic model because the symbols, you have to use some kind of symbols. For humans, the most meaningful symbols are terms.

Gabriel described the anatomical knowledge he considers most important as spatial and symbolic. He has worked with these concepts for many years, but the terms themselves derive from computer science and artificial intelligence. By describing anatomical learning as the construction of a mental image of human anatomy, including knowledge of three-dimensional structure and its identifying terms, he created an anatomy that leaves out the affective, relational, cultural, and bodily dimensions of anatomy education.

Gabriel has maintained that dissection still has a place in the medical curriculum, but his view of anatomy education subordinates lessons about death, the rite of passage into medical culture, and the reinforcement of knowledge created by tactile interaction with the body to the mental models physicians develop. This reflects the cognitive approach to physician knowledge. Marc Berg (1997) describes how medical practitioners constructed physician problem solving as a purely cognitive exercise, treating the physician's mind as an information-processing system that develops "symbolic mental representations" of problems (1997, 27). The cognitive view of anatomical knowledge deemphasizes the role of the student's body and emotions in anatomical learning and early physician training.

Some of Gabriel's ideas about the significance of language and structure in anatomical knowing developed from his explorations of artificial intelligence. Symbol manipulation that follows highly structured rules, such as rules of a game of chess, remains the easiest form of thought to approximate with a computer. Much artificial intelligence research has privileged abstract thought as the most significant aspect of human intelligence to emulate. According to this way of thinking, emotion and embodied action are peripheral to and distracting from learning. Such thinking has roots in European philosophical and cultural traditions, but may also, in Gabriel's case, come more specifically from the tools he has worked with and the knowledge practices they promote. Some critics of artificial intelligence have argued that the view of cognition adopted by early researchers in the field fails to acknowledge that cognition builds on embodied relations with the world. Dreyfus (1992), for example, argues that because computers do not develop as embodied beings interacting in the world, they will never know how to be intelligent. Some of Gabriel's dismissal of embodied cognition may come from his work with systems that appear to reproduce a mind without a body.

For Cassie, anatomy education begins with touch, with identification with another human body, and with wonder. For Gabriel, such considerations are secondary to the formation of mental models. Gabriel's view is far easier to represent on a computer. Indeed, I have heard several anatomists lament the loss of the physical and emotional experience of human dissection, which cannot be quantified in any meaningful way. The difficulty of gathering evidence about dissection's subjective lessons and their translation into clinical practice makes anatomists I have spoken with feel vulnerable to arguments about dissection's inefficiency as a learning tool. Verifying students' acquisition of language and structure is far easier than verifying their acquisition of in-depth anatomical perception and respect for patient bodies.

Mistakes and Memory

Dissection proponents argue that errors will increase as fewer physicians have deep knowledge of anatomy, but data about such errors remain elusive. Cassie argued that students with less anatomy training will make more mistakes:

> You're going to see an explosion in these errors. It's going to be an indirect cause and effect. It's true you can't [see cause and effect] directly;

in a court of law no lawyer would do that. But in a way I suppose you could. There will be cases when it's traceable back. Let's go to the example of the anatomical difference between you and me. Some people have this double brachial artery and you go through cutting it, you don't know what you've hit, because you don't know your anatomy [well enough] to know that a lot of people have a double brachial artery. And then the patient bleeds to death in front of your face and you'll say, "Yeah, but I've isolated the whole brachial. I don't know what's bleeding there." And it's your second brachial. [Such a patient will] bleed out in literally three minutes because that's how big it is.

The example Cassie gives is dramatic: a patient dies because a surgeon is unaware of an anatomical variation. Surgeons, however, build on and improve their anatomical knowledge during closely supervised residencies. Errors resulting from weak anatomical knowledge will rarely include fatal errors, but they will include costly ones, such as wasted time, unnecessary tests, and excessive referrals. Whether such errors will contribute to deaths, court battles, or the rising costs of health care likely will be difficult to separate from other clinical issues. Nigel Greene, an anatomy instructor, told me that student dissections often reveal that death certificates misstate the cause of death, though such errors typically are not clinically significant (a proper diagnosis would not have lengthened most of these patients' lives). Like Cassie, Nigel found these trends worrying.

Although anatomists fret about clinical errors that poor anatomy knowledge could cause, they also argue that dissection mistakes might help students learn. Richard Hunt, the retired anatomist, argued that mistakes stick in a student's memory:

It's . . . the hands-on thing, the hand-brain notion. Another thing is that you learn where a structure is because you don't want to cut it and, therefore, you dissect carefully. . . . If you want to have something stick in your head and you cut the facial nerve, you will forever remember what it was.

According to Richard, cutting a nerve critical to human function has an emotional valence that strongly reinforces memory. This contrasts with Gabriel's view of emotion as something to be managed lest it interfere with learning. A mistake represents a "microbreakdown," a moment that interrupts the flow of experience, leading to new modes of behaving (Varela

1992, 328). In this moment, emotions—frustration at the mistake, recognition of what this mistake would do to a living patient—lodges the structure firmly in the student's mind. The mistake itself is unimportant (the cadaver is dead, after all), but a mistake can mark a moment when the student must stop working and reflect on what happened and upon the effects such a mistake would have on an actual patient.

Although Richard described a dissection error as a learning opportunity, others might describe it as a lost opportunity to back up and try to get it right. The destructive nature of dissection—the fact that it is a one-way process—has inspired technology builders to imagine digital teaching tools by appealing to pedagogical logics common in mathematics, chemistry, and other sciences. A computer expert working on the Visible Human Project told me that a chance conversation with an anatomist inspired library officials to start the project. As the library official recounted the story:

> [The anatomist] says, "If you really want to use computers in medical education, you should do it in the subject of anatomy." Immediately, I figured that's why he's an anatomy professor. So, I says, "Why?" And he says, "Because you can't study anatomy. You take it apart and then what? You can't study it like you study mathematics. Or you study any of the sciences. [With mathematics and the sciences], you do the experiment. You read the book. You work the formulas. You can keep regurgitating it. You can't do that with anatomy because you're exposed to it once. You take it apart. Anatomy is three-dimensional. You do it from the top-down [meaning from the outside in]. You never saw it from the bottom up. It's different. . . . You can't back it up. You can't reset. You can't do any of that. So if you could do it on a computer, you could do all of the above."

Mathematical and chemical formulas are reversible. That is, one can solve the equation one way, then try it in reverse to see if the logic holds. Dissection, however, uses a real body whose destruction cannot be reversed. Students have no opportunity to go back if they make mistakes. A well-designed computer program, the anatomist argued, would allow users to take apart the computerized body, put it back together, change the angle of approach, and repeat the process as often as needed to learn how structures fit together, making dissection a two-way process. Dissection, in this view, comes to resemble solving a puzzle, an exercise that can require considerable spatial orientation skills but far less affective charge.

The arguments that a dissection mistake is a learning opportunity or that a digital dissection could be reversible present two different concepts of learning. The first argument suggests that students recognize that a slip of the knife while dissecting a cadaver would be enormously damaging to a patient's life and a physician's career if committed on a living patient. According to Richard, this recognition can be marshaled as a force for lodging an anatomical structure (and its significance) in memory. This resembles the logic of surgery education: in the operating room, surgeons discuss potential dangers, actual mistakes, and near misses constantly by orally rehearsing the stakes of a surgical slip. As I argue in chapter 4, this constant recitation of the high stakes of surgical practice becomes embodied in trainees as a powerful imperative to do no harm.

The argument that dissection should be made digitally reversible makes memory a function of repeated practice. This logic also works in surgery because residents are encouraged to practice as often as possible on as many patients as possible. Thus, surgical education in the operating room combines high-stakes practice with frequent and varied repetition. The logic of repetition also is common to mathematical and chemical learning, in which the ability to manipulate equations in multiple ways develops into mastery. But mathematical or chemical problem solving typically entails low-stakes manipulation of equations, often as preparation for higher-stakes activities, such as building a prototype or mixing chemicals. The logic of low-stakes manipulation of symbols dominates in simulation and other disciplinary models of education that encourage repetition as the right means to achieve embodied mastery.

Both cadavers and digital dissection programs provide a virtual enactment of medical practice. Dissection supporters locate laboratory work within the high-stakes milieu of clinical practice: a dissection error encourages the trainee to imagine the consequences of a similar error committed upon a living patient. In contrast, digital anatomy supporters reconstruct dissection as a form of symbol manipulation, making a case for the development of facility through repeated practice, regardless of relation to the problems physicians ultimately will face. In the first view, the cadaver becomes a privileged object-subject, a surrogate for the patient with a central role in a major rite of medical passage. In the second view, a digital cadaver is a self-contained object, a formal construction, like an architectural drawing perhaps, that can be decomposed and recomposed without reference to the external surroundings or to past or future.

The differences between cadaveric and anatomical technologies should not be viewed as exclusively about the objects in question. The anatomy laboratory as described in the previous chapter provides a setup intended to resemble a scientific or clinical laboratory. Anatomists work to call forth the cadaver's humanness by discussing the voluntary nature of donation, for example, and they often discuss the relationships of specific discoveries in their laboratory to clinical work. Anatomists also work to instill a particular form of clinical respect for human materials. In contrast, digital practice can take place anywhere with a computer and typically lacks the medicalized context provided by anatomists and the laboratory setting. Graphic models of bodies and instruments often look like cartoons, rather than like human bodies and surgical tools. Digital practice with these kinds of technologies also can evoke videogames, with their history of mindless digital violence at their worst and license to play at their best. Which method most effectively promotes learning of anatomical structures is unclear. Digital anatomy supporters argue effectively for the value of low-stakes practice through which a trainee can explore the meaning of mistakes (Satava 2006, 5). Used constructively, the ability to make a mistake to see what happens might provide trainees with new opportunities to think about clinical errors and medical ethics. But how such exploration would translate into clinical care—into the cultivation of a practitioner committed to doing no harm—is less clear.

Three-Dimensional Bodies

Anatomists often argue that cadavers provide a better model for teaching students the body's three-dimensional structures than do computerized or textual representations. Many anatomy proponents said tactile experience helps practitioners develop a sense for anatomy in three dimensions. Touch reinforces the visual understanding of the body's spaces.[7] Some anatomists and physicians argued, in a similar vein, that bodies are dense and that their structures are deeply interconnected. Laboriously taking the body apart gives students an appreciation of this density and helps teach three-dimensional spatial skills, one of the most important goals of anatomical teaching. For example, Dr. Harry Beauregard, a retired gynecologist, has said successful surgeons must develop the ability to extrapolate from two-dimensional images to the three-dimensional body (this skill also is fundamental to interpretation of radiological images). He said prosections—cadavers dissected for the student by an instructor—fail to provide the sense of connections that dissection can provide.

Jeremy Corso, a third-year medical student, discussed the difficulties of correlating pictures in a textbook to anatomical structures:

> You learn that three-dimensionality is drastically different from two dimensions. I can tell you we were going in to dissect and we had *Grant's Dissector*. It's this book that tells you what to do, and it has pictures and it even says, step one, cut here, step two, do that. And we would get totally lost because the body is just so complex, and there are so many variations that you don't always understand what structure you're looking at or how deep to go or what to do, and you really need a clinician next to you, or an anatomist to show you what you're looking at and where to go and give you some tips. You know, it's complicated. It's not just look at a picture or get a recipe and then execute it and find what you want.

According to Jeremy, dissection, like any complex craft skill, could be taught more effectively by a master teacher than by a book or a procedural guide. Jeremy had yet to develop the anatomical visualization skill that would allow him to dissect the body in layers. He struggled to understand just how deep to dissect to find structures of interest, a struggle that is typical of medical students and some beginning residents. Jeremy recognized that bodies vary enormously, so distinguishing canonical structure as presented by an atlas from normal and pathological variations in a cadaver or a living human body takes practice. Anatomical structures and dissection steps can be depicted or described, but dissection nevertheless requires expert guidance (see Pinch et al. 1996). Dissection exposes students not only to the body's regions and systems, but also to connections among tissues, muscles, fat, and fascia that may be clinically insignificant but might help form a three-dimensional understanding of, for example, the effect of an injury or the difficulty of penetrating a region surgically. Anatomical perception becomes embodied through action (Varela 1992). Medical students initially rely on experts' trained eyes and hands while they are training their own eyes and hands.

In contrast, some dissection critics argue that biomedical practitioners increasingly use medical imaging systems to diagnose diseases and guide practice. Often, these images provide full-color, real-time views of the living human body. The cadaver is a poor model to teach the dynamic anatomy of the living, they argue. Although cadavers permit some demonstrations of anatomical function, such as pulling on tendons in the forearm to observe how fingers move, critics believe that digital tools provide a better means of representing the body in action. To respond to the blossoming of image-based medicine, anatomists have increasingly incorporated such images into their courses. They represent a shift from an anatomical-structural view of the body to a physiological-functional view. The differences between the body as represented by the cadaver and the body as represented in a medical image reflect the many ways that bodies can be represented in biomedicine and beyond. Anatomists must attempt to anticipate which types of representations will most commonly guide future physicians.

Training and refinement of clinical perception occurs throughout medical training, especially as trainees come under the intense supervision of residency. Theoretically, computers could teach students procedural steps or visual cues to help them dissect. Practically, however, computers can determine whether a student has executed a task exactly, but they often cannot determine where and how a student has strayed, whether the student cannot see or has missed a step, or cannot see the proper anatomy (see Suchman 1987 on problems with procedural scripts). If anatomy teaching focuses on visualizing structures in patients' bodies, students may require extensive practice with real bodies. As I show in the surgical examples in the next three chapters, discerning structures in the living body takes years of expert guidance and practice to learn. Anatomists, medical school curriculum experts, and residency program directors have debated when trainees should get this practice.

Canonical versus Instantiated Anatomy

Debates about anatomy teaching all are underlain by a significant tension in biomedicine that transcends anatomical study. Ernan, the physician building digital anatomical teaching tools, captured this tension by distinguishing between "canonical" and "instantiated" anatomy:

> I still think at this point that there's no substitute for the cadaver. You get the actual feel of the structures. You actually see the spatial relations

between objects that you can't grasp with a two-dimensional object. You can see whether the tissues are soft or hard, loose or dense, and you get the tactile perception. The other thing about cadavers: it gives you an instantiated model, not a canonical model. . . . Actual cadaver dissection is instantiated. A lot is the same for you and me and for everybody else. But the variations are infinite. They are in the granularity, in the details.

According to Ernan, the canonical model represents typical anatomy, the anatomy that most of us share, whereas the instantiated model reveals the particularities of individual bodies. Cadavers are instantiated bodies, models of human anatomy, but models derived from deceased individuals rather than ideal types.

Many anatomists argue that dissection teaches bodily variations more effectively than digital tools, which tend to present a canonical view of the body. Cassie stresses that first-year anatomy students learn the basics and learn how to find things quickly:

They know now that the heart is in the chest, it's not somewhere under the pelvis. They know all that utterly basic stuff. But the fine details, above all, are the anomalies. Because we all think we look like the textbook, but of course, we don't. There are not two people that look the same inside. We're as different on the inside as we are in our facial features.

Digital modelers say they can build models showing any variation that exists, though I have not seen this claim put into practice. Anatomy laboratories are well equipped to show differences because students can compare variations among all the cadavers in the room. Several practitioners I spoke with said their anatomy professors used laboratory cadavers to teach anatomical variations and pathological problems, lessons they found fascinating and memorable. For example, I observed an anatomy class at Coastal University while students dissected the heart. One group of dissectors became frustrated because they could not find the heart, a seemingly simple task. With help from an instructor, they found a very enlarged and damaged heart that had become mired in clotted blood. The patient had suffered a dissecting aneurysm, a commonly fatal condition that causes the layers of the aorta to split and separate. The patient probably bled to death as blood leaked into his chest cavity. The instructor said the aneurysm likely was the patient's cause of death. Anatomical and pathological variations in bodies are normal findings in a typical anatomy laboratory; good instructors use them as teaching opportunities.

The advantages of the anatomy laboratory resemble the advantages of clinics in the late eighteenth century, bringing many bodies together in a clinical space, where practitioners can see variations, and the consequences of variations, caused by diseases or by anatomical structure (Foucault 1973). Having many instances of normal anatomical variations and pathological anatomy can reinforce for students the highly variable nature of the human body and the significance of paying attention to details, a vital aspect of biomedicine's inductive method of clinical diagnosis and problem solving.

The tension between canonical and instantiated bodies threads throughout many discussions about how to develop effective teaching technologies for medicine. An open-ended laboratory experience, for example, would entail exploration of very specific bodies, instantiated bodies, their pathologies, and their variations. A course geared toward exams, by contrast, would tend to teach a canonical body, one as close to normal as possible, possibly with some discussion of major anatomical variations. Medical students studying anatomy wrestle with the relationship between canonical and instantiated anatomy. For example, an anatomist on a list-serv for anatomy teachers argued in favor of making the discovery of pathology a key part of the gross anatomy laboratory. He wrote,

> Currently, when the students find cancerous lymph nodes destroying normal tissue, they get frustrated because they can't "see" what's expected of them. . . . We also get students frustrated by "anomalies" that are only minor variations. [By examining pathology], they will learn what is a variation and what is normal.

Students who hope to see "typical" anatomy will become frustrated by pathological and nonpathological variations that depart from the canonical body. They want the canonical body because that will be on the exams. Yet clinical work requires the ability to shift from canonical anatomy to instantiated anatomy and back. One surgeon I spoke with, for example, described starting each surgery with canonical anatomy in mind and continually revising it as details of the patient's specific anatomy come into view.

Cadavers also are the instantiated bodies of former human beings, so some teaching programs encourage students to develop respect for patients by first developing a connection with an individual cadaver, a connection based on touch and identification, as Cassie described above. This pedagogical model treats learning as a product of bodily action that engages multiple senses. This type of learning also often involves working in a team, which is a critical skill in medical practice. A pedagogical theory based on a cognitive theory of learning works from the notion that what matters is development of an abstract mental model that integrates anatomical language with visual-spatial structures. This model replaces learning through bodily action with learning through mental repetition. According to some anatomists, such as Graeme, the Australian anatomist, the results may be identical on exams, but dissection proponents argue that learning to treat patients involves much more than an exam can cover. The tension between the canonical versus the instantiated body in biomedicine has existed at least as long as students have had to learn normal anatomy for exams, while also needing to understand variations on normal anatomy in practice. But simulation and teaching technologies for medicine, which often are produced in collaboration with engineers and others who tend to work from abstract models, make this tension more acute.

The tension between canonical and instantiated anatomies helped encourage the researchers working on the Visible Human Project to section and image two cadavers that could be used to make models of real bodies, efforts that resulted in the image databases known as the Visible Human Male and the Visible Human Female. Many earlier computational modeling efforts began with models made using computer-assisted design, which builds graphic models from basic geometric shapes. Researchers rejected these models on the grounds that they were insufficiently faithful to the human body. As Thomas Laqueur (1990, 166) points out, what gets to count as canonical anatomy changes with historical and cultural movement. The Visible Human Project begins to shift the meaning of the canonical body because the bodies presented are as close to canonical as researchers could find and their use in anatomy applications is ubiquitous, but they remain the bodies of individuals, rooting the canonical in two specific bodies.[8]

Tensions between canonical and instantiated anatomy also have affected efforts to develop surgical simulators. For example, at the 2002 Medicine Meets Virtual Reality conference, an annual meeting that focuses on the technologies of modeling and simulating human bodies, two young engineers presented a paper in which they had designed a virtual model that doctors could navigate to practice surgical manipulations. The model looked vaguely intestine-like but did not reflect actual human anatomy. A few minutes into their presentation, Dr. Richard Satava, a leading researcher in the field of virtual medicine, stood up from his place in the audience. His body was tense, and he spoke with an anger that seemed out of proportion to the circumstances. Intestine-like is not good enough, he said. Physicians work on real bodies. Models need to be of real bodies to be effective teaching tools. In the early 1990s, debates about whether graphic models should begin from wire-and-foam mockups of body parts or from images of real bodies ended in favor of models made from real bodies. The engineers' model was a throwback, he said.

The historical debates that Satava invoked do not seem significant enough to account for his anger, but Satava strongly advocated the use of models made from images of real human anatomy and he was pushing back hard against a return to models lacking a basis in images of actual humans. Yet his argument that physicians work on real bodies echoes words I heard often while doing fieldwork among medical technology designers: no matter how technological physicians get, they still treat "real" or "human" bodies. The real body Satava described is, in fact, not a real body at all. Rather, it is a graphic model made from images of real bodies. But his anger suggested that he worried about the potential distance separating models from the bodies a physician treats. The word "real" asks us to look at what it is contrasted to, in this case a graphic model vaguely resembling an intestine. The model's purpose was to give physicians opportunities to practice surgical manipulation. The engineers reasoned that the material practiced upon would not matter if the model could teach a generalized type of skill. But for Satava, medical practice must remain linked to real human bodies.

Although Satava and other technologically oriented physicians advocate digital teaching technologies, they are uncomfortable with technologies that could lead training away from the instantiated body, the real body, the clinical body. The instantiated body, the individual and specific body, remains vital to clinical practice and currently is a significant part of how trainees learn. They learn to focus on details—anatomical, clinical, technical—that make each case, each body, unique, learning to inductively sort out these details to make a diagnosis. The epistemic anxiety that occurs when physicians sense that technologies are leading them away from the "real" body explains a significant tension in biomedicine that promises to become larger as treatment regimes such as decision protocols and evidence-based medicine, which aggregate and abstract information about bodies, become more powerful (see Timmermans 2003). Biomedicine needs both types of bodies, canonical and instantiated. Physicians must work from particular details of a case to the general physical state these suggest and back to the particular. The trend in medical technology development, however, is toward more abstraction, more aggregation, fewer "real" bodies. Encounters with instantiated bodies, either real bodies or programs created with built-in variation, get deferred to clinical work or to future computational developments. Some physicians discern a danger in new technologies that rely heavily on the canonical; they fear that the specifics of individual bodies and cases will be lost. Debates about dissection reflect these larger tensions. Dissection is always dissection of an instantiated body, yet computers tend to teach the canonical body.

Conclusion

Medical training enacts at least two bodies: that of the patient and that of the practitioner. A parallel exists between the practice object used to teach anatomy and the practitioner, who develops by learning with particular objects. Proponents of dissection argue that physicians' perceptual skills begin to be embodied in the anatomy laboratory. The act of touching the cadaver removes trainees from abstract concerns about bodies and puts them into very direct relation with a cadaver's physical properties. Some anatomists argue that the experience helps trainees develop anatomical perception. Also, as students touch cadavers and come to recognize their own bodies in the cadavers, they develop respect.

Proponents of digital tools argue that anatomical knowing is information processing: students must be able to match anatomical terms with an internalized, visual model of structure. This view is representational. What matters is not the cadaver or any relation with the cadaver, but the completeness and accuracy of the image formed in the mind. This representational view follows a theory of knowing that privileges abstract symbol processing, a common computational metaphor of mind. Moves to digitize anatomy also follow several rationalizing trends in medicine. Most obviously, digital anatomy promises to reduce the expenses of willed-body donation programs. Digital anatomy also follows the logics of digital technologies that change the relationship of bodies to time and space: digital anatomy applications are meant to take anatomy learning out of the laboratory and the classroom, making learning tools mobile and, possibly, marketable. This could represent the "enterprising up" of anatomical education (Strathern 1992). Further, digital anatomy makes dissection reversible, changing the pedagogical focus from high-stakes, emotionally laden, situated learning to disciplinary drill and practice with anatomical models that can be reset, rather than with body parts that can be destroyed. Finally, digital anatomy's focus on cognitive absorption of names and structures reduces or eliminates those aspects of anatomy learning that are difficult to quantify and, therefore, difficult to embed in a computer, including the affective and tactile lessons of dissection.

The craft-oriented, relational view of anatomy and the representational, information-processing view of anatomy index different areas of medical practice. Both teach anatomical terms and structural thinking. Dissection, however, relates to medicine's craft traditions, particularly surgical method and teamwork. And it encourages the scrutiny of anatomical and pathological signs (received by all the senses) as evidence for the inductive method of clinical diagnosis. Further, dissection allows medical students a first encounter with medicine's emotional demands. Digital anatomy speaks to areas of medicine driven by medical-imaging technologies that represent the human body on a two-dimensional screen, which is an increasingly important mediator for biomedical diagnosis and treatment. Further, digital anatomy allows students to explore bodies, to make mistakes and try again, and to practice as often as necessary to achieve mastery. As digital tools for teaching anatomy become more able to compete with dissection, anatomy instructors and medical school administrators running willed-body donation programs must ask what is gained when anatomical learning goes digital and what is lost.

three

CULTIVATING THE PHYSICIAN'S BODY

How a doctor thinks can first be discerned by how he speaks and
how he listens. In addition to words spoken and heard, there is
nonverbal communication, his attention to the body language of
his patient as well as his own body language—his expressions,
his posture, his gestures.

GROOPMAN 2008

"There is no syllabus," complained a first-year surgery resident. After grad-
uating from a Middle Eastern medical school, the resident, whom I will call
Dr. Amal Nassif, had been on a general surgery rotation for three weeks and
had not been in North America for much longer. We were sitting at a nurse's
station outside several surgery suites, waiting for anesthesiologists to finish
prepping the next patient. Amal's first weeks had been disorienting and
frustrating, he said. When he was on call, he was on call for four surgery
services, handling about forty-five patients. The next resident up the hierarchy from him handled only twenty. He asked how this could possibly
make sense, his voice a mix of confusion and anger. Residents, surgeons,
and nurses told him what to do but rarely explained their reasons. When he
asked senior residents and staff physicians whether this disorienting flurry
of activity was typical, they told him, "This is the shit I went through. Now
you've got to go through it."

I told Amal about a talented young surgeon, who told me that all the
surgeons he knew had doubts about their career choice at some point
during residency. Amal thanked me. Two weeks later, I encountered Amal at
the same nurse's station. His work was getting easier, he said, and made

more sense to him. He made a point of thanking me again for telling him that surgery residents have doubts. While we waited for another patient (a constant feature of surgical schedules), the surgery service's chief resident, a confident and funny woman named Dr. Julie Martinez, joined the conversation. If Julie had doubts, they were not evident. Amal decided to test my statement, asking his chief if she had ever wondered about her career choice. "Oh, yes," Julie said. Amal looked surprised. Her first days in the operating room were terrifying, she explained. She started to quake, imitating herself as a frightened beginner, and said she did not want to touch anything. When someone asked her to do something, she would think, "Me?" Other residents bragged about performing complex procedures and she only gradually learned that they usually had held retractors or done other simple tasks during these procedures. Only time and practice in the operating room had made her more confident.

When new residents arrive at the hospital, they start clinical work with little delay. They must rapidly grasp formal and informal social rules and learn to manage the enormous work demands placed on them. Much resident learning involves observing practices, attempting them under supervision, developing increasing autonomy, and, eventually, passing skills on to those more junior, a practice known as "see one, do one, teach one."[1] Many physicians I have talked with consider their first year of residency and their first year as staff physicians to have the steepest learning curves of medical education because both entail vast increases in knowledge and responsibility. This chapter discusses surgical internship and residency education, showing how practices in clinics, wards, and operating rooms accumulate, leading residents to embody behavioral dispositions of surgeons, and more broadly, medical professionals. I focus here on larger issues of medical embodiment, especially those related to the earliest years of clinical training and the cultivation of surgical affect and judgment. By making the embodiment of medical practices central to my analysis, I show how practices in specific sociotechnical milieux accumulate to remake the trainee's body in ways that allow the emergence of unique dispositions to act, to relate, to believe, and to feel that many medical practitioners share.

Embodying the Hidden Curriculum of Medicine

In contrast to the formal, programmatic syllabus that Amal craved, a vast amount of medical learning involves the adoption of values, styles of practice, priorities for treatment, and techniques that are rarely invoked as explicit curricular objectives. Instead, clinical trainees receive a mix of lessons that range from updates on the latest clinical science to demonstrations of technique to messages (both stated and unstated) about expectations for performance. Many of these lessons take place in the clinic and are determined by the needs of particular patients. Although clinical instructors often have well-defined expectations of the skills that trainees should develop, these are rarely articulated as they would be on a syllabus. Scholarly and popular depictions of medical training contain descriptions of the development of a physician's senses, diagnostic abilities, emotional composure, and competence. Bringing a focus on embodiment to these accounts can make the picture more complete. Specific medical practices, such as stitching or tying knots, clearly are techniques of the body. Less obvious, perhaps, are the ways that medical values, affects, judgment, and styles of interaction also become embodied with clinical practice.

Medical residency programs have been likened to Erving Goffman's "total institutions," such as asylums and army training camps, in which institutional rules govern every aspect of a person's life, from when and where one sleeps to what clothing one wears, what food one eats, and what comportment is expected (Goffman 1961a; Good 1994). People are stripped of their previous identities and often must undergo various forms of humiliation and mortification as part of a transformation of self. Such institutions remake a person's being in conformity with the organization's expectations for disciplined behavior (Goffman 1961a; see also Foucault 1977). The comparison is apt, especially for the grueling first years of residency as they were practiced during most of the twentieth century, when residency requirements entailed up to 120 hours of work a week, supervision that often was harsh and sometimes abusive,[2] and, until recent decades, actual residence in the hospital (the origin of the term "resident"). The comparison of residency to life in an asylum or army camp, however, misses residents' ultimate trajectory, as they engage in "prestigious imitation" (Mauss 2007, 53–54) of their supervisors, moving from relatively simple tasks toward full responsibility for the work and risks of healing. Medical trainees are expected to adapt to demands of the institution and to advance into the professional roles of its most prestigious leaders. They must master clinical practices and learn clinical judgment. Rather than remaining cogs in a disciplinary machine as inmates and soldiers often do, medical residents work toward increasing autonomy and responsibility as they demonstrate growing proficiency (Ludmerer 1999, 97–98).

The transition from medical school to clinical residency marks a shift from the formal schooling of the classroom to situated learning that occurs in a hospital. The transition from overwhelmed first-year resident to confident chief entails several existential transformations that continue long after a senior resident becomes a fully qualified surgeon with responsibility for treatment.[3] Medical residents are apprentices to many masters. In general, the education of apprentices has "as much to do with how to behave as it has to do with mastering specific tasks" (Coy 1989, 3). This form of education involves learning specialized practices that appear secret or mysterious to those on the outside and convey a sense of distinctive identity to the practitioner. Residency training mixes qualities of several kinds of apprenticeship, including a concern with rules, formal and informal, which often structure large organizations and strong relations with one or several masters, as characterizes craft apprenticeships (Goody 1989, 248). By definition, most residency training occurs through clinical interactions with patients, peers, and superiors. No formal sequence of learning occurs, as in a classroom setting with a formal program of instruction. Instead, many specialty areas have skills they expect residents to master before they advance to new levels, but verifying achievement of these goals takes place largely under the purview of clinical instructors. Clinical reformers, who are pushing for more standard measures of residents' progress, have criticized this as training that focuses more on time in residence than on skills acquired (Satava 2008, 147).[4]

Many lessons of clinical instruction represent the aspects of learning that practitioners call medicine's "hidden curriculum." Definitions of the hidden curriculum vary. Hafferty and Franks argue that the formal teachings of medical school courses, especially those covering ethical and social comportment, can be undone by negative behavioral lessons modeled by senior clinicians (Hafferty and Franks 1994). Using a more positive definition of "hidden curriculum," Kenneth Ludmerer, in his essential history of U.S. medical education (1999), explicitly contrasts medicine's "hidden curriculum," which he describes as "noncognitive," with the formal curriculum, which emphasizes knowledge and reasoning.[5] The hidden curriculum becomes instilled through student experiences as they learn medical "attitudes, values, character, and professional identity" (70). Both sources describe how trainees observe and listen to supervisors and peers, eventually mimicking their affective and technical practices and behaviors. These practices and behaviors become habitual, incorporated into the trainee's ways of knowing and doing, ultimately becoming impossible to separate from one's self.

Ludmerer describes medicine's hidden curriculum in cultural terms, saying that supervisors model "habits of thoroughness, attentiveness to detail, questioning, listening, thinking and caring" (1999, 361). He identifies four major aspects of the hidden curriculum: developing a compassionate bedside manner; adopting a view of patients as either humans or objects; learning professional "attitudes, values, and temperament"; and absorbing tacit cues from their instructors about what to downplay or ignore in clinical work (Ludmerer 1999, 70–71). Most physicians I encountered occasionally reflected upon aspects of the hidden curriculum in conversations with me and with their trainees. But an instructor's formal account of bedside manner or ethical behavior may bear little resemblance to what a trainee actually learns. Many of the subtleties of a positive clinical encounter remain impossible to verbalize. Once mastered, these skills become part of the professional persona of a "physician," developing into largely taken-for-granted dispositions to act in culturally specific ways (see Bourdieu 1977). Indeed, "hidden" is something of a misnomer because although physicians in teaching hospitals rarely cite the qualities Ludmerer describes in so many words, I found that they continually invoke them in stories and aphorisms, especially when they tell tales about their own training. Physicians in teaching hospitals reinforce the ways of acting that they model for their trainees with morality tales about proper ways of being and doing in medicine. These tales can be located somewhere between formal lessons and tacit behaviors, accompanying clinical activities with a susurrus of commentary of immense pedagogical value to those capable of listening.

The definitions of the hidden curriculum that Hafferty, Franks, and Ludmerer provide are represented as products of unspecified (and often unspecifiable) interactions of trainees with patients and supervisors. Yet, many of the behaviors Ludmerer describes involve bodily actions, such as expressions of understanding conveyed through words and body language that accompany a physician's discussion of bad news with a patient or family. As defined by W. L. Heinrichs and S. Srivastava (n.d.), two surgeons, the hidden curriculum clearly entails learning of bodily techniques. "This execution of steps to achieve individual, small goals often occurs rapidly and without comment, being lost in the choreography," they write. These definitions of the hidden curriculum stand in contrast to the formal clarity of a syllabus. They show clinical learning as it unfolds in the situated milieu of the hospital and as it is governed by unspoken normative codes commonly found in apprenticeship teaching systems.

Techniques learned at all levels of medical training reveal how much of technical training in medicine contains lessons about the social and affective requirements of being a doctor. Byron Good, for example, picks up the sensory and affective components of medical training when he quotes a medical student, who says, "I'll find myself in conversation. . . . I'll all of a sudden start to think about, you know, if I took the scalpel and made a cut [on you] right here, what would that look like? [*laughing*]. . . . Very often that happens. And it's a frightening thing" (1994, 73). Good shows that, as anatomy students become aware of the internal dimensions of bodies, they experience perceptual shifts that change the ways they look at bodies. But considering embodiment more broadly opens this quotation up to further analysis. First, the student describes this process of looking as initiated by the scalpel. This student's knowledge of the body's interior develops while he dissects. Seeing is inextricably bound up with dissecting. The student's knowledge of anatomy gets articulated as the student exposes structures in the body.[6] Second, the student's momentary experience of confusion of bodies to be cut up inside the laboratory and bodies to be left untouched on the street makes him laugh, even as he describes it as frightening. The student is learning to cut and to see in the laboratory, embodying new techniques for opening, examining, and knowing bodies.

When the student imagines himself dissecting bodies on the street, he begins to articulate new divisions in the world: between spaces where you cut and spaces where you do not cut and between bodies you cut and bodies you do not cut. Though this sounds self-evident, the spatial and social separations that authorize human dissection are profound. In these two spaces and with these two kinds of bodies, the student knows he should have very different physical, affective, and perceptual relations. Yet the affective intensity of the laboratory has bled into his everyday life. These experiences, which involve the student's body, his imagination, and his emotions, have encouraged him to worry about what separates patients' bodies from other bodies. These lessons—all contained in one upsetting fantasy—begin with the student imagining himself picking up a scalpel, a fantasy prompted by actual cutting in the laboratory. The relations of fantasy, reality, emotions, techniques, senses, and bodies in this story are complex, but the student's embodied experience—the techniques of the body that he learns for performing dissection and managing his actions and emotions—remains central.

The embodied skills that physicians must learn are perceptual, social, and affective. They also involve the development of higher-level abilities, such as intuition and judgment. T. M. Luhrmann, whose ethnography of psychiatric training includes observations applicable to medical training generally, describes how residents learn to recognize disease states from clusters of symptoms and disease patterns. "Intuition is the capacity to recognize patterns in body and behavior that are relevant to clinical problems, to see what is wrong with a patient, to judge the severity of the problem, and to choose an intervention that leads as quickly as possible to the patient's recovery" (2000, 34). Luhrmann's description of diagnosis shows how residents develop diagnostic intuition through repeated encounters with patients whose symptoms must be matched against disease classifications, known as "nosologies." Repetition of this matching process makes these clusters of symptoms coalesce into a correspondence between learned category and disease state. What Luhrmann describes as intuition begins with pattern recognition, which entails the construction of a perceptual syntax that gives coherence and meaning to behavioral signs. Intuition is a function of the progressive embodiment of clinical observation and medical practices, but as the word suggests, intuition also reflects a sensory embodiment that offers possible answers even when the reasons for these answers are not perfectly articulable. The accumulated and sedimented experiences and practices that make up this form of knowing also are not fully available to conscious review (see Merleau-Ponty 2002). Intuition thus becomes a technique of the body.

Hafferty and Franks, Ludmerer, Good, and Luhrmann show how the experiences of practice in a clinical context remake young physicians' values, intuitions, and perceptions. These scholars reveal medical training to be a cumulative process as trainees learn from mimicking more senior practitioners, wrestling with the meaning of dissection and other activities, and repeatedly identifying patterns among symptoms. These examples appear to be different aspects of the same process of cultivating medical professionalism, diagnostic skills, and perception. Examining them as aspects of medical embodiment, however, reveals the ways these seemingly diverse aspects of professional development emerge from the accumulation of practices that come to define the physician's relations with superiors, with medical ways of knowing, and with patient bodies. Much of what has been labeled the "hidden curriculum" in biomedicine consists of consciously or subconsciously adopted techniques of the body.

"Good Hands"

Surgical residencies take the general form of most other medical residencies, although surgeons have long considered themselves to be a breed apart from other physicians (Lawrence 1998). Surgery is a medical specialty that historically has been tied to craft work because of the physical techniques surgeons employ.[7] Since the early twentieth century, surgery has become one of medicine's most technological specialties (Stevens 1999). The definition of the word "surgeon" emphasizes the field's connection to craft by combining the Greek *cheir* (hand) and *ergon* (work) to portray the connection of hands to surgical action. The term captures the deep connection of surgery to physical action, though the emphasis on hands neglects the extent to which the surgeon's entire body participates in doing surgery.

Surgeons often use the phrase "good hands" to describe other surgeons' abilities. Several surgeons told me that the phrase rarely means technical skills when applied to medical students and beginning residents because they have yet to develop technical abilities. Dr. Anna Wilson, a hand surgeon, indicated that, with juniors, the phrase indicates someone who is adept at working within the social and organizational structures of the operating room by reading up on a case beforehand, showing up on time, and knowing when to ask questions and when to challenge the senior surgeon. Juniors who demonstrate that they understand surgery's unstated social and organizational rules, especially those who earn reputations as "stars," typically have more opportunities to operate, giving them more possibilities of becoming technically superior. With senior surgeons, the phrase typically applies to surgeons as a form of praise but sometimes is used as condemnation of another skill that may be lacking, such as good bedside manner.

I asked Dr. Nick Perrotta, a general surgeon, what "good hands" meant to him. He held up his hand and replied, "I don't mean this," indicating manual dexterity as he rubbed his fingers together. "Good hands," he said, means common sense: the ability to intuit the right thing to do even when not taught explicitly. He reminded me of a procedure he had performed that morning, during which he had used a tightly focused, high-pressure jet of water to dissect around a liver tumor. A very junior trainee on his first rotation held a suction device intended to keep the operative site clear of blood, but he kept placing it below the incision, allowing blood oozing from above the site to obscure Nick's work. Placing the suction above the spot where Nick was dissecting would have made sense, but the surgeon had to tell the student to move the suction several times. The student lacked "good hands," Nick said. Although "good hands" can be ascribed to talented technicians, Nick's example reveals the extent to which "good hands" is a metonym for the much broader combination of craft skill and situational awareness that makes up surgical ability. "Good hands," meaning the kind of common sense the trainee seemed to lack, is a foundation for good surgical judgment.

Nick's equation of "good hands" with common sense indicates that surgical embodiment goes far beyond technical skill. Surgery is embodied action, action that creates unique physical relationships between patients and surgeons. Surgeons argue that proficient technical skills are simply necessary for the job of doing surgery and that judgment is more important. This formulation suggests that the two are unrelated phenomena, as though judgment does not accrue from years of physical practice in the operating room. Separating technical skill from judgment makes technical skills appear to be purely physical labor, whereas judgment and intuition sound exclusively mental. These separations seem to replicate the split between mind and body that often characterizes Euro-American thought. But a look at the examples and the statements of physicians in this chapter and the rest of this book shows that surgeons recognize the existence of a much more complex interplay between physical and mental action. Nick's equation of "good hands" with common sense is just one example.

Developing Wisdom

Surgeons often dismiss the physical and technical aspects of their abilities as representing only a fraction of what they do. Several told me they became technically competent without any preexisting craft skills, such as the ability to sew. One group of surgeons I talked with collectively agreed that physical technique represents only 20 percent of their work. Some studies indicate that visual-spatial abilities may be more important for surgical success than nimble fingers (Groopman 2008, 141–42). These separations of body from mind and eyes from fingers reflect the profound fragmentation of bodies that characterizes much of biomedicine. Making hard distinctions between the components of embodied activity can mislead. The fragmentation of bodies reflects Euro-American cultural biases that privilege abstract, visual, and mental work over bodily labor. But separating mind from body and body parts from one another neglects the ways in which a practitioner's entire body participates in medical learning. Further, such divisions neglect the ways in which bodily techniques accumulate with experience, becoming increasingly connected to higher-level technical and sensory abilities, as well as to seemingly cognitive abilities such as judgment.

Surgeons simultaneously, and contradictorily, downplay the significance of the physical techniques of surgery while acknowledging the importance of technical skill. Two surgeons have created a pyramid of surgical learning that provides a useful schematic for thinking about the cumulative process of medical embodiment. Rather than separating physical from other forms of labor in the operating room, the pyramid represents judgment (and, ideally, wisdom) as emerging, rather than separate, from skills and information. Information, particularly the enormous amount of anatomical and clinical data that medical students cram incessantly, rests at the pyramid's base. Skill building follows information acquisition, the surgeons argued. With practice and experience, the trainee develops judgment. According to these two physicians, wisdom sits at the cumulative pinnacle of medical learning (Heinrichs and Srivastava n.d.). The pyramid simplifies a complex learning process that contains much more recursivity than the hierarchical pyramid suggests, but it gives a sense of the bottom-up process of medical learning. Each lower level gets subsumed under the higher levels, so that information, skills, practice, and experience come together at the service of judgment. As they develop, these skills begin to aggregate, becoming "a unity of action that is so reliable that it becomes invisible" (Latour 2002, 252).

At the highest levels of their craft, as surgeons in teaching hospitals demonstrate, tacit knowing and consciousness intertwine. As Richard Sennett describes this process, skilled craftspeople work with "the tacit knowledge serving as an anchor, the explicit awareness serving as critique and corrective" (2009, 50). Complex abilities emerge from repetition. Practitioners grapple with particular skills for years, developing facility and, later, more complex aspects of skill, such as fine motor coordination or the ability to determine a successful or unsuccessful attempt by sight. Over time, practitioners embody these developments in the individual package called a "surgeon." Separating medical practices from the physician's identity becomes increasingly difficult as knowledges, practices, and experiences become lodged within the practitioner, that is, as they become body (Bourdieu 1977).

The situated clinical learning that Amal, the first-year resident, initially found so disorienting takes place within a highly structured social milieu that puts beginning residents at the bottom of a powerful hierarchy. Clinical work requires more teamwork and greater deference to hierarchy than most medical students have previously experienced. During clinical rotations, supervising staff members typically require interns and junior residents to meet with patients, take patient histories, and present cases during rounds in which all members of a service gather to discuss diagnoses and treatment plans. When taking case histories, interns must present themselves to patients as medical professionals. Deviations from accepted standards meet with disapproval. For example, when a young resident, who evidently had finished a rotation late the night before, arrived at weekly rounds on a general surgery service at Urban Hospital unshaven, unkempt, and, evidently, unwashed, his supervisors greeted him with ribald teasing and speculations about his carousing. The teasing contained a powerful didactic message: Physicians should always present themselves professionally. The moment made me look around the room to note just how clean-cut and clean-shaven everyone else was, even those wearing surgical scrubs. Early on, trainees learn to present themselves as doctors by mimicking the tone, demeanor, dress, and professionalism of their mentors. From the first days of residency, trainees are encouraged to present themselves professionally, to enact the role of a physician before they embody it (DelVecchio Good 1995).

Case presentations teach trainees to bring the masses of information they memorized in medical school to bear upon clinical problems. While observing service rounds on a general surgery service, I watched a new resident present her first case. The resident recounted the details of a scoring system for pancreatitis, a painful inflammation of the pancreas that can cause severe complications. A surgeon asked her what she should do with a patient with Grade 2 pancreatitis and whether Grade 2 or Grade 4 is more serious. She did not know. A young surgeon in the group lectured her about the grading system, saying it can provide a diagnostically useful measure of how sick a patient is. A senior surgeon asked whether one would operate on a Grade 4 patient who had been taken to the intensive care unit. The resident said that, based on the fact that the Grade 4 patient is sicker, the answer should be "yes." The senior surgeon, laughing, said, "Well, you're wrong." A patient under intensive care with Grade 4 pancreatitis must be stabilized before undergoing surgery. The surgeon's use of mortification emphasized that the resident still had to learn that wrong answers have clinical consequences. Apprenticeship systems of training often include degradation of beginners before they rise to a new status (Haas 1989, 88). Thus, the surgeon mobilized the resident's affect to encourage her to embody the lesson.

Clinical trainees must begin to make practical, clinical sense of the information they spend years memorizing in medical school. "They have to make a transition from just collecting information to synthesizing and interpreting information," a chief resident said. That is, they must shift from "knowing that" to "knowing how." Knowing how in this sense means understanding that scoring systems and other abstract diagnostic measures have clinical meaning and clinical consequences. The scoring system is one means of helping physicians make judgments about the severity of a case and the patient's sickness. But understanding the scoring system's significance requires expert help. The surgeons pushed the new resident to connect abstract categories to a specific case. The resident had to learn to weigh the patient's symptoms against his ability to withstand major surgery. The senior surgeon's laughter seemed to ride a contradictory line between mockery and a softening of the critique of the resident's embarrassing performance. This worked to engage her emotions. His laughter also told the resident that she had a personal stake in the answer. The surgeon did not explain why one does not operate on a pancreatitis patient who needs intensive care, sending an implicit message that she should find out for herself and be prepared to answer such questions later. For the resident, the presentation marked a transition from the abstract principles and formalized knowledges of the classroom to the situated details of clinical cases, details that both patient and physician have a stake in getting right.

Surgeons describe the opportunity to do surgical work as a "carrot" given to juniors as a reward for exhibiting good social and organizational skills. Dr. Jill English, a chief surgery resident, said, "I spend more time making sure that they're good students than helping them decide if they want to do surgery or not." When I asked what she meant by "making sure that they're good students," she clarified with an anecdote:

For example, this morning the girl that was sitting next to me [in a meeting of the surgical service], we had asked her to present a patient today, and she forgot. And she just rolled in this morning after being post-call yesterday and having the whole day to do it. "Who was I supposed to present, and what was I supposed to do?" So I made it very clear by my facial expressions that I was distinctly unhappy with it, and then she didn't go to breakfast with the team. She spent the time looking at the chart, learning as much as she could, to present the patient. And I'm harder on her because she wants to go into surgery.

The education that trainees receive in the hospital includes inculcation in medical hierarchies and in the expectations and values of clinical teamwork: forgetting to prepare a case is unacceptable. The chief resident supervises the residents on the service. And, because an unprepared trainee reflects poorly on her management of subordinates, Jill made certain that the junior who forgot to prepare her case understood her displeasure.

Jill's comment about her facial expression captures a key element of the hidden curriculum in clinical teaching: much of it is nonverbal, ranging from facial expressions and gestures to taps on a misplaced hand when it blocks a surgeon's view. Especially in the past, this training sometimes included verbal and physical abuse, though these practices have declined as surgeons' teaching has come under greater scrutiny by hospitals and educators (Cassell 1991; Heinrichs and Srivastava n.d.; Ludmerer 1999). Jill's use of facial expression to indicate her displeasure suggests that medical embodiment involves, in part, sensitizing trainees to superiors' body language. The watchfulness required to parse supervisors' language and gesture forms part of trainees' adoption of their demeanor. They must become attuned not only to what patients' bodies tell them, but also to what their supervisors' bodies tell them.

Clinical rotations give trainees broad exposure to many facets of clinical work and help them choose a specialty. Many come to the hospital knowing very little about the hospital system. As Jill described the experience of beginning trainees:

They've never seen how it works in the hospital. And that's with respect to everything. How rounds go in the morning. How to write orders. Or how to write prescriptions. Or knowing that you have to pee before you go to the OR because your case is going to take a long time.

Residents typically teach juniors basic techniques, while staff physicians teach deeper clinical knowledge, such as the indications of particular diseases or the steps of a surgical procedure. As hospitals have become more concerned about liability and errors, they have encouraged more extensive supervision of trainees (Kohn et al. 2000; Ludmerer 1999). Having a superior suggest an appropriate time to urinate shows how profoundly disorienting early clinical work can be, as well as how much trainees may come to rely on more senior practitioners for direction, even with their own basic bodily functions. Further, it shows the extent of the bodily discipline expected of surgeons (see Moreira 2004).

Several surgeons told me that they allow beginners who demonstrate their social and technical preparation to advance from observing, holding retractors, and cutting stitches to more complex practice, such as stitching up an incision in the patient's skin at the end of a procedure, more rapidly than those who appear less motivated. At the end of a long surgery, I watched Jill patiently show basic knot-tying to a medical student doing a brief clinical rotation. She would not let him tie a knot on his own, saying later:

It's time. I'm not mean. I would let him do it if we had all the time in the world. But, you know, [the attending surgeon] has a schedule. And the fellows can only stand there for so long.

Financial pressures in the United States and backlogs of cases in Canada (another form of financial pressure) have increased demands upon operating teams to move more patients through the system, giving juniors fewer opportunities to practice than in the past (Ludmerer 1999). The time crunch puts an extra burden on residents to practice some skills, such as tying knots, on their own. Pressures to increase patient "throughput" also are driving interest in teaching that occurs outside the operating room, such as the development and use of surgical simulators.

Clinical work often begins with seemingly menial labor. Trainees call this work SCUT, an acronym with several meanings, including "some clinically useful training." Clinical work is situated in the hospital; opportunities for practice are contingent upon the hospital's patient population at any given moment. Amal's statement about the lack of a syllabus reflects the disorienting qualities of early clinical work. A syllabus is a synopsis for a course of instruction, a linear depiction that structures learning, revealing the instructor's objectives and dictating how learning should proceed. But a resident's education takes place in the hospital, in a sociotechnical milieu under pressures that increasingly put treatment, research, and pedagogy into tension (Ludmerer 1999). The day-to-day accumulation of clinical abilities that occurs in the hospital would be very difficult to capture as a linear set of learning goals. For most of his education prior to residency, Amal followed required programs organized and directed by others. In the first weeks of residency, without a syllabus, he felt thrown into a morass of clinical activities. He did not know how to set priorities or decide what he had to learn and what he could ignore. The formal knowledge he learned in medical school had become jumbled with practical techniques and new information. Although residency education bears little resemblance to their previous education, Amal and most other residents begin to find their way after a few weeks.

Overwhelmed junior residents must look to those more senior for guidance. A few weeks after our initial encounter, Amal pointed to several lengths of suture wrapped around a desk handle at the nurse's station and said that Julie, his chief resident, had taught him more about tying knots in a single half-hour session than he had learned in hours of practicing with a kit he received when he started work on the service. "Put that in your book," Julie joked. Further, Amal said, one of the staff surgeons had taught him the significance of wound care. "Without that, how would I have known about wound care?" he asked. He was rapidly learning which residents and physicians seemed most interested in and capable of teaching. This is one of the inconsistencies that medical education reformers want to fix: residency education is highly contingent upon the skills, time, and commitment of staff physicians. A good instructor can make a career; a bad instructor can destroy one (see especially Cassell 1998). Senior residents teach juniors technical skills and survival tactics. During residency, trainees build on these basic skills to gradually embody complex procedural knowledge and, eventually, clinical judgment.

Higher-level skills, such as surgical judgment, cannot be taught exclusively by verbal means. Rather, these skills develop with years of practice. Like other tacit skills, judgment, intuition, and clinical wisdom only fully "'make sense' when they have already been mastered" (Goody 1989, 247). Nevertheless, residents and fellows actively observe and listen to senior residents and surgeons, trying to parse the embodied abilities that supervisors enact. Jill, who was just beginning her year as chief resident, told me that she had mastered much of the technical work of surgery and was observing how senior surgeons use judgment to make operative decisions:

> The hardest thing, I think, about surgery is knowing when and when not to operate. It's not the operating. Now for me, yeah, I still have to learn. Not my way around the OR. It's more intra-operative decisions, especially for the bigger surgeries. . . . I need to know . . . how to change my plan in the OR. Beyond that, I need a diagnosis and treatment plan. You need to be sharp enough to figure out what the problem is. And then you need to be smart enough to know whether or not to do something about it.

As Jill described it, she had to know enough—about anatomies, about procedures, about contingencies—to know when to intervene and when to change course. She listened carefully to senior surgeons during rounds (meetings of the surgical service), working to understand how the surgeons she respected made these kinds of judgments. Given the complexity of factors that surgeons often must consider before making a decision to operate, it is difficult to imagine a neat decision-making algorithm that could cover all variables and contingencies. Medical judgments are subtle and often are not easily explicable.

As I discuss in the next chapter, decisions not to operate are decisions to prevent injury and discomfort in patients who are poor candidates for surgery. These are some of the most difficult decisions that surgeons make, especially when the patient is too unstable to risk surgery but could die without intervention. They go against a surgical training that values action over inaction, decisiveness over uncertainty, and confidence over timidity (Cassell 1991, 1998; Katz 1999). To a person, the surgeons I spoke with said they valued good decision making over technical bravura; they valued judgment over virtuosity.[8]

As with other professions that involve imitation of those in positions of authority, residents and fellows spend a great deal of time scrutinizing the actions of their superiors, determining which qualities they want to emulate and which they will avoid. Here, I quote at length from an interview that I did with Dr. Mihir Banerjee, a general surgeon who had just completed a surgical fellowship and was starting his career on a hospital staff. Surgical residents often add a fellowship to their training. Fellowships give fully qualified practitioners opportunities to master a subspecialty or to hone their expertise with a particular surgeon or group. Mihir said he had learned more as a fellow than at any point in his training because he worked autonomously but always with a senior surgeon nearby to share ideas and back him up. The discussion reveals the mix of judgment, affect, and style of interaction that Mihir was working actively to learn from his superior, a man his peers described as a "surgeon's surgeon":

MIHIR: I think he has a lot to teach in terms of bedside manner, a lot to teach in terms of clear judgment decisions. He has the very adult ability to cut through the crap to see the critical issue or the decision point. It's his strength and sometimes his weakness. He doesn't get sidetracked by the little details. He's a big-picture kind of guy and sees where things are going and sees where a patient is going. He leaves a lot of little details for others to pick up, which is fine. He's very good at putting the perspective on a thing. He's very good at taking that step back and seeing the bigger picture and seeing where things are actually going and what actually needs to be done without getting caught up in the little things. He has very clear operative decision making.

RP: I've been in the OR with him twice. He said something that struck me. He said that once you decide what you're going to do, everything unfolds from there. He then showed that anatomically. It makes perfect sense, but it's not totally intuitive [to me].

MIHIR: Yes, that's definitely a strength. It's a strength outside of the operating room and inside the operating room. The other thing is, he's unflappably calm no matter how bad things are going. And that's something I would love to learn from him. I try to emulate that, but it's not my strength. I don't have his confidence. I don't know that he's always had it. He certainly claims he did, and he's certainly more confident than I am. When you're operating with him you feel very secure that anything you do wrong, he could probably find a way to fix. And when you're training, that's an enormous asset. And I hope that at some point someone will say the same about me. But I know when I am stressed, I get a bit snappish, and I get a bit short with people, and I get frustrated. It's one of my weaknesses that I'm trying consciously to fix.

Mihir discusses the senior surgeon's bedside manner and clinical judgment in a breath, fluidly mixing observations about his affective style and decision making.

The young surgeon described these characteristics in terms of his superior's bodily presence in space. The senior surgeon "sees" where he is going, can get "perspective," and can "step back" to get a sense of the big picture. This bodily description of surgical judgment is both metaphorical and actual. In surgery, one must remain constantly aware of the spaces peripheral to the exact spot where one is working because potential dangers and complications can lurk there. Judgment and clear decision making in surgery emerge from a precise sense of one's location and direction of movement relative to the patient's body. One must also be mindful of potential problems as the operation proceeds. Thus, the ability to plan a surgery and prepare for contingencies rests on a base of knowledge, skill, and experience that allows a surgeon to focus on a single point of action while remaining aware of the larger surgical situation as it unfolds in time and space.

Despite my comment about decision making, Mihir's remarks about judgment rapidly gave way to affective issues, such as his supervisor's calm and confidence. Mihir wanted to emulate his supervisor's clear decision making and his calm, but he found himself lacking, especially when stressed. No one had to tell Mihir that calm in the operating room can be an asset for all involved; he knew it in his body, particularly in the feelings of security that the senior surgeon's calm inspired in him. Mihir's comments illustrate the intensity with which young surgeons try to emulate the abilities that their superiors demonstrate, as well as what they need to practice to develop their own versions of those abilities. Scholars studying education, especially in apprenticeships, use the word "scaffolding" to describe how experts structure activities so novices can participate (Goody 1989, 235–36). The procedural scaffolding senior surgeons provide can be augmented by affective scaffolding, the creation of a calm, secure environment where a junior can feel confident that the consequences of a mistake can be managed. Providing a sense of security in the operating room is vital to the patient's safety and the trainee's development.

Senior surgeons must impart an extraordinarily complex mix of technical, affective, improvisational, and procedural skills, many of which are difficult or impossible to articulate verbally (Pinch et al. 1996). As Mihir says of his superior:

Articulating exactly what you want someone to do is a difficult thing when teaching operating. It's one thing that [he] does not do well. He has this very innate sense of how to do things, and he sometimes finds it very difficult to articulate what he's doing, or how he's doing it, or why he's doing it that way. It's so obvious to him that he can't explain it.

In other words, a very talented surgeon is not necessarily a gifted teacher. This disparity made Mihir's superior "a very difficult person to learn from at the junior level." However, the difficulties would be lessened with a student who is sufficiently advanced to learn from example and depend less on explicit teaching. Mihir said of the same surgeon:

He is easier to learn from at the senior level than at the junior level. In fact, he has very little time or patience for teaching junior residents because they are so far behind, or so far away from him in terms of their understanding of what is going on that it is difficult for him to dumb it down a bit. He doesn't have the patience to do it.

"Innate" means a quality one is born with, but the word increasingly has come to mean internal, embodied, and resistant to analysis. Mihir's comments about his supervisor's innate abilities suggest that, whether through natural ability, years of practice, or some combination, the expert surgeon often struggled to articulate to others the skills that are self-evident to him.

Situated clinical teaching occurs inside and outside the operating room. I followed Nick Perrotta, the general surgeon, as he and a resident visited several patients who had just been admitted to the hospital. I raced after Nick and the resident as they zipped through the halls. The resident gave a quick rundown of each patient's reasons for admission. One woman had come to the hospital several times for pain accompanying the passage of gallstones. Nick examined her briefly, looking in her eyes for jaundice. During the examination, he slowed notably, explaining clearly and carefully the tests he planned to do, punctuating his explanations with pats on the patient's knee. Then he went to find the woman's daughter. The daughter looked exhausted and crumpled. She was angry, saying her mother had been to the hospital many times for the same kind of pain. Nick reassured her several times that he would get answers. Nick said the pain might have been caused by irritation from the stones or by a tumor. Then he caught himself and said, "If it's a tumor, it's a very small one."

"Very small," the resident echoed, evidently for emphasis. The daughter looked frustrated. Nick said everything would be all right, offered her a cup of coffee, which she declined, and gruffly patted her shoulder. As he talked with the patient and her daughter, Nick was calm and reassuring. I also observed an ability, which I noted many times, to make statements about his abilities that would sound arrogant coming from most other people, but which, from him, seemed self-assured. Even when doing what one anesthesiologist described to me as "teaching by boasting," Nick's manner was of such confident good humor that it rarely grated. Whatever combination of nature and nurture encouraged these traits to emerge, Nick's bedside manner stood out as unusually assured among physicians I observed. Nick structured the interaction so the patient and her daughter would feel reassured about his ability to diagnose and treat the patient's symptoms. Affective scaffolding can help trainees in the operating room and can reassure patients and their families in the clinic.

Nick described practice in the operating room as the only means he knew of becoming a good surgeon and likened it to improving at sports. He talked about finding "the zone," a sports metaphor describing the point where one has seen most of what can go wrong in an operating room. At that point, he said, the surgeon can handle problems with relative ease. Nick said most surgeons get into the zone, if they ever do, at the point during their careers when they have done a thousand or more of any given procedure. I often saw him in the operating room on days when he was not scheduled to operate because he had an emergency or had added a case or because he needed equipment not found in his usual operating suite. "All surgeons are workaholics," Nick said, certainly including himself. He was also the only surgeon I met who said he loved his years of residency. Nick's comments reflect the extent to which surgeons' bodies become the primary instruments of surgical action, forged and honed through practice.

From first case presentations to learning when to operate and when not, surgical internships, residencies, and fellowships are grueling tests of a trainee's stamina, fortitude, and ability to navigate the social and organizational demands of hierarchically organized hospital work, demands that often are poorly spelled out or require setting and revising priorities. There is no syllabus, but residents teach each other a great deal during lessons tacked onto the end of a surgery or during informal "corridor talk," moments when unspoken social knowledge that never ends up on lesson plans gets conveyed (Downey et al. 1997). Years must pass before tying knots, examining patients, and making case presentations develop into bedside manner, calm in the operating room, and the decision-making skills of a surgeon working in the zone. Advanced surgical skills, which Amal had yet to develop and Nick had long since acquired, undoubtedly include exceptional technique and good judgment in the operating room. These also include affective abilities that have been called part of the hidden curriculum, such as the ability to comfort a frightened patient or to inspire calm and confidence in others. Embodied dispositions to act in ways consistent with biomedical modes of perception, action, and thought accumulate with years of clinical practice.

Shifts in Surgical Worlds

In recent decades, changes in medical institutions have begun to alter existing methods of medical teaching. These include pressure to move patients through the hospital more quickly, efforts to prevent errors, and broad shifts in many areas of North American business and government toward more bureaucratic measures of control. For example, an influential Institute of Medicine report on errors in medicine called for more systematic training (including the use of simulation), the development of performance standards for health professionals, and better design of drug protocols and devices to limit confusions that often occur in clinical settings (Kohn et al. 2000). These institutional changes have begun to move this modified master-apprentice system toward more external measures of abilities and outcomes.

One change the surgeons I worked with discussed incessantly was the reduction in resident work hours to eighty hours a week, a reduction of up to forty hours a week on some medical services. The push to change resident work hours began after the 1984 death in a New York hospital of eighteen-year-old Libby Zion. Though she died from a lethal combination of prescription and illicit drugs, a series of inquiries found that resident exhaustion was among the causes for Zion's death. This led New York State to limit residency hours in 1989. In Canada, residents' organizations in Ontario and Quebec negotiated duty hour limits starting in the mid-1990s. Starting in 2003, the U.S. Accreditation Council for Graduate Medical Education required hospitals to limit residents' hours to eighty hours per week, along with other restrictions on twenty-four-hour shifts. The changes in American residency hours were announced while I was doing fieldwork in

2002 and, after hearing many stories about the grinding brutality of resident sleep deprivation, I was surprised that several surgeons I spoke with were more concerned than pleased with the changes.

The effects of exhaustion on residents working as much as 110 hours a week have been well documented. They include inability to learn or absorb new information, reductions in professionalism in treatment of patients and interactions with colleagues, increases in mistakes and cutting of corners, and psychological and interpersonal effects in residents' personal lives (Papp et al. 2004). Charles Bosk, in his 1979 account of errors in surgery, quoted one resident who was upset about a patient who had died in his care. The resident believed he missed the obvious symptoms of a heart attack because he was too exhausted to recognize them:

> You can't really do this job unless you get some rest. I stress rest because we're so tired we're not people, we're robots. You'd be surprised how depressed cerebral function is when you're really tired. And when you're here every day thinking about surgical problems, you don't notice other things. Look—I know all the signs of heart failure. Christ, she was frothing at the mouth. . . . I know the signs, but they're not in the front of my mind, you know, because I'm thinking about pararectal abscesses [abscess adjacent to rectum], or wound infections, and you don't always put together what is under your nose. Today's thing, that's our fault. Last night she should have had an emergency heart consultation, but it was so late, we were so tired, we thought that it could wait until morning. (99)

The resident uses striking Cartesian language about his "depressed cerebral functions" to describe his inability to connect what is evident to his senses to his knowledge of the symptoms of heart failure. Reading this resident's words, one of many similar stories, one might conclude that physicians would welcome reductions in work hours, but debates about how changes in hours might affect patient care have continued since the reductions took effect.

Proponents of cuts in work hours argue that well-rested residents have a better balance of work to personal life, reduced stress levels, reduced tendencies to make errors, and better decision-making skills (see Zare et al. 2004). Skeptics, especially among surgeons in teaching hospitals, worry that reduced hours have harmed young surgeons' commitment to sacrifice themselves to care for patients. When discussions of work hours first began in the 1980s, the American College of Surgeons, a major educational and lobbying organization for surgeons, argued that "lack of familiarity with a patient, not fatigue, is the major cause of errors of judgment" (quoted in Barden et al. 2002, 531). Surgeons also have argued that residents who work fewer hours complete their training with less experience in the operating room, though findings have been mixed (Barden et al. 2002; Carlin et al. 2007; Spencer and Teitelbaum 2005). Others have found that residents spend less time in clinics after reductions in hours (Spencer and Teitelbaum 2005). One surgeon replied to an article about changes in working hours and summed up the surgical ethos that he felt was at stake: "For almost 100 years, the expectation of surgical education has been constant availability, ownership of patients, all the things that we pride ourselves in, and now we are coming to what has almost turned into shift work" (Enej Gasevic, quoted in Carlin et al. 2007, 330). Surgeons argue that the ability of residents to be available to patients forms part of their style of care. The values of continuity across the term of a patient's time in the hospital resemble a surgeon's commitment to remain at a patient's side during surgery.

The surgical residents I spoke with all supported the eighty-hour week, while senior surgeons were more ambivalent, citing worries that their patients might lose continuity of care with the move toward shorter shifts. Dr. Emily Gold, a general surgeon, described what she saw as the effects of limiting residency hours on one young surgeon:

> When she's here, she's excellent. She's a very good surgeon. Good resident. Very good to be on call with. She handles emergencies very well. But when her shift is done, she's done. That's how nurses work, and even anesthetists. But surgeons, to me, I guess I'm old-fashioned. And if there's a complication, you deal with it.

According to this surgeon, young residents leave when their shift ends, rather than sticking around when the need arises. Emily said she could see a change in trainees' commitment to ensuring continuity of care, a change that erodes the professional distinctions surgeons make to separate themselves from other medical practitioners. Emily suggested that the change goes deeper than a scheduling revision. Older surgeons used to remain in the hospital to deal with problems; younger ones hand cases off to another crew. Unstated are the class implications of comparing surgeons to other medical professionals, including nurses, who have long been treated with less respect than physicians, and anesthesiologists, who are physicians, but not physicians who have ongoing contact with patients. Emily and others worried that changes in residency hours make surgeons more like workers performing a job and less like professionals dedicating themselves to the art of healing. Some told me they would not allow a resident with a shift-work mentality to work on their service.

The term "shift work" came up often in these discussions and reflected a worry related to professional class that surgery might come to resemble a factory production system staffed by workers engaged in repetitive tasks while longing for a whistle's blow to set them free. Surgeons' comments index three fears about the work they do. First, physicians have long denigrated surgeons as medicine's craft workers, reminding them that, until the mid-nineteenth century, surgical work was performed by butchers, barbers, and others who worked on bodies with their hands (Lawrence 1998). This is another reminder of the Cartesian dualism that has long privileged minds over hands, which includes privileging a physician's diagnostic skill over a surgeon's technical skill. Although surgeons themselves cite their decisiveness and orientation to action as virtues, they also downplay their physical skill in favor of good judgment as a measure of surgical success. Second, surgical work, like much of medical work, often is repetitive. Indeed, the clinical pattern recognition that Luhrmann discusses requires repetition. But surgeons are quick to argue that their work requires higher-level judgment, decision making, and improvisational abilities, distancing their work from the repetition that occurs on a production line. Third, hospital staffs face many efficiency efforts motivated by industrial management principles derived from factory work, such as a focus on increasing patient "throughput" (moving more patient bodies through the operating room). All of these concerns reflect anxieties about surgeons' status as professionals.

European and American workers who use their hands have long been held in less esteem than those whose work is primarily intellectual. This division has separated physicians from surgeons. Over the course of the twentieth century, however, North American surgeons have raised their standing relative to physicians by tying their work to technology and to the rapid development of engineering (Stevens 1999, 55). The focus on surgery's technological achievements encourages surgeons to downplay the craft aspects of their work. Though changes in residency hours might genuinely challenge hospitals that have relied upon residents' labor, the surgeons I spoke with did not mention financial concerns. Instead, they seemed most worried by changes that reflect upon their sense of professional identity. Part of this identity rests upon surgeons separating themselves from craft workers who "only" work with their hands. Another aspect of surgeons' identity entails a commitment to sacrifice their own bodies (by working shifts that last for thirty-six or more hours or by staying by the patient's side for as long as a patient is on the operating table) (Moreira 2004, 122; see also Herzig 2006). Limiting residency hours challenges many senior surgeons' sense that their trainees must develop an embodied commitment to practice surgery.

Emotional Surgeons

Mihir, the new staff surgeon, praised his supervisor's ability to give patients hope while simultaneously criticizing him for sometimes being unwilling to admit defeat when a patient's death was imminent. Mihir wanted to find a line between comfort and realism, but he had not yet achieved a balance that felt right to him. Mihir works in a surgical subspecialty that treats unusually sick patients, a significant number of whom will die or receive terminal diagnoses while in his care. Regular contact with dying patients may make Mihir particularly attentive to the nuances of relating to very sick patients, but many other surgeons I spoke with also described their struggles to construct an emotional stance toward patients consistent with professional care. This is one of the most difficult and neglected aspects of the hidden curriculum to embody because it entails learning how to manage one's own emotions and how to read, sometimes from unarticulated cues, what a patient needs. No textbook or formal program can teach such things. Interacting well with patients requires another form of medical judgment, one that depends upon a physician's ability to sense a patient's emotions and the physician's own response.

The struggle to find good ways to relate emotionally to suffering patients came through clearly during an informal discussion I had with a group of surgeons and an educational technologies expert about whether physicians can allow their emotions to play a role in patient care. Dr. Richard Hunt, a retired surgeon, argued for a stronger role for physician emotion in medical care, but everyone present, especially two mid-career surgeons, Dr. Ramesh Chanda and Dr. Anna Wilson, both of whom are compassionate individuals, struggled to articulate their beliefs about patient relations:

RAMESH: Do you think that getting involved emotionally, first of all, whether it's against the ethics, but even if it's not, does it in some way cloud your judgment?

RICHARD: Yes.

RAMESH: It does. And you have to be emotionally distant from the patient to make good judgments?

RICHARD: Supposedly.

RAMESH: I mean if you have to amputate the leg of this fellow and you get emotionally involved . . .

RICHARD: You feel badly. Then you have to just coldly go and do it.

Ramesh made a distinction between emotional and rational judgment. These separations are ubiquitous in European and American philosophical traditions. They tend to imply that emotion pollutes reason (Lutz 1986).[9] These distinctions also pervade biomedical training. Richard sympathized with this view, but he nuanced it by giving patient care a temporal dimension: there are times when it is important to feel for a patient and times when one must act "coldly."

The discussion continued, and the group became enmeshed in a debate about the right words for a physician's ideal emotional stance. In the late 1950s, the sociologist Renee Fox wrote a classic essay, which has been widely read among medical students, about emotional socialization and the need to develop what she called "detached concern" (1988) The discussion echoed Fox's words, which may not have been coincidental. The group continued:

ANNA: How's this? Is this an appropriate phrase: "Detached compassion"?

RICHARD: Uh, yeah, except what's the matter with "attached compassion"?

ANNA: Well, that you get too far into it, then you're . . . I don't know. I'm just looking for the right word to express what's appropriate.

Anna argued for compassion, saying that physicians would simultaneously need emotional detachment or distance. Richard suggested that some emotional attachment on a physician's part might be appropriate, but Anna balked, arguing that a physician might get "too far into" the emotions that can accompany medical treatment. Her language suggests that closeness might make distance or perspective difficult, again invoking a desire to separate emotion from reason. But she clearly struggled to find the right words to express the kind of emotional balancing that physicians must do regularly when doing clinical work. Richard kept seeking the correct term:

> RICHARD: You want to be compassionate, but you want to be objective.
> ANNA: You want to be more human than nonhuman.
> RICHARD: How about "compassionate objectivity"?
> ANNA: OK, I like that.

Anna sought a phrase that would balance clinical judgment with humanity and compassion. But as she began to articulate the effects of attachment ("you get too far into it"), she backed away and said she was just looking for the right words to express the correct stance. The words Anna and Richard traded are significant. "Compassion" means being moved by the suffering of others and can include identifying with their feelings. "Detached compassion" appears to be an oxymoron and suggests that a physician must maintain distance in the face of suffering. By settling upon "objectivity," the physicians evidently agreed that "detachment" suggests too much distance from compassionate care. "Objectivity" in this usage suggests rational thought freed from individual, possibly emotional, coloring (see Daston and Galison 2007). The right words for a physician who is moved by the suffering of others, but who remains composed and professional, are intuitively easy to understand but difficult to articulate and even more difficult to practice.

Anna's comment about being more human than nonhuman reflects the difficulty with detachment. Clinical medicine builds upon scientific work, but patient care is not, strictly speaking, scientific work. The uncomfortable combination of detachment and compassion, or compassion and objectivity, reflects physicians' wrestling to position themselves between the abstract ideals of science and the art of healing. Physicians often say they seek a clinical stance that is free from bias, but the reality of patient care suggests that the best physicians must develop a stance that uses the best available treatments, while acknowledging the patient's and their own situatedness within human social relations. The opposite of this is an automaton that "will not be put into motion by others" (Despret 2004a, 118). The clinician who remains unaffected by clinical practice and patient suffering also will be less able to affect the situation in positive ways.

After listening to the physicians, Sue Hopwood, an educational technologies researcher, questioned the distancing effects of this view of objectivity:

SUE: Why is there such a problem with objectivity, though? It seems to me you have to have some empathy or compassion. Your compassion allows you to make a wise decision about that patient.
RICHARD: Not necessarily.

Later, Sue returned to this theme:

SUE: Yeah. I can see that it's important for the physician, this business of detachment. That might be the only way to survive the profession. But you were saying it's put in terms of objectivity about the patient.

Sue acknowledged that detachment may be a necessary coping strategy for physicians, but she pointed out that detachment as a coping strategy and objectivity about the patient may not be identical. Returning to her first remark about compassion, she questioned whether objectivity must preclude compassion and empathy. Sue asked what is perhaps the most important question of the discussion: Is a physician's need to withdraw from difficult medical problems to survive emotionally the same as bringing objectivity to treatment? Richard's response, "not necessarily," suggests that he does not see the value of compassion or empathy for good clinical decision making. Rather, he separates compassion and action: physicians should be compassionate toward their patients because their patients need it, but they also should undertake potentially traumatic clinical work "coldly."[10] Sue argued that wise decisions emerge from understanding the patient's plight, that is, from understanding the person as a human being who may be afraid or suffering or otherwise in need of solace.

Many patients, including me, have experienced the feelings of fury and helplessness that callous or indifferent care provokes. While doing fieldwork I saw physicians young and old who were passionate about their work and powerfully affected by their patients. The difficult emotions physicians must wrestle with became clear to me during a casual conversation with two surgeons, one of whom was retired. While chit-chatting over lunch, the subject of residency training came up and the retired surgeon, whose residency was forty years in the past, began to recount a story about a woman who arrived in the emergency room while he was on call. She had uncontrollable bleeding, and nothing he did slowed the bleeding enough to save her life. As he told this story, the surgeon teared up, allowing himself to feel grief at the woman's death and his own inability to save her life. The memory of this woman's death had stayed with him for decades.

In the hospital, physicians find themselves asked to reconcile scientific values and the emphasis on objectivity with their charge to ease human suffering. Vinciane Despret (2004a, 2004b), in a rearticulation of William James's theories of emotion, argues that emotions mediate between actions in the world and human responses. Despret argues that emotions create a hesitation, an indeterminacy between action and response, a space to unfold new questions, new possibilities for relating, new ways of being. "When emotion is linked to a broader plan that consists of producing a new relationship to the world . . . it is no longer just what *is* to be known but what *causes* knowing" (2004a, 210). Viewed this way, these physicians' affective experiences—the intense relationships among residents and senior surgeons, the difficulties of articulating the connections between compassion and objectivity, the painful memories of helplessly watching a woman die—all produce medical ways of relating to patients and knowing their conditions. When physicians learn the complexities of interacting with patients and with one another, they are not learning a set of rules that can be applied or lumped together under the heading of "comportment" or "bedside manner." In the sense described by Despret, the emotions a physician experiences while practicing can lead a practitioner to hesitate, to think about which of a master surgeon's abilities they wish to emulate or improve upon, for example, or whether a better means might be found to stop uncontrollable bleeding. These emotions produce new ways of relating in the world.

Embodiment, Affect, Judgment

According to Despret, emotions are "ways of defining and negotiating social relationships and the self in a moral order" (2004a, 249). Emotion is, I argue, necessary for the formation of judgment. Amal, for example, hungered for the formal clarity of a syllabus, a document that would tell him what he should learn and in what order. As a beginning resident, he was angered and overwhelmed by the responsibility of caring for forty patients on the ward. His anger pushed him to ask why someone at his very junior level had responsibility for so many patients. His frustrations led him to ask which senior residents and surgeons could provide the best instruction.

Over time, he began to create new categories, organizing learning around social structures rather than formal lessons as he began to learn his job.

In this section, I discuss judgment as a surgical ability that becomes embodied with experience. Surgeons describe judgment as one of the most important abilities they must develop. Judgment about when to operate came up often in my discussions with surgeons and it underlies the surgical saying, "The surgery was a success, but the patient died." That is, technical proficiency cannot necessarily save a patient if the surgeon has made a poor judgment about whether the patient could withstand surgery.

To consider judgment in biomedicine, I begin with a brief philosophical detour. Kant defines judgment as "the faculty of thinking the particular as contained under the universal" (2007, 15). For Kant, judgment is an evaluation that requires weighing a specific situation against general rules arrived at through rational analysis. Merleau-Ponty rejects Kant's conception of judgment because he says it presupposes the existence of a self-contained rationality, a "mind" (the thing that thinks) that is strongly divided from the senses (the things that passively receive information) and from the world (the thing that provides information). For Merleau-Ponty, perception (including a subject's socio-historical formation, which often remains tacit) reflects a "logic lived through" (2002, 57), that is, an accumulation of bodily experiences that cannot be fully understood through conscious evaluation. Treating judgment as separate from embodied experience neglects the broader ways in which the embodied subject inhabits the world. Knowing that emerges from experience in the world always overruns consciousness. We always know more than we think we know.

Merleau-Ponty's critique of the category of judgment stems from his observation that our perceptions are never wholly transparent to us. Perception, he argues, using concepts that fit well with constructivist perspectives of science studies, develops within a historically and culturally situated "setting" (see Csordas 1990). Perception grows with engagement in the world. He argues that our entire knowledge of the world builds first from our location within that world and the particular forms that our perceptions and our histories (including our linguistic and cultural histories) take. "All consciousness is, in some measure, perceptual consciousness," he writes. "If it were possible to lay bare and unfold all the presuppositions in what I call my reason or my ideas at each moment, we should always find experiences which have not been made explicit, large-scale contributions from past and present, a whole 'sedimentary history' which is not only relevant to the *genesis* of my thought, but which determines its *significance*" (2002, 459).

What one perceives is structured by an entire "sedimentary history," including one's sociocultural history, which structures one's responses while remaining largely outside consciousness. Because perceptual histories are never wholly transparent, Merleau-Ponty rejects the notion of an executive, all-knowing rationality that judges a particular empirical situation.

Though these charges need not be incompatible, rationality often gets equated with dispassionate observation and, in bodily terms, with distance. If one adheres to the view of rational inquiry that values detachment, then, empathy becomes "too close" or "lacking perspective." As I have argued throughout this chapter, the development of advanced medical abilities, including judgment, relies on the gradual embodiment of specifiable and unspecifiable perceptual abilities, techniques, and knowledges. Many of these embodied abilities develop in contexts in which emotion plays a significant role. Consider Amal's anger and frustration; the trainee's embarrassment about being ridiculed for her lack of knowledge; Mihir's attempts to rein in his emotions when under duress; and the discussion group's debate about detachment and compassion. Despret argues that emotion becomes "an undetermined experience that split[s] up the world, mind and bodies in a radically different way" (2004a, 125–26). Emotions challenge physicians and trainees to interact with the world in new ways, revealing that trainees have something important at stake in clinical interactions. Amal and other trainees learn to manage competently when on the ward or when making a diagnosis. Mihir recognizes that managing his emotions will help him manage the surgical team. The discussion group seeks the right words to help them relate to patients with an appropriate balance of affect and reason.

Physicians use the word "judgment" to acknowledge that clinical work contains uncertainties and moral implications that require subtlety and an ability to read the situation that goes well beyond matching symptoms to diagnoses. In an ideal situation, the benefits of medical action are weighed against the possibility of unnecessary disfigurement, pain, or even death. Yet physicians do not treat judgment as beginning from universal principles beyond the medical imperative to limit harm to patients. Medical judgment resembles diagnostic intuition, in the sense Luhrmann (2000) describes it, as an ability to interpret medical signs and make good treatment decisions within a context in which physicians must grapple with human suffering. Judgment develops with accumulated experiences of medical practice and in communication with formal diagnostic and treatment categories. Thus judgment becomes an emergent property of experiences of observing other physicians, doing clinical work, and attending to outcomes of clinical actions in a context in which one's emotions, body, and being often are implicated.

Many medical decisions, whether to attempt surgery on a risky patient, for example, contain too much uncertainty to be made from some preset algorithm. The surgeon must make decisions that reconcile the injunction to "do no harm" with specific treatment recommendations for particular ailments. Further, many medical aids to judgment, such as the scoring system for grading the severity of a case of pancreatitis described earlier, represent a more complex interplay of agencies, objects, and knowledges than are contained in philosophical examples concerned with the mental categorization of judgment. The scoring system represents an attempt to codify judgment: if a patient is too sick to withstand surgery, then a senior surgeon should make the judgment to wait for the patient to stabilize. A less experienced surgeon ideally could arrive at a similar conclusion using these scoring criteria.

The two surgeons who created the pyramid of surgical learning argued that experience is the necessary step toward developing judgment (Heinrichs and Srivastava n.d.). Jill, the chief resident, was one of many surgeons who said that judging when to operate and when to wait is a vital skill. At the beginning of her fifth year of residency, Jill continued to carefully observe senior physicians to learn more about surgical planning and the larger issues of surgical treatment. The abilities that Jill describes—knowing how to improvise, knowing how to construct operative plans, and knowing when to hold back—are at the heart of surgical judgment. Some judgments are relatively simple. Other cases are much more difficult because physicians must consider the complex interplay between the urgency of surgery, the patient's overall condition, and the patient's medical history. Over time, surgeons accumulate extensive experience by evaluating and watching others evaluate just these factors. These complex judgments rest upon simpler evaluations of the patient's condition and history. They also rest upon the interplay of sensory, affective, and cognitive aspects of physicians' clinical experiences. The reasoning processes that physicians undergo build upon their experiences with particular cases as much or more than they emerge from reflection on textbook cases or fundamental principles. Inductive ability, as surgeons like Jill describe it, evolves from practice and observation. Much of this experience develops from learning particular ways of relating to bodies, that is, from embodied action.

Conclusion

The transition from medical school to residency is a transition from a formal program of coursework to a situated medical apprenticeship. During residency, trainees learn to apply the knowledge they have absorbed through textbooks, lectures, and exams. Residency education resembles the remaking of self that occurs in total institutions. The hierarchical and institutional structures, the mortification of subordinates, the powerfully enforced norms of dress and comportment, and the affective intensity of the experience encourage trainees to embody the norms and practices of physicians. What becomes embodied has less to do with rules for physician behavior than with dispositions to act in ways consistent with being a doctor (see Bourdieu 1977). A trainee learns medical skills as part of a larger transformation of self that is required to become a doctor.

The concept of the "hidden curriculum" implies either culturally informed ways of acting located in the larger milieu of medical work or emotional learning lodged "inside" individual practitioners. The formulation of the lessons of the hidden curriculum as cultural or emotional seemingly locates these lessons outside the scope of medical practices and suggests that they are resistant to formalization. But, by focusing on physician embodiment, I have depicted surgical residency education as intensely physical, relational, and emotional. Technical problems become entangled with affective challenges and clinical consequences. The trainee's body, as it observes, acts, and feels, moves to the center of medical learning.

By attending to bodily aspects of residency education, the accumulation of small, daily actions a resident makes becomes connected to the development of higher-level abilities, such as judgment. By examining how medical knowing becomes embodied through practice in the hospital, the cultural and emotional aspects of clinical learning become more clearly related to technical and formal knowledge. Judgment and compassion become emergent properties of accumulated information, skill, practice, and experience, including emotional experience.

four

·····

TECHNIQUES AND ETHICS IN
THE OPERATING ROOM

The surgery was a success, but the patient died.

Sometimes wrong, but never in doubt.

SURGICAL APHORISMS

A surgeon I know describes what she does as "controlled violence." These two words define surgery as the use of physical force to promote healing or improve function. The phrase also tersely captures the ethical stakes of surgery. The Hippocratic Oath and its most common paraphrase, "First, do no harm," is medicine's first and most important moral code. Surgeons, in particular, must balance the physical forces used to invade and alter patients' bodies against the possibilities of doing harm. To explain, I build from the distinction raised by a medical student cited in chapter 1, who became more comfortable with her first cadaver dissection by observing that violence done to a body cannot always be equated with harm. According to the *Oxford English Dictionary*, "violence" is an Old French word describing the use of physical force that causes injury or damage. Etymologically, the connection of violence to the morally neutral "physical force" suggests that sometimes "violence" has a strong moral connotation, but not always. In contrast, the morally laden Old English word "harm" means evil, whether in intent or effect, as perpetrated upon a person or thing. The difference between violence and harm is "ethically vast, but practically narrow"[1] and often rests upon the surgeon's first word, "control."[2]

Medical historians and sociologists have shown how operating rooms are spaces of control that augment and constrain the surgeon's power (Hirschauer 1991; Schlich 2007). The patient's consent, the training surgeons undergo, and the highly structured spaces and hierarchies of the operating room authorize surgeons to use physical force to promote healing. I argue that control in surgery includes surgeons' abilities to direct their own bodies and to manage others' actions. I locate surgical ethics partly in technique, in practices that surgeons use to perform surgery and to prevent harm, that is, in the embodiment of control. Techniques of the body used to perform surgery become ethical practices.

Surgeons describe themselves as medicine's action-oriented practitioners, and many say they value the direct connection between action and response in surgery (see Cassell 1991, 1998; Katz 1999). This self-description contains a number of assumptions about surgical care. Surgeons share a deep sense that they intervene to heal. They assume that pathology is located in the body's structures, and their job is to act upon the body to repair it. They work from the understanding that the body is a biological-anatomical entity, a wondrous machine but a machine nevertheless. But not even the most mechanistic of surgeons imagines the human body wholly instrumentally (see Rabinow 1996). For example, drilling a screw into a patient's bone could be imagined as a purely physical skill, akin to drilling a screw into a piece of wood, yet few would argue that the experience of drilling into wood and drilling into living bone is the same. Damaging a piece of wood and damaging a human body cannot be equated. Surgeons use physical force to intervene, but they also must exercise extraordinary control to prevent harm. As I show, control in the operating room is a guiding principle that informs surgeons' technical, pedagogical, and verbal activities. Learning to treat bodies requires the development of an ethic of care, a set of practices that guide hands and treatments in ways that limit harm.[3] This approach makes ethics the embodied product of education in a situated clinical milieu, rather than the adoption of the formal principles common among ethicists (for important anthropological critiques of the abstractions of biomedical ethicists, see Cohen 1999; Das 1999; Kleinman 1997, 1999). By treating ethics as embodied, I show how ethical treatment can be situated within clinical practice, rather than as a product of contemplation of abstract principles. In this sense, ethics are techniques of the body.

The gulf that separates master surgeons, who daily make decisions that could mean life or death for their patients, and nervous beginners, who do not know where to stand or what to touch, seems so impossibly vast as to be unbridgeable. In this chapter, I focus on the cultivation of surgical residents' skills in the operating room, documenting how surgeons teach techniques for controlling violence using physical and verbal guidance. As trainees accumulate skills and experiences over years of eighty-hour weeks, they ideally learn to judge when a particular surgical action might risk more than it achieves. Eventually, residents move into the ranks of attending surgeons, those with responsibility for deciding who operates and who gets operated upon. Senior surgeons teach residents the methods and meanings of surgical actions, often by subtle means, such as nearly subliminal guiding, storytelling, and jokes. Further, they encourage trainees to work beyond the limits of their abilities without crossing into unsafe practices that might harm the patient. Surgeons working with residents repeatedly demonstrate to trainees that control as technique and ethic is at stake at every level of surgical work.

Remaking the Body

No one would dispute that the surgeon's body plays a central role in surgical action. But the relationship of embodiment to practice in surgery remains understudied. Ethnographies of surgery typically take one of two approaches.[4] The first focuses on the social relations of surgeons, including operating-room hierarchies, means of reinforcing roles, evaluations of competence, and the social and institutional difficulties created by surgeons' power (Bosk 1979; DelVecchio Good 1995; Goffman 1961b; Katz 1999). Ethnographies of surgeons' social relations describe common character traits of surgeons, such as their confidence, decisiveness, heroic self-image, and macho attitudes (Cassell 1991, 1998). These accounts typically contain few detailed descriptions of surgical operating practices and tend to examine surgical subjectivity as already constituted, as though surgeons are born, not made. Ethnographies taking the second approach contain a wealth of detail about how the sociotechnical practices of surgery make the operating team a "surgeon body," a many-armed, multiskilled operator united by the attending surgeon (Hirschauer 1991; Moreira 2004). These sociological contributions make the forces and agencies of the surgical system apparent by showing the relationship between a surgeon's structural position in the surgical team and his or her power. They also have the curious effect of both heightening the senior surgeon's hierarchical power (as the entity coordinating all those arms) and flattening the distinctions one can make among senior surgeons and other members of the team, including their technical abilities and reasons for being in the operating room. Inspired by Foucault's work on fields of power, these ethnographies remove surgical power from any notion of innate qualities possessed by surgeons, making it largely a function of one's position in a system (Foucault 1972; Schlich 2007).

The concept of surgical embodiment brings practitioners' social and technical training together with the structuring effects of other bodies and instruments in the operating room. Surgical embodiment includes the accumulation of socially informed technical practices beginning with the development of craft in the sense used by Mauss of "skill, presence of mind and habit" (2007, 58). The embodiment of techniques and values leads to the formation of *habitus*, embodied dispositions that guide action (Bourdieu 1977; Mahmood 2005; Mauss 2007). In this analysis, the development of the ethical subject occurs through regular practice of ethical techniques (Foucault 1986, 2005; Mahmood 2005). By examining surgical practices as they are situated within an environment that gives them meaning, I show how trainees learn control over their actions so they can apply physical force without causing harm. The embodiment of technique also involves developing judgment about when and how to proceed surgically. Bringing focus to training—to the changes in skill and power that occur over time— allows me to show how the surgeon-subject "is constituted in real practices" (Foucault 1984, 369). Surgical training cultivates surgical subjectivity, surgeons' ability to act, and their technical, institutional, and moral authority to do so. The endpoint of surgical education is incorporation, not only of the skills of a surgeon, but also of the ethics, values, and meanings of surgery. This discussion of embodiment in surgery brings the effects of surgical environment together with the embodied effects of habitual practice by looking first at space, time, and costume in the operating room and then examining in detail four interactions involving three staff surgeons. These interactions reveal how surgical habitus—the embodied guiding principles and values of surgeons—develops through years of supervised practice that cultivate the techniques and ethics of surgical control.

Disciplined Spaces

Space, time, and costume in the operating room create a positive pedagogical economy that reinforces bodily discipline and social hierarchy. The operating-room hierarchy places surgeons at the center and all others at the periphery, gradually moving residents from small tasks to full participation at the center of the surgical action (see Lave and Wenger 1991).[5] Sociologists and anthropologists have debated the relationship between instrumental requirements for surgical preparations, such as draping, and ritual or symbolic significance of surgical spaces, costumes, and rituals, but they have said little about the identity-structuring effects on surgical trainees of operating rooms, scrubs, masks and gowns, and scrubbing of hands (Hirschauer 1991; Katz 1981, 1999).[6] Erving Goffman exempts surgical trainees from his analyses of surgery (1961b), but elsewhere he shows how institutional isolation, dress, and disciplinary practices remake subjects in institutionalized settings (1961a). Surgical training is both disciplinary and professional, in some ways resembling the remaking of the subject that occurs in total institutions, even if its ultimate goal is embodied technique, rather than unthinking obedience (Goffman 1961b, 1961a; Good 1994).

Surgical suites in hospitals typically are separated from the rest of the hospital. The separation of staff and visitors begins at the entrance. The passage from the "staff only" signs on doors leading to operating suites to the tightly restricted area surrounding a patient leads through several zones of increasing sterility. Staff members monitor each zone more tightly than the last. Nurses at a station called a "control desk" restrict access to operating suites, a circulating nurse watches over the operating room, and the entire operating team watches over the sterile area to ensure that only those with permission and preparation enter. Medical students earn the right to occupy the innermost zone by learning how to scrub and by demonstrating social skills that convince the surgeon of their readiness to approach the patient.

Everyone entering the operating suites must don scrubs, shoe coverings, and head coverings. Scrubs effect a shift in the operating-room personnel's status as individuals become professionals and then part of a team. Staff and residents enforce surgical discipline and hierarchy from the moment one enters. On my second day observing surgeries, for example, I forgot to don a disposable cap before entering the corridor outside the operating rooms. A surgeon who did not know me barked at me to do so in a manner that, in most situations, would be inappropriate coming from a stranger. But surgeons have the authority to yell at wayward medical students—and anthropologists—when they violate the rules of the operating suite. It was a lesson I never forgot and the type of lesson medical students receive almost daily.

Those who occupy the sterile area around the patient must undergo a highly routinized scrubbing procedure before donning surgical gowns and gloves. These sterilization rituals "exaggerate the discontinuity in the operating room," separating the operating room from the rest of the hospital and the outside world (Katz 1981, 345; see also Douglas 1966). Scrubbing and gowning are part of the bodily discipline that newly arrived students and residents must master. Sterility rules are second nature to experienced surgeons and nurses, but they take time and practice to become embodied habits. These technical lessons also have a social component. In a series of interactions typical of medical students, I watched a resident, Dr. Amal Nassif, in the first weeks of his training at Hilltop Hospital as he wrestled with sterility. Once gowned and gloved, Amal stood still at the center of the operating room, uncertain what to do next. Margaret Edwards, an operating-room nurse, warned another nurse to keep an eye on him, saying he was very "green" and seemed to have "Helping Hands Syndrome." He wanted to reach a gloved, sterile hand out to help a nonsterile person, which would contaminate him and require him to scrub again. Later, Margaret growled at Amal that he would face real trouble if he forced her to scrub twice. After several such remarks, Dr. Cory Nguyen, the surgical fellow, told Amal to place his hands on the patient's draped legs, where they would remain safely sterile and out of the way. Amal kept his hands in place until the attending surgeon gave him a retractor to hold. Amal's frozen helplessness is common among operating-room newcomers. And the nurse's term "Helping Hands Syndrome" suggests that the urge to extend a sterile hand is common enough to have its own mock diagnostic category that requires regular nursing vigilance.

Scrubbing and maintaining sterility are ritualized technical skills (Katz 1981, 1999). Maintaining strict separation of sterile and nonsterile is easy to understand, but difficult to practice. Moving, touching, and even standing become fraught for new operating-room inhabitants in crowded spaces filled with equipment and the purposeful bustlings of sterile and nonsterile personnel. These lessons in sterility and comportment locate new students at the bottom of the surgical hierarchy and defamiliarize them with their bodies by placing them in unfamiliar surroundings with unfamiliar rules, rules that dictate where they stand and what they touch. Scrubbing and sterility rules have a clear instrumental purpose. But their defamiliarizing effect on new trainees places them in the hands of more senior personnel who, as in the case of the nurse's admonishments, show them what is at stake technically and socially if they contaminate themselves or others (Goffman 1961b).

During a surgical procedure, everyone in the operating room also must wear surgical masks. I have watched surgery staff chastise unknown medical students and visitors, including visiting physicians, for not wearing masks. But physicians and nurses who are more senior have more liberty to play with the rules than do juniors. For example, when a nurse who had a sterile instrument table open in the operating room chided Dr. Johnny Sawyer, a chief resident, for not wearing a surgical mask, Johnny pulled his scrub shirt up over his mouth, bugged out his eyes, and hopped ape-like toward the table. His performance showed that he was senior enough to play with sterile zones without incurring more than mild rebuke from the nurses. Erving Goffman (1961b) says such actions by surgeons create "role distance," momentarily separating them from the gravitas of their roles as healing professionals. But surgeons and nurses tolerate such antics only when performed by colleagues and senior residents, suggesting that one must earn the ability to step out of one's role. Johnny's gorilla act showed that he could play with the boundaries of sterile zones and challenge the nurse's authority in ways a first-year resident could not. But Johnny never touched the table.

Time also plays a role in surgical embodiment. Time focuses attention on the operating area. Breaks between surgeries are relatively relaxed; focus and attention increase in several preoperative steps. Surgical time intensifies when the patient goes under an anesthetic, time surgeons must use wisely because patients recover more quickly when they spend fewer hours in a state of what anesthesiologists call "controlled poisoning" (Schlich 2007). Surgeons make the patient's time on the operating table their own time at the operating table. Surgeons almost never leave the operating table during critical phases of the operation, often not leaving until assistants wheel the patient into the recovery room, even when surgeries take seven or eight hours. While nurses rotate into and out of the operating room and junior trainees might be called away to work on another case, senior residents and fellows, who often supervise opening and closing the patient's body, remain at the patient's side as long or longer than the attending surgeon. Bodily discipline and focus are crucial to surgeons. Ignoring one's bodily needs reveals an embodied commitment to remain by the patient's side (Moreira 2004, 122).

When the critical moments of the procedure end, the surgeon often opens the conversation to nonsurgical topics, a distancing move that ends the focused time of the operation as the patient (in successful surgeries) returns to consciousness (Goffman 1961b, 125; Katz 1981). Limiting time under anesthesia clearly is important for patient safety. Surgeons in teaching hospitals add to the patient's time when they teach, making time part of the care-for-education trade that residents, physicians, and patients accept in academic medical centers. Over the past thirty years, external forces, such as pressures on teaching staff to do lucrative clinical work, have eroded teaching time (Ludmerer 1999).

When surgical schedules fall behind, as they often do, senior surgeons press everyone, especially anesthesiologists, to hurry patients into the operating room. Mounting pressure on surgeons to, in terms borrowed from industry, "increase patient throughput," heightens tensions for the entire operating team and further limits a surgeon's teaching time (Ludmerer 1999).[7] Surgeons have very little time to review anatomy or procedure with trainees or to allow a resident to correct a noncritical mistake, such as retying a slipped stitch. These time constraints also increase pressure on trainees to limit the inevitable fumblings of a beginner.

Learning in the operating room occurs through bodily imitation guided by the structuring effects of the environment. Byron Good's analysis likening medical schools to "total institutions" clarifies that external controls over everything from inmates' clothing to haircuts to schedules serve as continual reminders, at the subconscious, bodily level, of the institutions' principles (Good 1994; see also Goffman 1961a). The operating room is a "symbolically structured environment" that "exerts an anonymous, pervasive pedagogic action" (Bourdieu 1977). In the operating room, space, time, and costume make a surgeon's actions and attitudes meaningful. Obviously, the surgical environment serves important instrumental functions related to sterility, patient safety, and work organization (Collins 1994a). In this environment, however, a trainee's costume, participation in increasingly restricted surgical zones, and subjection to the time demands of surgery also become components of remaking a trainee into a surgeon.

Teaching Control

Control has different meanings at different levels of surgical training, entailing different kinds of technical and ethical lessons. Many types of control exist in the operating room, including the cybernetic control of anesthesiologists, who must maintain patients in an unconscious state, often with artificially lowered blood pressure, without letting them awaken or slip into death, and the bureaucratic control contained in nurses' accounting for each small piece of equipment (sponges, needles, suture materials). I focus exclusively on surgeons' embodied control, the ability to use one's body as an instrument of surgical action while utilizing techniques intended to avoid harm. I recount four surgical interactions to show what control means in each. These individual surgeries exemplify lessons I observed in many teaching surgeries.

Senior surgeons I have interviewed cite experience accumulated over years of practice as the most important factor in their ability to make good decisions about when and how to treat patients. They cite common sense and a willingness to work hard as qualities they look for in beginning trainees. They actively seek residents who make rapid decisions, and they joke about internists and physicians in other specialties, who they say spend too much time contemplating each treatment decision (Katz 1999). Surgeons also have little patience for those who proceed too eagerly. They joke among themselves about technically proficient peers who fail to restrain their eagerness to operate. The adage "The surgery was a success, but the patient died" signals the dangers of focus on technique to the exclusion of critical judgments about a patient's ability to withstand surgery.

A senior surgeon's decisions not to operate reveal what control can mean at the peak of one's surgical career.[8] I followed Dr. Nick Perrotta, a liver surgeon, and Dr. Julie Martinez, a fourth-year resident, on surgery rounds. After visiting several patients and family members, Nick and Julie stood in the corridor to confer about three more patients on the ward. Julie told Nick that another surgeon had recommended major surgery on a woman who had suffered a stroke. No, Nick replied. He pursed his lips, and his normally gregarious facial expression closed, a look I came to interpret as displeasure. He wanted to do something, but surgery on such a risky patient would be unwise. Another patient, a seventy-year-old woman, also was a candidate for surgery. "How does she look?" Nick asked. "Ninety," the resident replied. This rapid-fire discussion of the patient's relative age condensed all the evaluation work Julie had already done to determine the patient's fitness for surgery. No again. Nick decided to try to ease the patient's discomfort by doing a palliative, minimally invasive procedure, but further intervention would be too risky. Nick said matter-of-factly that a third patient was going to die and again declined to operate. His lips remained tightly sealed.

These are some of the hardest decisions surgeons make, going against the desire to do something to help the patient and against surgery's general orientation toward action. In several months of observing rounds and discussions on this surgery service, I observed that quizzing of residents and surgery fellows often focused on whether the patient met clinical criteria for surgery. In general, less experienced surgeons were more eager to operate. In an interview, Nick said he draws on his experience with thousands of cases to make critical decisions, often weighing the risk of death in the operating room against potential pain and potential benefits after the operation. Nick said it helps that he has a busy practice; he has years of experience with patients and pathologies and no urgency to operate on marginal cases. He can choose to make decisions based on what he believes to be in the patient's best interests.[9] Though Nick's decisions do not rest on technical skills in any simple sense, his ability to exercise good surgical judgment rests on decades of experience with hundreds of patients.

This also is a teaching moment for Julie, who observed how the information she provided went into her supervisor's decision making. She watched Nick weigh the patient's condition and risk against the possibilities of pain or palliation. More subtly, she saw what was at stake in her reports of a patient's condition: information she collected formed the basis for life-or-death decisions. Nick's ability to draw on accumulated practice to make difficult decisions is one endpoint of surgical training. Nick had to exercise control over his own orientation to action. His questions to Julie opened up the subtleties underlying the facts of the case, showing some reasons, such as a patient's preexisting problems or poor overall condition, why surgery would have been inappropriate for these patients, even when a textbook evaluation of the patient's condition might have indicated surgery (see Katz 1999). Nick also revealed what was at stake in these evaluations: a risky patient could face complications, unnecessary pain, or a hastened death if he were to proceed too aggressively. Ethical decision making at Nick's level includes delicately balancing a patient's condition against the possibility that surgery might do more harm than good.

Surgery and the Left Hand

The stakes in a medical student's or resident's earliest days of training are not nearly this dire. Dr. Anna Wilson, a hand surgeon, described the development of technical skill as the "composite of exposure and desire":

> I really view it as a package. You don't expect someone very junior to possess good judgment in the context of experience because they don't have it. So I think, early on, it's attitude. It's eagerness. It's poise in the sense of being able to modulate when is a good time to ask a question; when is it appropriate to be, not confrontational, but challenging; and when is it better to recede in one's role in the hierarchy. And, as far as the technical end, it's eagerness, willingness to learn, willingness to try, and then it's the acquisition of technical skills, relative to experience.

As Anna indicates, decisions to let juniors act often involve more social than technical evaluations (see Bosk 1979; DelVecchio Good 1995). Anna's word "poise" indicates that social skills can be expressed verbally and bodily. Clearly, trainees learn skills commensurate with their experience. Refining those skills means that social lessons contained in situated technical lessons evolve as trainees progress. The ethical stakes also evolve. At all levels of practice, however, limiting injury remains paramount. For beginners, this means primarily following superiors' directions; for more senior residents, it means balancing their skills against increasing responsibilities and technical difficulties; for senior surgeons, it means making decisions that weigh the risks and benefits of surgery in terms of the patient's life and future health.

When I observed her at work in 2001 and 2002, Anna had nearly two decades of surgical experience. As a teacher of medical students, she has learned to break her work down into discrete actions to explain them to students. In several conversations with medical students, she noted that instruments such as scalpels, scissors, and probes act as extensions of her hands and that the physical sensations of surgery remain relatively transparent to her when all goes smoothly. Michael Polanyi says our awareness of muscular movements remains tacit when we perform a skill: "We are attending *from* these elementary movements *to* the achievement of their joint purpose, and hence are usually unable to specify these elementary acts" (1966, 10). To teach such actions, a surgeon must be able to communicate what he or she is doing (Pinch et al. 1996). But, although the trainee may have a conceptual understanding of the required action, knowing surgery means knowing how to do surgery. When all goes well, a surgeon can take her skills largely for granted, a quality Martin Heidegger calls "handiness," a state of being that occurs "when we take care of things, using them but not paying specific attention to them" (1996, 69–70). The actions of the surgeon's hands are, thus, handy. But a surgeon cannot assume trainees have mastered surgery's physical skills, regardless of their level of seniority. The surgeon, who has legal and ethical responsibility to ensure that the patient gets the best care possible, must manage trainees' unhandiness to prevent errors that could harm the patient.

I watched Anna teach a medical student how to use a drill during a complex wrist surgery. The patient was an athlete who damaged his left wrist while lifting weights. His forearm was suspended upright using a device with pulleys. An arthroscopic examination of the narrow spaces between the wrist bones showed that several torn ligaments had loosened the strong arch of wrist bones, allowing them to rub together, fostering arthritis. The arch is a structural feature, analogous to an architectural arch, which allows such weight-bearing activities as handsprings and push-ups. The tiny ligaments could not be repaired. Anna decided to shorten the man's ulna—one of the two bones in the forearm—to keep it from banging into the arch and aggravating the injury. Surgeon and resident made a large incision in the man's forearm, cut out a one-inch segment of bone using a small saw, then joined the ends with a metal plate. They anchored the plate by drilling screws through four holes in the plate and into the bone.[10]

Jeremy Corso, a third-year medical student doing a summer internship under Anna's supervision, held retractors and helped stabilize the wrist. Jeremy had observed and assisted in surgeries for several weeks, and Anna decided to let him place the final screw. Jeremy moved to the patient's side next to the operative site, then flashed me a look of terror. Johnny, the chief resident, braced the patient's wrist from one side. To better position Jeremy's body, Anna insisted that he hold the drill in his left hand instead of his right, even though he is right-handed. Anna's decision to make Jeremy use his left hand provided an important teaching moment, even though it was dictated entirely by the spaces around the patient's body. Anna helped

Jeremy hold and guide the drill. Braced by Anna and Johnny, Jeremy successfully placed the screw.

Several days later, Jeremy and Anna discussed the procedure during a group coffee. Jeremy said he was frightened, but he put on a brave face:

> I'm right-handed and [the surgeon] was like, "Use your left hand." And I was thinking, "Why?"

Anna replied, "Because he was doing this." She held out her right hand, as though holding the drill, and twisted her body around, so her right hand wrapped around her left side, leaving her wrist bent at an awkward angle. Anna did not tell Jeremy that his body was twisted when the drill was in his right hand. Rather, she demonstrated it and made a joke of it. Her mimicry showed Jeremy's improper position and became another teaching moment, indicating that Anna wanted Jeremy to use his entire body to help keep the screw aligned. The drilling lesson was a "situated action," an action that occurred in "the context of particular concrete circumstances" (Suchman 1987, viii). But the choice of hands clearly made the experience more significant for Jeremy. Anna's demonstration also revealed what could have happened if Jeremy had used his right hand: with his body twisted, he would have been unable to properly align his arm, the drill, and the screw. The chances of improperly angling the screw would have increased dramatically.

Even after Anna's physical demonstration, Jeremy remained focused on the issue of handedness:

> JEREMY: I wanted to [use my right hand] because my dominant hand, I felt would be, I really, honestly felt I would have been able to screw it in better, but yet she insisted that I do it with my left.
>
> ANNA: You were getting that hazing. It's mostly in fun, but it's also pushing your boundaries.
>
> JEREMY: And it's all for a good purpose, to ultimately do it right, learn it.

The interaction indicated that surgeon and student framed the procedure very differently. Jeremy focused only on his body and its right-handedness. Anna examined the entire operating field, particularly the patient's body and the tight spaces around it, then judged which hand to use. Her next statement sounded like a non sequitur but actually was a crucial part of the interaction: she called her instructions "hazing" and said she was pushing

Jeremy's boundaries. The hazing of medical students by surgeons and staff reinforces the rigid hierarchy of the surgical team (Bosk 1979). It also continually reminds students how little they know. Pushing Jeremy to try something beyond his abilities had a similar effect. As with learning to scrub and maintain sterility, Anna introduced Jeremy to a new area of practice by taking him out of the comfortable familiarities of his own body's right-handedness and into the anxiety not only of drilling a screw into a patient's arm, but also of using his left hand. The interaction makes clear that the drill was not the only piece of equipment unfamiliar to the student. Jeremy's left hand also was "unhandy."

Asking Jeremy to use his left hand not only correctly positioned his body in relation to drill and patient; it also effected the boundary-pushing Anna desired. The situation furthered the student's defamiliarization with his body, subtly reinforcing Jeremy's position as neophyte and Anna's power as the person who knew how to operate, the person who had learned to judge the surgical situation and her trainees' skills. Jeremy's final statement, that Anna pushed him so he would learn correct technique, shows that he understood the dual goal of education and treatment. Anna articulated her purpose quite clearly: she wanted to push Jeremy to a new level of practice, regardless of whether he felt prepared to advance. She pushed him past the limits of his abilities, testing his willingness both to try something new and to let her assess his readiness.

Later in the discussion, Anna explained the contextual work she and Johnny did for Jeremy:

> Did you notice what we did with you? I mean you were probably so conscious of what you were doing, but both [Johnny] and I were right on you. It's almost like learning to ride a bike. I was guiding your hand. [Johnny] was over there [bracing the patient's wrist]. We were giving you all this silent feedback, like giving you the counterpressure and stuff, so you wouldn't fail. So that's the part where it's that baby step and then you slowly withdraw the support.

Anna acknowledged that two frames—hers and the student's—were at work. Anna framed the drilling experience so Jeremy could set the screw correctly and so he would begin to understand how to position his body. This resembles accounts of framing in other high-risk professions that involve complex multipart tasks in which the responsible expert, such as an attending surgeon or ship's pilot, rotates juniors through discrete tasks, teaching them a complex procedure by breaking it into its elements and simultaneously managing the larger, high-risk activity (Hutchins 1993). Framing by supervisors thus contains any mistakes juniors make.

In this case, Jeremy focused on hand, drill, screw, and bone, and remained unaware or only peripherally aware of the support he received, while Anna watched Jeremy, guided his hands, watched him embed the screw, and monitored the resident's counterpressure. She acknowledged that Jeremy could only focus on his own body, whereas she enlisted four bodies—Jeremy's, Johnny's, the patient's, and her own—to help Jeremy set the screw properly. She made Jeremy's hands into another type of instrument, an extension of the drill. In effect, the surgeon wielded the student's hands. As Jeremy continued to practice, Anna would gradually pull back her support until the student wielded the drill instead of the surgeon wielding the student.

Within Anna's frame—in the operating room—there was little room for trial and error. What did Jeremy learn by placing the screw? After his summer internship, Jeremy wrote a brief report about his work, saying he would have benefited from spending more time reviewing anatomy and surgical procedural manuals before each surgery. He got some physical practice and experience in the operating room. But his drilling experience worked on at least two other levels:

> I was appreciative of the opportunity to hold retractors, cut stitches, and on one occasion, screw a K-wire through a bone, and on another, more precarious opportunity, to use my left (non-dominant) hand to apply a screw through a metal plate and into a bone. [Dr. Wilson] said I should use my left hand because the angle was better, but perhaps it was out of a secretive desire to turn me into a southpaw like her and [another doctor]. =). [emoticon in original]

Somatically, Jeremy experienced the correct feel of drilling. He said using his left hand improved the angle of the drill. But he described the positioning as being related to hand and drill, remaining within his narrow frame, focusing on the point of contact and not on his entire body's relation to the drill, the patient's body, or the bodies of surgeon and resident. His statement was technically correct, but insufficient, as Anna's body-twisting mimicry revealed. Jeremy also jokingly misrepresented the left-handed surgeon's intention, saying she secretly might have wanted to make him a "southpaw." The joke contains an important truth about surgical training: Jeremy would have to learn to use his nondominant hand proficiently if he planned to pursue surgery as a career. Surgeons talk often about this aspect of their embodied skill, saying that their colleagues' use of a nondominant hand can reveal far more about their technical ability than their use of the dominant hand, showing how profoundly surgical training alters one's relationship to one's body. Surgeons must learn control in their entire bodies, and they must make decisions based not on their natural bodily preferences but on what the situation in the operating room dictates. Learning embodied control in the operating room means learning to understand one's position in relation to all the bodies in the operating field, especially the patient's.

This interaction defamiliarized Jeremy with his own body, taking him out of the comfort of using his right hand. Defamiliarization is critical to these early lessons of surgery because the student must relinquish his body to the surgeon, who decides what he will do and how he will do it. Control at this level means allowing supervisors to structure and guide the beginner's every move to the point of taking physical control of a trainee's hands to guide his actions. Anna framed the interaction so Jeremy could not fail. Trainees do make mistakes in the operating room, but senior surgeons do everything possible to limit the damage they can do. In this interaction, Jeremy had to relinquish his body and his convictions about his capabilities to Anna's guidance and judgment. Thus, ethical technique for Jeremy required deference to his superior's decisions. Anna, on the other hand, had to balance Jeremy's need to learn, his lack of surgical technique, and her mandate to protect the patient. For Jeremy, the beginner, ethical technique meant giving up some control of his body, while for Anna it meant exerting control over underlings' bodies and practices. The surgeon drilled the physical and social lessons of surgery into the student's body just as surely as the student drilled the screw into the patient's forearm.

Guiding Eye and Hand, Building Confidence

On another day, Anna guided Dr. Ken Miller, a second-year resident, through a wrist surgery. Anna described Ken, out of his hearing, as skilled with his hands but lazy, often lacking basic knowledge of anatomy and procedure. Ken had an air of confidence in the operating room that made him appear more senior than he was. While waiting for a patient suffering from wrist pain, Anna quizzed him about symptoms of carpal tunnel syndrome, a painful swelling of tissues in the tightly constricted spaces at the base of the palm.[11] Ken hesitated but answered correctly. She asked him which nerve becomes compressed, causing wrist pain. The median nerve, he replied tentatively. "That's very good," Anna said, mildly sarcastically, then asked him which branch of the median nerve. He did not know the answer. She told him to review the anatomy.[12]

When attendants wheeled the patient in, Anna made certain that an anesthetizing nerve block in his arm had taken effect. She chatted in Spanish with the muscular patient for a moment while anesthesiologists put a mask on his face. As the patient slipped under general anesthesia, Anna absentmindedly stroked his wrist, and I could not decide whether she was comforting him, ensuring that he had no feeling in the wrist, palpating the injury, or thinking about the procedure. She told me he had symptoms of carpal tunnel syndrome but in the wrong location, farther back in the wrist, inches away from the base of his hand. She showed me a swelling on the wrist but did not speculate about its cause.

With Ken looking on, Anna drew a line on the man's hand to indicate the path of the incision and to mark the major landmarks on the palm. She gave Ken some heuristics for finding the landmarks. She described how she learned to do carpal tunnel releases and how the procedure had changed. As Ken cut into the skin, purple tissue bulged through the incision. Resident and surgeon were surprised. "What's that muscle belly doing there?" Ken asked. Anna did not reply, but she instructed him to open the tough layers of tissue in the man's palm. Further dissection revealed an unusual anatomical variation of the *palmaris longus* muscle. The muscles in the forearm, which enable hand movement, are thick, purple muscles toward the elbow and become thin, white tendons as they approach the wrist. In this case, the patient's *palmaris longus* was reversed; the muscular portion crowded the wrist, and the long tendon stretched toward the elbow. The muscle pressed on nerves in the man's forearm, causing pain. Fortunately for the patient, the muscle is not critical, and is sometimes used as a "spare part"[13] to replace other muscles. Anna decided to remove it.

As Ken dissected the base of the man's palm, Anna repeatedly warned the resident that his scalpel was straying too far "radially," toward the man's thumb. Straying reflected the resident's lack of experience and, possibly, his weak anatomical knowledge. Anna told the resident a story about a hand-surgery fellowship she did at a Harvard-affiliated hospital. She said Harvard surgeons gave very subtle directions: first, they would nod or point. Then they would quietly say, "I think you'd better move," which meant, "Move now." Anything more urgent, and the resident or fellow was in deep trouble. She called these understated instructions "Harvard speak."

This situated teaching moment contained at least four lessons. The first teaching moment was quizzing, when Anna asked Ken to verbally recite what he knew of wrist anatomy. Quizzing makes medical trainees perform their knowledge, reinforcing the importance of massive amounts of memorized knowledge that a physician must recall on the spot. Quizzing—known as "pimping" among medical students—pushes students to study anatomical and procedural knowledge continually, to keep on their toes, and to keep reviewing such knowledge until it is available whenever needed, that is, until it is durably embodied. Anna's sarcasm when Ken provided weak answers gave him an unstated social cue. Knowing that the median nerve runs through the carpal tunnel is barely adequate. Details matter. Anna expected him to do better. Anatomical knowledge gets relearned and reinforced throughout a surgeon's career. Anna told me that she often reviews the anatomy of regions where she operates infrequently, bringing the subtle bends and twists of nerves and vessels back into awareness. Ken, too, should have reviewed the patient's anatomy before he operated. Quizzing challenged any comfortable assumptions Ken might have made that anything less than precise knowledge would do. Medical students often report worrying that, if they miss an instruction or skip a lecture, they might be faced with a patient who suffers from some condition covered by the missing lesson. The fear reflects concern that some gap in their knowledge could lead them to harm a patient. Anna's quizzing sent Ken the message that his weak knowledge was unacceptable. If he were to continue to show up with insufficient preparation, the sanctions would become more severe.

The second situated lesson was drawing on the patient's hand. Surgeons often use sterile pens to draw the basics of the procedure on a drape or, more often, directly on the patient's body. Anna said that drawing creates common ground between her and the residents working with her:

> I do draw a lot, particularly for complex procedures. It's for me as much as for them because it sets what their level of understanding is coming

into it. If I said, "Well, let's just see what they know," that's not really fair to either of us because we would be constantly feeling each other out. If I say, "Here's the distal radius; these are the points that we're going after; this is what I'm looking for, it may not be obvious to you." But if [they] have this in mind, then [they've] got something to work towards.

The drawing meant that Anna did not have to guess what Ken knew, and Ken did not have to guess what she expected. It gave Ken a path to cut along and made Anna's knowledge explicit. The drawing created a path for the incision and a map of surgical procedure in relation to anatomical land-marks. It brought the wrist and its unusual pathology into the social inter-action of surgeon and resident, becoming a mark of human intervention analogous to the *picada*, the dirt track, that Claude Lévi-Strauss says opens the wilderness to human understanding and exploitation, socializing the natural (1973, 272). The drawing formed part of both Anna's and Ken's rehearsal of the surgical procedure, bringing surgeon, resident, and wrist into the same conversation. The meaning of Anna's trace is complicated. The stroke of a pen inscribes years of surgical practice, procedural knowl-edge, and anatomical knowledge on the patient's body. The line was a "material-semiotic actor" (Haraway 1990, 200) that revealed the opening into the wrist and signaled to the resident what he eventually would have to know.[14] The drawing showed where the skin would be divided, and it separated the surgeon from resident, revealing the gulf of knowledge be-tween them. Ken had to cross the line with his scalpel and, later, with knowledge he would accumulate during his residency. For Anna, control in this moment meant using her knowledge to show Ken what to do and to remind him that learning proper anatomy and procedure contains practical and ethical implications for future practice.

The third form of teaching contained in this interaction was the story about "Harvard speak." Storytelling is an important part of medical teach-ing, conveying social information about medical practice and social struc-tures (Bosk 1979; Hafferty 1988). Intimately connected to the narrative art of case presentation, storytelling is critical to teaching in biomedicine, orient-ing students and residents to the field, and establishing tacit boundaries and social controls (Hafferty 1988, 345). Storytelling reinforces physical teaching for students less adept at understanding nonverbal cues. In this case, the story reinforced the meanings of silent pointing and verbal cues. It told Ken where his attention should have been and how seriously he should have taken Anna's verbal reminders. Storytelling powerfully structures lessons taught in the operating room. The stories, adages, and jokes surgeons repeat invoke the "principles of morally acceptable behavior" (Foucault 2005, 327) that discursively shape the surgeon's habitus. Anna told Ken that he should follow her guidance and listen carefully to her words.

Anna's repeated reminders about straying provided a fourth lesson. During a discussion about surgical teaching that occurred after this surgery, Anna explained how she guides students nonverbally and verbally:

> I do a lot of manual guiding, guiding them with my pointing instrument, my freer. And I'm constantly guiding, and they're mostly not aware of it because it's becoming part of the field. But if they start drifting, then I may have to say something if they don't pick up the visual cue. I'm . . . guiding, almost like a pointer. Sometimes it's pushing the tissue or getting it in the right plane. Sometimes you have to say, "No, move your knife over here," if they're not quite so clued in.

Much of the guiding Anna and other surgeons do is nonverbal. As with Jeremy's use of the drill, she expected Ken to focus on the task and remain relatively unaware of the guidance. Unlike Jeremy, who required bracing and guiding, Ken worked more autonomously and required only visual cues and verbal reminders. Thus, Anna first used nonverbal indications to guide him. She used an instrument at the edge of his field of vision to urge Ken's hand to stay in the correct path. This was a largely subliminal cue because the instrument became part of Ken's larger perceptual field. The pointer became part of Ken's "outer horizon," contextual or background information that structured his perception of the area of focus (Dreyfus 1992, 240–41). This guiding also gave Ken the sense that he was acting autonomously. Verbal guidance was a last resort that occurred when the resident failed to recognize the visual cue. Verbal cues are less than optimal because they remind residents that they are not acting alone.

Surgeons typically teach by demonstrating a procedure, then turning it over to residents to try under their guidance. Residents then teach it to their juniors, a teaching practice known as "See one, do one, teach one." Nonverbal guiding is a form of steering a resident, letting the resident do as much as possible autonomously before making corrections. Tacit guiding often gives residents the impression that a procedure is easy—until they try it by themselves. Confidence and decisiveness are among the traits surgical residents learn during their training (see also Cassell 1991; Katz 1999). Reasoned decisiveness becomes important in a world of medicine where doctors must manage pathologies, diagnoses, and outcomes that often are far from certain (Fox 1957; Katz 1981). Speed matters to surgeons, and second-guessing one's decision can be a problem. Steering residents by physically guiding or pointing in their visual field makes residents feel as though they are proceeding unguided. Guiding gives students and residents the illusion of working autonomously and competently, the illusion of possessing skills they have not yet acquired. Residents come to believe a procedure is easy, in part because the attending surgeon encourages them to believe that they have accomplished the procedure easily and largely alone. This method allows surgeons to maintain control over the resident's actions without giving the appearance of doing so. This helps residents develop the confidence and decisiveness needed to practice surgery. Excessive surgical confidence often is mocked with the adage "Sometimes wrong, but never in doubt."

All four lessons reveal that what is at stake for a resident is the relationship between knowledge and action. Quizzing, drawing, the "Harvard-speak" story, and the warning about straying all revealed that to act in a properly controlled manner, a resident eventually must combine technical skills, which Ken had, with knowledge of anatomy and procedure, which he lacked. Control for Ken meant being better informed, knowing anatomically and physically how not to stray. Ken's confidence was a virtue, one to be fostered, but it had to be tempered with deeper knowledge. Ken was more advanced than Jeremy and worked more autonomously. But the lessons in the making of a surgeon—lessons about studying, straying, and what it meant to cross the line—clearly told Ken what he had to do to advance. More subtly, they indicated that learning anatomy and procedure formed part of the resident's ethical responsibility to master surgical knowledge.

Attending to the Vast Difference

During another teaching surgery, I observed Julie Martinez, the chief resident, perform her first minimally invasive hernia surgery. Though Julie had four years of surgical experience, she was just learning to repair hernias. Hernias occur most easily wherever there is an opening or weakness in the abdominal wall that bits of tissue might slip through, as is the case with the inguinal area of a man's groin, which allows passage of the spermatic duct and affiliated blood vessels through the abdomen to the testicles.[15] In the case of an inguinal hernia, bits of tissue, usually intestine, pass through the weakened abdominal wall and must be pulled back into place before the surgeon patches the hernia. This particular patient had two herniated areas, one on each side of the vessels running through the abdominal wall.

Dr. Tom Berg, the staff physician, helped Julie place ports inside the man's abdomen. Once, Tom had created a space in the abdomen, he inserted a camera. He used the laparoscope with his hands and indicated the two herniated areas of the man's abdomen as depicted on two monitors suspended over the patient's legs. He then pointed out the blood vessels leading from the patient's abdomen to his testicles. Julie put up her hand, palm out, and leaned back as though pushing her body away from the vessels. "Stay away," she said, mock seriously, evidently referring to a previous interaction. The gesture physically enacted the danger of coming too close to a blood vessel and the need to steer clear. Julie performed the instruction to stay away from the vessels. The gesture was not literal—she would never make this particular move to avoid harming structures. Instead, it was embodied: she had incorporated the instruction and its meaning. Natasha Myers (2007) has shown how biologists contort their bodies to mimic the complex folds of protein molecules, using gestures and movement to understand and teach structure. In both instances, meaning resides in the body in ways that cannot be reduced to linguistic or cognitive understanding.

Tom pointed to a structure that he called the "vast difference," which actually was the *vas deferens*, the tube that carries sperm to the urethra. Though many medical mnemonics for anatomical structures are sexual, this one was particularly potent because it plays on gendered anatomical differences between men and women.[16] Tom then pointed to a few more blood vessels, saying Julie should be extra careful to avoid them because they would bleed excessively if nicked. This narration of anatomy created common surgical and epistemological ground in the patient's body, grounding abstract anatomical knowledge in the specifics of the individual patient. The narrative resembled the line Anna drew on the patient's wrist because it constructed the common space within which resident and surgeon were working. The construction of a three-dimensional work space is particularly important for minimally invasive surgeries because surgeons use anatomical landmarks to navigate three-dimensional anatomy as depicted on a two-dimensional screen. Physical methods, such as pointing and marking tissues, also are more difficult with minimally invasive surgery. Narrating the procedure is an important part of the discursive framing of surgical action, creating an operative site marked by anatomical landmarks and procedural steps.

Tom asked Julie if she wanted to do both sides of the hernia. "I can start, but if you get exasperated, you can take over because I haven't done any," Julie said, clearly indicating the state of her skills to her supervising surgeon. Tom told Julie to make a large flap out of the abdominal wall, into which she would insert a piece of mesh that would reinforce the wall. He said, "You want to start your flap way up high towards this vessel." Teaching minimally invasive procedures is more difficult than teaching open surgery because supervisors typically cannot point out structures or guide students with a pointer. They also have less direct control over residents' actions, making it more difficult to prevent them from making mistakes.[17]

Julie worked with tiny scissors and a harmonic scalpel that were threaded through small holes in the abdomen. "I think your hands are reversed," Tom said, "but let's see how you do." Julie's hands looked tangled up with each other as she held the long handles of the laparoscopic instruments. Either Tom did not think this was a big problem or he wanted her to discover for herself what would work best. In an environment of genuinely disciplinary control, such as the eighteenth-century military drills that Michel Foucault (1977) describes, trainees have strict constraints placed on their movements. But surgical practice must help trainees develop confidence and autonomy. Within the limits of safety, supervisors can allow trainees to sort out some bodily actions on their own. These actions eventually develop into the "regulated improvisations" of the habitus (Bourdieu 1977). The ethical imperative to do no harm, as it becomes embodied in surgical practice, encourages surgeons to control their actions in this relatively autonomous setting.

As Julie dissected the flap, Tom described the landmarks and the procedures: "You're going to take that line down along the ligament later," he told her. "And you're going to make three quarters of a square. . . . This is how far laterally you're going to get. Maybe another inch. . . . Use the back of your scissors to push the fat away and develop the plane. . . . You want to cover your defect. . . . There's your vessel, up and to the left. . . . You want to get that peritoneum out."

While Tom narrated the procedure, Julie worked silently to create the flap. She cleared away crumpled peritoneal tissue that crowded into the defect and escaped through the abdominal wall. As she pulled the tissue out of the herniated area, she began to see the hernia more clearly. Her concentration was total. She bobbed her head to either side of the camera, as though to get a better view, even though moving her body could not have changed her relationship to the images on the two-dimensional screen. Only moving the camera would have helped. Julie's bobbing suggests that she had not yet embodied the relationship between the two-dimensional monitor and the patient's three-dimensional abdomen, a relationship surgeons develop after years of practice doing minimally invasive surgeries.[18] I have never seen a more senior surgeon do this. The movement was extraneous. Experienced surgeons still their bodies to prevent inadvertent movements of instruments, making their own bodies the most significant instruments of surgical control.[19] Tom did not call attention to Julie's excess movement; she had enough to do to manage instruments and procedure. Stillness would come later.

Julie nicked a blood vessel and blood leaked into the abdominal space. She muttered a curse.

"That's OK," Tom said. "We'll just put a clip on it." He asked a nurse to find a clip. He exhibited the extraordinary calm that I have observed when something dangerous occurs during a surgery. The nurses could not find a clip, which annoyed him. "The patient is bleeding," he said. "We should not have to go look for it. It should be in the room where we're doing lap case."

Surgeons are renowned for having explosive tempers, but the only times I saw surgeons get angry was when slowness or lack of attention or knowledge could have endangered the patient.[20] In this case, Tom did not express anger at Julie. Rather, the surgical staff's failure to stock clips angered him. The anger appeared mostly tactical, a means of saying, "This is serious." When a nurse finally hustled the clip into the room, Julie placed it on the vessel, then sheepishly asked Tom if he would like to handle the second herniated area.

"Let's not worry about it," he reassured her. "It's part of surgery. You do something wrong, and you fix it."

"I had lost the vessels," she said.

"You have to ask yourself: What could go wrong here?"

This brief exchange speaks volumes about surgical training. Perfect control may be a goal, but it is also an impossibility. Surgeons slip. And they learn to fix their mistakes rapidly and without fuss. Julie's response was exemplary. She reviewed her error, marking her mistake in a way that would make her less likely to repeat it. She also revealed the danger of focusing too narrowly: she lost sight of the blood vessels and nicked one. Tom told her to check the larger area for potential danger; this was one reason to name the vessels as they came into view. What was at stake for Julie was neither the need to give control over her body to the surgeon, as with Jeremy, nor the need to develop more anatomical knowledge, as with Ken. Instead, Julie had to embody greater facility with the tools of minimally invasive surgery, and she had to learn to widen her frame to consider what might go wrong in the area surrounding the spot where she worked. Julie had to master bodily control over her movements and her instruments. She also had to develop a wider perceptual sense of the surgical field as depicted on the monitor.

Each of the interactions with trainees that I have described reveals the progressive widening of frame expected of trainees, from simple actions to actions informed by anatomical and procedural knowledge to a broader horizon that keeps the entire anatomical region in awareness. Anna told me that one of her teachers constantly warned students that "there is always a snake in the grass." This told trainees that they would have to learn to note potential dangers, such as an unexpected anatomical variation or a partially obscured nerve or blood vessel, which might lurk at the edge of their visual horizon.

Tom instructed Julie to pull some fat away from the abdominal wall. "Grab the fat hand over hand," he told her. "You see that white part? That's the fascia." Then Tom pointed to several structures that came into view on the monitor. "That's his testicle and that's the vas. Obviously that stays."

Julie let the piece of tissue she's grasping slip. "Oof, that's frustrating," she said.

"You're doing fine," he replied. "There's the [spermatic] cord there. You want to leave the cord. Please. It's a man thing."

Tom reminded Julie several times in a few minutes that hernia repair is not a simple procedure. More important, he engaged in a delicate dance of caution and trust as Julie finished the first hernia repair. After she nicked the blood vessel, he let her continue. But he stepped up his reminders of the anatomical danger areas, noting repeatedly that they form part of a man's sexual apparatus and that damage to them could impair the patient's manhood. Tom gendered the joke and subtly tied it to himself by emphasizing that "it's a man thing." As a man, he had empathy for the male patient and the potential danger to his reproductive organs if Julie made a more serious slip. This also reinvoked the potential dangers of surgery: nicking a blood vessel usually is a minor mistake, but damaging a man's spermatic cord, which includes the vas deferens, testicular blood supply, and several critical nerves, would be much more serious. Future generations were at stake. This reminded Julie of the patient's personhood, as well as reminding her of the trust the patient had placed in the surgical team. Gendering the jokes heightened their charge. Although Tom's remarks were genuine cautions to Julie to be more careful, they were done in a lighthearted way. Tom's joke revealed the dangers without dwelling on them in ways that could have further rattled Julie's composure (Goffman 1961b, 117–18). Jokes in the operating room often focus on the moments of greatest danger, typically occurring after such dangers have been surmounted and order restored (Katz 1981, 348).

Jokes like Tom's also serve a pedagogical purpose: they virtually reopen the moment, giving the trainee a chance to glimpse the danger it contained for the patient's well-being or the resident's career, then they leave the moment of danger in the past. The joke has the double effect of revealing and minimizing the danger, teaching it as a hazard a well-trained surgeon can learn to avoid.[21] After Julie's slip, Tom verbally reasserted the need for control and the consequences of a slip. The joke reminded Julie of the ethical stakes: slips cause harm. Maintaining control of one's actions and one's awareness of the outer horizon can limit that harm.

Julie placed the mesh and tacked it into place with several screws that anchored themselves like tiny corkscrews into the abdominal wall. Tom then decided that he would repair the other side. He did not explain why, but he narrated his actions for Julie. He picked up a cautery to dissect the abdominal wall. Julie had used a scissors to do this. Tom told Julie that this kind of dissection could be done with either instrument, but he typically found it easier to use the cautery. He had left the choice up to her, teaching technique as open-ended choices, rather than rigid rules. "This side is going to be easier," he said. "There are the vessels."

"Stay away," Julie said, repeating the same pushing away gesture she had made earlier, though her earlier mistake gave the repetition more irony.

Tom pulled tissue away from the abdominal wall and explained, "This is what I was saying. You just separate and then the plane starts to open up. You see what I'm saying?"

"Totally," Julie said. This kind of teaching allowed Julie to see how to do correctly what she had wrestled with earlier, giving her a close-to-real-time lesson in how to do it correctly.[22]

"OK, I just need to do a little bit more medially so I get a really good view of the defect," Tom said. "Here, I have to see, so I get a view of Cooper's ligament. I get as much fat out as possible, so we get good adherence between the mesh and the abdominal wall. Medically, I'd like to see the defect better." He described his decision-making process as it happened, including that he would like to do more work on a particular area near the defect, but he had to avoid the area around the ligament because many nerves ran through it.

At this point, Dr. Emily Gold, another staff surgeon, and close colleague of Tom's, wandered into the operating room, sat in a rolling chair, and scooted it up to the side of the operating table, almost, but not quite into the sterile field, where she could see the laparoscopic monitors the surgeons were using. Only a senior surgeon could get away with this kind of move without being chastised by the staff. Emily examined Tom's work on the screen, then made a remark that I could not hear.

"That's a compliment," Tom said.

"That's because it's Dr. Berg's side. Mine looks like I did it open," Julie said, referring to the bleeding she caused, noting that it looked like an open surgery done through a large incision in the abdomen, rather than through small holes that bled much less. Julie's self-denigrating joke again invoked her less-experienced role. Emily replied that she herself was just beginning to get comfortable doing laparoscopic hernia operations and would like to do a dozen or more in a row to really master them.

Whereas Julie's joke distanced her from the senior surgeons, Emily's reassurance narrowed that distance, showing that these are difficult skills that require regular and repeated practice even by experienced surgeons. Ken, the second-year resident, required needling to bring his knowledge in line with his confidence; Julie needed reassurance to bolster her confidence. Ken's excess of confidence and Julie's lack of it may reflect gendered responses to intense training situations (a topic that could use more research). In both cases, the attending surgeons used their own knowledge and expertise—their positions as qualified senior surgeons—to create social distance from or closeness to the resident. Anna, Tom, and Emily continually modeled their knowledge, skill, and attitude for residents, demonstrating calm professionalism as they worked through unanticipated difficulties, becoming irritated only when actions by a junior or other member of the team could have harmed the patient.

Tom let Julie embed the final tacks in a mesh that he pressed against the patient's abdominal wall. Julie struggled to place the tacks properly so she could anchor them securely.

"It takes coordination," Tom said.

"I should have played more videogames," she replied.[23] Whether through videogames, surgical simulations, or surgical practice, Julie signaled that she needed practice with the fine motor control that minimally invasive surgery requires, repeating assertions about her lack of experience, while also noting what she needed to make up her deficiencies.

"Don't get the bladder, please," Tom told Julie, then proceeded to tell two stories about other surgeons who nicked the bladder while tacking a mesh over a hernia, saying it caused some painful urination but adding that the problem went away quickly. The stories had two effects: they told Julie that others make mistakes and that the consequences could be painful but minor. Tom's comments showed the relative stakes of various errors: nicking a blood vessel typically is a minor mistake, putting a small hole in the bladder causes the patient short-term pain, and damaging nerves or reproductive organs can be devastating.

During this surgery, Tom, Emily, and Julie engaged in jokes, discussion, and gestures that revealed the dangers and difficulties of repairing a hernia using minimally invasive techniques. Tom used gender to heighten the humor and add urgency to his warnings about potential pitfalls. Julie replied with humor to reinforce this message and to show deference to the two senior surgeons. And Emily used her own experience to reassure Julie of the procedure's difficulty and to bolster the resident's confidence. Three issues were at stake: protecting the patient, teaching the resident to avoid danger by widening her frame, and ensuring that she maintain confidence after a mistake. Widening the frame and physically learning the procedure became technical skills and ethical principles that the senior surgeons modeled for the resident, showing her the meaning of control at her level of training.

Training Techniques and Ethics

The cultivation of a surgeon begins during a student's premedical education and during the early years of medical school. Anatomy and the anatomy laboratory certainly play a role in this preparation but so, too, do courses with content unrelated to surgery that present students with quantities of information seemingly too vast to absorb and with a hierarchical relation to instructors. In these courses, the sheer quantity of information to be learned isolates students from nonclinicians and encourages them to find fellowship with their cohorts (Becker et al. 1961). These courses also send a message to students that medicine entails far more information than one person can master, fostering the values of disciplined review and practice, as well as consultation and lifelong learning. The values of teamwork and constant study and practice intensify and become specific on surgical wards, where interns may spend a few weeks on a clinical rotation or may elect a surgical residency and career. The operating-room environment, from spaces and schedules to surgical rituals and clothing, all emphasize surgery's separation from other types of medical practice, reinforcing its hierarchical structures and the values of control of one's body and behavior.[24]

Up to this point, I have focused on how surgical practice cultivates techniques and ethics of control. Here, I show how a focus on embodiment brings these issues into view. Surgical training clearly involves learning "techniques of the body" (Mauss 2007). Marcel Mauss argues that learning technique begins with "prestigious imitation" (2007, 53–54), actions that, even when strictly physical, are imposed by an authority in whom the trainee has confidence: "It is precisely this notion of the prestige of the person who performs the ordered, authorized, tested, action *vis-à-vis* the imitating individual that contains all the social element" (54). Many of the ethnographies of surgery cited above show how the surgical milieu, from the operating-room setup to the hierarchical structure of the team, locates the senior surgeon at the center of surgical action (Goffman 1961b; Hirschauer 1991; Moreira 2004). The surgical milieu, along with the wisdom of technique that accumulates in senior surgeons' bodies, grants them prestige enough to be imitated by juniors. Building on Mauss, Pierre Bourdieu argues that the structuring effects of the environment build particular organizing principles, habits, and ways of being into the minds and bodies of cultural actors (1977, 72). Subjects absorb and adopt the lessons of the social world as "meaning-made-body" (75). Other scholars contend that practicing beliefs and behaviors instills the techniques of ethical practice; practices make the ethical subject (Foucault 1986, 2005; Mahmood 2005). Practices that accumulate in the ethical subject's body become permanent dispositions to speak, think, and act (Bourdieu 1977; Foucault 2005). These dispositions, structures of speaking and acting, become durably installed in the ethical subject (Foucault 2005, 322).

These foundational works on practice within symbolically structured environments reveal how verbal and physical practices that take place within structuring environments take on significance and serve as bodily enactments and reinforcements of meaning. Understanding the process of subject formation through bodily learning, however, requires attention to the temporal dimension of this formation, especially within complex and lengthy hierarchical apprenticeships such as surgical training. Surgeons teach by example and by framing trainees' practice to teach techniques of bodily control and protect patients from harm. The specific practices trainees engage in, such as using a drill to put a screw into a bone, may be identical at every level of skill (even when levels of ability are demonstrably different), but at each level, the meaning of control changes. Studying the formation of surgical embodiment shows that controlling violence involves different actions and requires different knowledges at each level of surgical training.

Opening up the connection of techniques and ethics in the cultivation of surgeons requires scrutiny of four aspects of surgical training. First, the endpoint of surgical education clearly is the creation of a competent senior surgeon who can act autonomously, make decisions for the benefit of his or her patients, teach juniors (at least in academic practices), and perform procedures with appropriate skill and caution. Mauss's prestigious imitation is the endpoint of surgical education. The skills that senior surgeons exhibit and the judgments and decisions that they make are so far beyond beginners' abilities that they are almost impossible to discern in the work beginners do, such as holding retractors and cutting stitches.[25] Of necessity, training begins with small, carefully framed tasks. As small skills lead to larger ones, what begins as imitation of those more senior gradually becomes embodied. True imitation of the surgeon's craft occurs only when the trainee becomes the surgeon (Polanyi 1962, 1966).

Second, examining control of violence as the technical and ethical material to be worked on in surgical training reveals that its form changes dramatically over time.[26] For Amal, the first-year resident, control means maintaining sterility and staying out of the way; for Julie, the chief resident, control means mastering minimally invasive techniques and widening her perceptual horizon; for Nick, the master surgeon, control means choosing not to operate when he fears he will do more harm than good. For surgeons in academic practice, control also means constructing an operating environment and surgical field in which trainees can learn while keeping patients safe. The surgeon's craft builds from simple techniques to complex relationships of technique, procedure, and anatomy to more complex exercises of wisdom and judgment. At each level, good practice requires the embodiment of control.

Third, the means by which trainees learn control appropriate to their level also requires examination. In this context, ethical practice means embodying techniques that limit harm. Constant practice, most of it in the operating room, helps trainees achieve physical control of their actions. Supervisors structure practice so trainees work up to and beyond the limits of their abilities while receiving guidance so they do not harm patients. Guiding by superiors protects patients and creates frames in which trainees' actions can be contained and led to a proper outcome. Guided training provides confidence and a sense of competence that initially is somewhat illusory. Practice makes trainees' illusory competence increasingly real. This supervision continually reinforces the message that harming patients is unacceptable.

Finally, the mode by which trainees are incited to exercise control must be interrogated. That is, if control of decisive and confident surgical action is at stake in surgery, trainees must continually be incited to exercise their obligation to practice control. They must understand that they are doing violence by invading and altering patients' bodies, but that violence must not become harm. In the intense moments of finding (and sometimes crossing) the line of danger in surgery, surgeons often reveal exactly what trainees require to perform the task at hand and to avoid danger in the future. These lessons are contained in stories, jokes, occasional outbursts, and other performances that reveal the dangers—to patients and careers— of mistakes. Thus, trainees are continually incited to embody knowledges and techniques that make dangerous practice routine. What counts as dangerous practice for beginners changes dramatically over the course of surgical training.

During surgical training, all four aspects of training for control are contained in most interactions: the senior surgeon ideally embodies the endpoint of training. The surgeon also models control and helps trainees to exercise control appropriate to their abilities. And the structuring environment and the practices of those in it act in concert to reinforce control as technique and ethic of surgical practice: this is what trainees work on from the moment they enter the operating room. Even after surgeons become fully qualified to take responsibility for patients, accrediting agencies, and, in principle, surgeons' own ethics of professional practice, encourage them to continue learning new technical and social practices for providing care. Surgical training mixes repetition designed to durably embody particular skills with teaching intended to instill an ethical stance toward the meaning of those practices as techniques that limit harm.

Conclusion

Healing in surgery is rooted in carefully crafted action. Medical students and residents, whose education in medical thought and perception begins during the first days of medical school, arrive in the operating room prepared to receive the social lessons of technical training in surgery. Teaching surgery involves a unique process of acculturation that entails, first, defamiliarizing the trainee with his or her body, and then installing new schemes of perception and thought—the embodied practices of a surgeon. These practices include techniques for controlling one's body and limiting harm. When surgeons practice "controlled violence," control becomes a technique and an ethic of surgical training and practice. Control also becomes an impossible-to-meet ideal. This ideal makes surgeons attend to their bodies' readiness to undergo the rigors of working in the operating room. For example, one surgeon I know does not drink caffeinated coffee on operating days because it increases the natural tremor of her hands. Another surgeon lost forty pounds because he struggled to maintain his grueling schedule when he was heavier. Further, most surgeons read up on the latest developments in techniques and technologies, and attend continuing medical education courses. Learning is a continual part of a surgeon's craft.

The ideals of control also are guiding surgery's future. The operating room is a space of enclosure—a space where the sum of productive forces is greater than its component parts (Deleuze 1992). The highly disciplined spaces and procedures of surgery are gradually opening up, becoming fragmented, and being divided as new technologies provide means of operating on patients from a distance, or with a remote surgeon in consultation with the surgeon holding the scalpel. Control in surgery relates to control in laboratory and industrial settings (Schlich 2007). Though the nuances of the term's meaning in laboratories and operating rooms bear further investigation, the desire for control also is a driver for changes in surgical education and practice.

Within the context of operating-room practice, surgeons make decisions based almost exclusively on the biomedical limitation of harm. For example, I have watched surgeons reject a voluntary organ donation on the grounds that the prospective donor was medically unfit. But I have not seen surgeons make operating decisions based on larger social and ethical concerns. Though physicians certainly discuss broader ethical worries, such as disparities in treatment for poor and minority patients, developing a consistent, embodied approach to resolving such concerns would require broader social consensus than exists now about the right actions to take. Teaching the ethics and techniques of limiting harm within a strictly biomedical frame is obvious. When the frame widens to include treatment decisions with broader social implications, exploring the meaning of "do no harm" becomes much more fraught.

Control as an ethical imperative in surgery can be expected to continue as an ideal of surgical education and technology development. As surgical training moves out of the operating room and into spaces like simulation centers, surgical educators likely will reinforce the value of constant practice as the means to achieve control. Conversely, the use of verbal and physical guidance within a structured environment will probably decline in importance. Exactly how these developments will change surgical training remains to be seen. Much depends on how surgery's risks—what is at stake for patients and practitioners—become embodied in future surgeons.

five

SWIMMING IN THE JOINT

With whose blood were my eyes crafted?
HARAWAY 1990, 192

My body is wherever there is something to be done.
MERLEAU-PONTY 2002, 291

A retired gynecologist I know, citing nineteenth-century surgeon William Halsted, said that anything he can see, he can operate on. The statement appears to be self-evident. Indeed, "exposure" is a surgeon's term for interventions that make an injury or pathology available to vision and action. But what happens when new technologies reconfigure the relationship of hands, eyes, tools, and patient body? This chapter examines surgeons' "specific embodiment" (Haraway 1990, 190), the technical and perceptual skills surgeons develop and deploy as they work to see and to act upon patients' bodies in the operating room. I interrogate examples of open surgeries and remotely mediated surgeries to show how action produces and shapes a surgeon's embodiment, the clinical perceptual skills and techniques unique to surgeons. These surgeries exemplify moments when the relationship between action and embodiment comes into view, revealing how new technologies can lead to new perceptual experiences, but also how those experiences emerge from the broad cultivation of a surgeon's craft.

Learning to see in surgery involves the crafting of much more than eyes. Surgical sight emerges from a link between seeing and acting that is so tight that seeing should not slip into the representational language of a medical gaze or of disembodied cognition. Rather, sight comes into being as one part of the embodied work surgeons do when they interact with tools and other bodies in surgery. Sight and touch intertwine; they "belong to the same world" in each individual's body and "yet they do not merge into one" (Merleau-Ponty 1964, 134). For example, most of us can sense the roughness of a tree's bark when we see it and most of us can envision a tree's bark when we touch it: these sensory experiences overlap, but they are not identical. All senses come into play during sensory interactions in surgery in ways that typically are taken for granted.

When new technologies enter the operating room, new relationships between perception and action emerge from the surgeon's embodied skills. The examples I recount make clear that minimally invasive technologies and techniques foster new relationships between practitioners' and patients' bodies. They also represent a new form of surgical embodiment. I examine two essential aspects of these phenomena: first, how embodied skills and experiences shape surgical perception; and second, how mediating technologies interact with embodied skills to create new perceptions. Medical students begin to learn the body's three-dimensional spaces in the anatomy laboratory. Surgical trainees put their three-dimensional spatial sense to work when they do open and minimally invasive procedures.

Medical ethnographers writing about anatomical and surgical dissection have described the visual (Good 1994) and representational (Hirschauer 1991) aspects of dissection. Surgeons, fully aware of the physical aspects of their work, often default to the language of mental models. The emphasis on visual and mental aspects of anatomical and surgical dissection downplays the significant ways in which surgeons engage all of their perceptual faculties to make structural changes to patients' bodies. The language of representation is inadequate for describing such interactions. Focusing on embodiment allows me to open up how surgeons and trainees at various levels come to acquire surgical means of perceiving and acting, especially perceiving and acting with technological mediation. I show how a surgeon's body must be crafted from social and technical interactions as they unfold in the operating room. Neither an open operative site nor an operative site depicted on a monitor is an image the surgeon views. Rather, the interplay of perception and action that takes place at an open or mediated operative site constructs the site as a three-dimensional space that the surgeon inhabits.

Sensing and Acting

I begin with two examples of open surgeries that reveal the broad embodiment at work in the operating theater. In these cases, surgeons see with their bodies. These two moments occurred during the same surgery. The patient was a middle-aged man with a Klatskin's tumor at the top of his bile duct. When I arrived in the operating room, Dr. Marcos Alexander, the hepatobiliary fellow, and Dr. Jill English, the chief resident, already had made a long incision across the abdomen and had retracted ribs and reflected muscles and intestines to reveal the liver. I stood behind the anesthesiologist's drape and looked over at the operative site. While Marcos and Jill worked to expose the tumor, the patient started to bleed heavily into his abdomen. The operative team kept working silently, looking for the source of the bleeding. Jill accidentally rubbed her head against the handle on the overhead lamp and a nurse started to swap out the handle to maintain sterility. "This is not a good time," Jill told the nurse in a monotone. "We've got some bleeding. We need the lamp now." The surgeons had nicked the patient's vena cava, the largest vein in the body, which returns all blood from the body to the heart. Dr. Nick Perrotta, the attending surgeon, told the anesthesiologist to call his chief, saying with typical surgical understatement, "We've got a little bit of a problem."

The vena cava travels between the liver and the rear wall of the abdomen. It runs deep at the back of the curved abdominal space that cradles the liver. The upper abdomen was rapidly filling with blood. The surgeons could not clearly see the vena cava's path to the patient's heart. Nick reached into the cavity, spent a moment exploring the space, then removed his hand and showed Marcos how he believed the vena cava ran. He held his palm upward and pushed his curved hand up and to the left, as though he was following the vessel's path as it ascended into the chest. He instructed the fellow to reach in and feel it. Marcos mimicked him, also tracing a curve to the left. They repeated the same movement of the palm until they agreed that this was indeed the curve the vessel followed. Nick said several times that the curved instrument would have to move to the left and not straight upward, where it would cause damage. Having traced the vena cava virtually, Marcos blindly slipped an instrument under the liver to lift it. Nick stitched the opening and, a very few moments later, they closed the hole and continued the procedure.

These surgeons could not see exactly what they were doing in this space. They could feel the path the retractor would have to take, and they could demonstrate using hand gestures that they had felt it. The demonstration had two purposes: to communicate the venous anatomy's path to each other and to rehearse the movements needed to slip the instrument under the liver. The gesture drew upon and captured both surgeons' years of experience working in this abdominal space. Nick and Marcos used touch and gesture to virtually make the abdominal space present to their bodies before they literally inhabited the abdominal space to repair the injury. After this gestural practice, they lifted the liver and stitched the cut vessel. The movement involved simultaneously imagining and practicing, learning with their hands. In this case, knowing was based on accumulated practice and gestural signals. Both surgeons understood the vena cava's path with their bodies. But they could not, in the strictest sense, see it.

The second moment came later during the same surgery. At a critical moment of this difficult bile duct resection, the anesthesiologist's machines broke down. Blood pressure and other anesthesia monitors extend the patient's body by making it emit signs that speak for the patient (Hirschauer 1991, 290). Particularly during long, difficult operations like this one, monitors tell surgeons and anesthesiologists alike whether the patient's body has destabilized. Low blood pressure is the ideal state for this type of operation, so the anesthesiologist must pharmacologically keep the pressure down while watching to ensure that it does not dip too low. If the pressure drops, the surgeons must step away to give anesthesiologists time to raise it. Late in this long operation, the blood pressure readout plunged. Glancing at it, Jill asked, "Is this a real number?" The anesthesiologist insisted that the numbers reflected a problem with their machines, not with the patient's body. The team proceeded. Nick asked the anesthesiologists repeatedly if the patient's blood pressure was OK. Each time he asked, he placed his hand inside the abdominal cavity and lifted his eyes to the monitors. The anesthesiologists insisted that everything was fine, while they rushed around trying to get their machines to work. They used a manual backup to ensure that blood pressure was adequate, but the surgeons could not see the numbers. The team completed the last steps of the resection, as well as the rest of the operation, without the benefit of a monitor the surgeons could see.

After the operation, I asked Nick for his account of what happened. "I could feel the aorta beating under my hand," he said. Each time he placed his hand inside the abdomen, the strong pulse from the aorta told him that the patient's heart was pumping blood through his body adequately, defying the numbers on the screen. The machine and the patient's aorta told him two different things. "I would have preferred the numbers," Nick said, wanting numerical proof of what he could feel with his hand. The monitor also could offer a precision about the patient's blood pressure that Nick's hand could not. Without a working monitor, Nick used his hand and its ability to understand the pulse beating through the aorta, rather than the information provided by the machine. Touch, bolstered by the anesthesiologists' reassurances, told him what he needed to know to continue the operation.

In both moments during this surgery, the surgeons continued to work effectively despite the loss of direct visual perception. Both surgeons had long since embodied the relevant abdominal anatomy and intervention techniques. Thus, both surgeons' bodies had already synthesized the look, feel, and motions of this region of the body. Merleau-Ponty describes perception as taking advantage of "familiarity with the world born of habit, that implicit sedimentary body of knowledge" (2002, 277). With the implicit knowledge of the patient's body born of carefully honed and frequently practiced techniques of the body, the two surgeons were able to utilize touch, gesture, and language to overcome their inability to see. Seeing for both Nick and Marcos involved tracing the vessel's path in gestures and rehearsing the correct movement until both surgeons were satisfied that Marcos could slide the instrument under the liver without doing any damage. In the first instance, knowing meant being able to trace the vena cava's path with one's hand. In the second, knowing meant trusting one's body despite the evidence given by one's eyes.

From Foucault onward, writers about medicine often have discussed the medical "gaze," an amalgamation of sensory cues and an organization of medical spaces, logics, and apparatuses of knowing that could tell physicians what they would see if they could open the patient up at autopsy (Foucault 1973). The concept captures the historical shift in the late eighteenth century from diagnosis based on taxonomical nosologies of disease toward diagnosis based on signs of disease as they are presented in human anatomical structures. Foucault's concept of the gaze (*le regard*) represents a broad sociohistorical construction of perception that is quite close to the sense in which I discuss learning to see and act in surgery. But the term too easily comes to represent the slippage from vision to thought common to European philosophical trends since Descartes and Locke (Rorty 1979). The physicians and many technology designers I encountered while doing field-work tended to sublimate bodily knowledge under the visual and cognitivist label of "mental model." But, although these surgeons might have an abstract understanding of the three-dimensional structures of venous anatomy, a too-rapid shift into visual or cognitive language elides other aspects of embodied knowing, such as touch and gesture, which occurred during two critical moments of this surgery. The rehearsal of the necessary movement by the surgeons and their performance of it for each other are more significant aspects of surgical knowing in the first instance. Touch clearly dominates in the second. Practiced physical skill and gestural communication are important aspects of surgical embodiment for the successful completion of this surgery.

Crafting Operative Sight

Removal of a Klatskin's tumor is an open surgery, so surgeons accessed the tumor through a large incision in the patient's abdomen. The remaining surgeries I examine all were done using minimally invasive surgical techniques. Minimally invasive surgery also is known as keyhole surgery, minimal access surgery, and, depending on surgical specialty, arthroscopy, laparoscopy, or endoscopy. All minimally invasive techniques involve threading a camera into a natural or artificial hole in the patient's body and performing the work while watching instruments on a monitor. The dozens of techniques surgeons use today began to develop in the 1970s. To perform these techniques, the surgeon inserts a camera and instruments into "ports" or holes in the patient's body. The surgeon operates while looking at a monitor located somewhere nearby. Unlike traditional open surgeries, the technology distances the surgeon's eyes and hands from the operative site. Putting the action on a monitor is the first, critical move toward surgical simulation, robotic surgery, and other kinds of remote surgical work (Satava 1997, 19).

The perceptual skills required to work in minimally invasive space differ significantly from those of open surgeries, leading to a new form of virtual embodiment that emerges from a new configuration of bodies and technologies during these surgeries. Surgeons have no direct manual contact with the insides of the patient's body. They cannot use their hands as probes, as Nick did when feeling the patient's vena cava. And they have a less direct kinesthetic "feel" for the body as transmitted through the instrument. Further, they must continually extrapolate from a two-dimensional image to an interaction of bodies and instruments in three dimensions, sometimes "constructing" a three-dimensional space by orally identifying anatomical structures as they appear on the screen. The early years of practicing with these technologies reveal the difficulties surgeons had learning and mastering them: gallbladder removals that now take forty minutes to an hour took longer than open gallbladder removal in the early 1990s, and after some cases involving severe complications made the minimally invasive procedure controversial (Zetka 2003, 28). However, patients who have undergone such a procedure typically require just a few days of recovery time, as opposed to weeks in a hospital, benefiting patients, hospitals, and insurance providers, whether public or private.[1]

I begin with a long narrative of a single surgery done by Dr. Tom Berg, an attending surgeon; Dr. Cory Nguyen, a surgical fellow; and Dr. Amal Nassif, a first-year resident. This surgery reveals in detail how sociotechnical action in the operating room crafts surgical perception. In teaching hospitals, where treatment and training occur together, crafting sight involves mutual articulation, that is, simultaneously crafting the operative site and helping juniors hone their craft. In this case, the patient had an esophageal hernia, a pathological widening of the abdominal tissues surrounding the opening where the esophagus passes from the chest into the abdomen. His stomach and other abdominal tissues had crept through the hernia into his chest, where they became stuck. The surgical team had to remove the abdominal material from the chest and narrow the opening connecting abdomen and chest.

Amal and Cory wheeled the patient into the operating room. The staff enlisted the patient's help to shift him onto the operating table and start anesthesia. After he lost consciousness, Cory worked with several nurses to position his body and tilt the table so his head would be higher than his toes. This encouraged the stomach to descend out of the chest with the help of gravity. Positioning patients on an operating table is itself a minor art form with important consequences: careful placement of limbs and bolstering with cushions can prevent nerve injuries caused by the improper position of an unconscious person. Positioning also can be used to improve access to some anatomical structures. In this sense, making the surgical body available to perception and action begins before a surgeon picks up an instrument.

The team separated the patient's nonsterile mouth from the rest of him with a drape and placed more drapes over his entire body, leaving his abdomen exposed. Draping "visually reduces" the body and brings the surgeon's focus to bear on the abdomen (Hirschauer 1991, 284). Cory and Amal sterilized the exposed skin with iodine, which made the yellow-brown abdomen look like something other than a man's belly. Scholars describe the process of reducing the body to signs as objectifying, separating the person from the operative site (Hirschauer 1991; Young 1997). These same ethnographers note that surgeons tend to describe their patients by the affected body part. I observed this in an emergency room, where there often is no time to get to know a patient's name. But more commonly, I have heard patients referred to by their surnames and, typically with "Mr." or "Ms." appended. Although physicians do refer to unconscious patients in the third person (the conscious person is absent), the surgeons I observed shifted comfortably between considering the person and considering the body of surgical intervention. Objectification occurs, but I have seen significant nuance in surgeons' treatment of conscious and unconscious patients on the operating table.

Before the surgeons could see the man's interior, they had to create a space for themselves. They inflated his abdomen with carbon dioxide, swelling the belly. Inflating the belly lifted and separated organs and tissues that normally remain collapsed, creating a space where light and instruments could reach. Neither positioning the patient nor inflating the abdomen made the injury visible, but both were conditions of possibility for seeing the injury.

Cory and Tom agreed upon locations where they would place small holes in the patient's abdomen, which would act as ports of entry for the camera and instruments. They used landmarks on the body itself to extrapolate the positions of internal organs, judging their entry points based on the best spots to visualize the hernia with the least potential for damaging the man's insides, correlating internal and external anatomy. Surgeons typically use standardized locations for ports, in part to give them a constant point of reference in the body. Surgeons working in the abdomen usually place the camera through the belly button and point it upward, creating a standard perspective on abdominal anatomy. Thus, from the first placement of ports, the surgeons constructed the abdomen as a familiar space, similar to other abdomens they had worked in.

Though surgeons know the usual anatomy of a region and use techniques such as port placement to standardize the space, they must guard against the assumption that they will find what they expect. Several academic surgeons I interviewed estimated that a third to half their surgeries contain anatomical anomalies, some of which are pathological. Some non-pathological anomalies, such as a heart lying in the right side of the chest, require surgeons to radically revise their usual steps or to improvise variations on standard procedures. The ability to shift between a canonical understanding of normal anatomy and the instantiated anatomy of the patient becomes profoundly important in these cases.

After placing the ports, Cory inserted a hollow tube called a trocar into the abdomen and threaded the camera through it and into the abdominal cavity. The abdomen's interior appeared on the screen. Its walls were stretched taut by carbon dioxide and looked pink and white with red marbling. Cory pointed the camera at the abdominal wall and, by poking the abdomen's exterior, reassured herself that she could insert the next two ports without damaging blood vessels or organs. Tom inserted a clever instrument that was straight when he slid it into the port. He then turned a screw to fold it into a triangle once it was inside the abdomen. Once folded, this instrument became a liver retractor. Tom handed Amal the retractor, which Amal held for the remainder of the operation. When he absentmindedly let the retractor slip, blocking the camera, Tom corrected him impatiently. Each step of the operation up to this point had contributed to making the abdomen into a three-dimensional space surgeons could work in. Though each step had a purpose related to opening the operative site, seeing and creating the space could not be disentangled.

Cory used the camera to find the hernia, which resembled a wadded-up bit of purple and white cloth stuffed through a hole in the smooth, curved wall at the top of the abdomen. Tom remarked that the "defect" appeared small. Cory gently tugged at the abdominal tissues to pull them away from the hole. She inserted a harmonic scalpel into the abdomen. The scalpel looked like a blunt pair of needle-nosed pliers under magnification. But wherever it clamped onto tissue, ultrasonic waves disrupted water molecules in the tissue, causing the tissues to smoke and then to part, as though cut by a very slow knife. Cory used it to separate diaphanous purple and white tissue where it adhered to the abdominal wall. She spent about twenty minutes detaching tissues and pulling them apart with a slow, monotonous rhythm.

"See where the stomach is?" Tom finally asked Cory. "That's your edge." The stomach looked like a solid line of whitish tissue encased in the diaphanous material Cory was detaching. The edge marked the dividing line between tissue to be cut and tissue that must not be cut. All Cory's work had been to separate tissues adhered to the abdominal wall and pull them far enough back into the abdomen that she could expose the stomach. Surgical perception in this moment entailed a complex process of placing a camera, separating tissues, tugging on them, and, finally, stating that the stomach had come into view. To borrow terms from the study of scientific images, separating adhered tissues to reveal the stomach "upgraded" the image, making difficult-to-discern distinctions among tissues much clearer (Lynch 1988, 161). Tom's statement that the stomach was the edge "defined" the scalpel's path by verbally sharpening the separation of abdominal wall, adhered tissue, and stomach that the fellow had created with the scalpel (161).

Though I have used the language of scientific visualization to describe the creation of the edge and Tom's acknowledgment of it, thinking of this work in representational terms captures only one aspect of the work. Tom used language and the patient's body itself to guide the actions of Cory's hands. Stefan Hirschauer writes that his informants described surgical dissection as "making anatomy" (1991, 301). This construction puts the emphasis on the visual practices of exposure that anatomical and surgical dissection share. But examining anatomical and surgical practices beyond their visual qualities reveals important differences. Anatomists dissect largely to create a representation of the body as it might appear in an atlas, that is, to make the anatomy visible. In contrast, a surgeon wants to see tissues, but making tissues visible is subordinate to doing the repair work of surgery while protecting tissues from unnecessary damage. Treating surgery as the creation of representations misses a basic point: although surgeons point out anatomical features to trainees, they make anatomy visible to treat it, not to see it. To forget this (and surgeons tell horror stories about colleagues who waste time doing extraneous dissection) puts the patient in unnecessary danger, taking the temporary objectification of the patient's body too far. An anatomist dissecting a cadaver can open a body's anatomy to visual inspection; a surgeon must intervene as little as necessary in order to effect treatment.

Cory continued detaching tissues. On the screen, she visibly plucked at the tissue with the scalpel.

"Not so much force," Tom told her. "Let the energy do the job." Cory did not need to tug. Tom instructed her to respect the harmonic scalpel's ability to part tissues cleanly. Used properly, the scalpel can provide a cleaner edge than other instruments. But Cory had to practice with the scalpel enough that holding it and not tugging would become a habit; she had to develop a feel for the instrument.

Finally, Tom's tone shifted. "The stomach is coming down. Much better," he said. "Ahhh, much better. We're winning. Slowly but surely; that's the way we have to be."

Tom told Cory to move her instruments to the left. She moved.

"Your left," he corrected. Left and right are problematic concepts in minimally invasive surgery. Anatomically, surgeons orient in relation to the patient's body, so left in reference to the patient signifies the patient's left side. With minimally invasive surgery, however, the incision acts as a fulcrum, so if the surgeon moves his or her hand to the left, the instrument tip will move to the right. This resembles rowing a boat: The rower places his or her hands forward and pulls back in order to pull the oar blade from back to front. But rowing is movement primarily in two directions, forward and backward, whereas minimally invasive surgery involves 360 degrees of movement around the fulcrum. Minimally invasive surgery alters the basic spatial orientation embodied in the concepts "left" and "right" because moving one's hands to the left moves the instrument tip to the right. Learning to sense and to act in minimally invasive space is, first, learning to orient oneself in a new space.

"It's a hard operation," Tom told Cory and Amal. "There's always a moment in the operation where you feel you start to turn a corner, but it's hard work." Turning the corner freed Tom to explain the operation to Amal. He told Cory she was doing a good job of continuing to separate tissues in small snips. He explained to Amal that bits of the peritoneum (abdominal tissue) were pushing up into the chest and attaching to tissues there.

Tom referred to something that had appeared on the screen that I could not discern, "That's the esophagus, that paler thing." Then he corrected himself. "No that's just fat. But the esophagus is going to be just deep to that," meaning that the esophagus lies behind the fat, deeper in the body. Adhered peritoneal tissue crossing the hernia blocked the view of the esophagus, making it difficult to see. Further, the camera and its light were inside the abdomen, peering through the hole into the unlighted chest, much as one might see a few feet into a cave while holding a flashlight at its entrance. Working at the upper end of the abdomen, across the diaphragm, and into the darkened chest cavity beyond made this operation difficult.

Tom knew where the esophagus was, but the body's beiges, reds, and grays briefly tripped him up. The patient's esophagus was where it ought to be, but fat obscured it. Surgeons become habituated to precision: distinguishing fat from muscle is part of the articulation work a surgeon does, verbally in this instance, but often with an instrument.

"Start at the base of the left crest," Tom instructed Cory. She started working on something in the lower right section of the image, which indicated that the left crest was the patient's left. "See that structure right there? I think that's your vagus nerve." I could not see the nerve: the tissue looked like undifferentiated reds and whites. I knew that the nerve was paler than the surrounding tissues, but this did not help. Unlike an anthropologist, a surgeon must know how to read the distinctions among these tissues because damage to the vagus or any other major nerve could be devastating.

"That's definitely esophagus, so we're going to work around it, and that will help us finish the rest of the dissection," Tom said. During these few minutes of cutting and tugging, the esophagus had gone from being difficult to differentiate from surrounding fat to a clearly delineated structure on the screen. Spatially defining the esophagus gave Cory an edge to work with as her dissection of the adhered tissues continued. Further, it gave the abdominal space a three-dimensional structure. Anatomically, the esophagus passes from the chest through the diaphragm. The hernia was a pathological expansion of this natural opening. The esophagus made the defect possible. Once exposed surgically, the esophagus gave structure to the tissues crumpled around it.

"That's your aorta posteriorly," Tom said. Cory asked whether one of the whitish structures that had become visible was the vagus nerve. "I don't think so," Tom replied. "The vagus is almost embedded in the wall of the aorta. . . . It's hard to explain because I don't have a free hand. I'm trying to explain with words." Tom had done this procedure and practiced upon this anatomy often enough that he knew where the vagus nerve ought to be. My anatomical atlas (Netter 1997) depicts the vagus as a series of white branching nerves, descending along the aorta and onto the esophagus, like a white vine climbing down a pair of red trunks. The living vagus on the computer monitor in the operating room lacked the clean boundaries and color contrast of the illustration. Again, the distinction between anatomical and surgical dissection is salient: anatomists remove fat and other tissue to clearly delineate nerves and their branches from other tissue. They may even inject vessels with dye to create more contrast. Anatomical illustrators tend to further exaggerate distinctions among tissues for pedagogical effect, often making a "cartoon," in the words of one anatomist. Surgeons, in contrast, need to know locations of these anatomical features, in this case to avoid them, as well as to identify them in living tissue, even if they are diseased, damaged, or displaced. But the fine dissection done for anatomical illustration usually is unnecessary in surgery and would be tremendously time-consuming and possibly dangerous to a living patient.

"I don't think we'll see the pleura," Tom said, referring to membranes that envelop the lungs. "I don't think we put a hole in it or you would see the lung. You don't always see the pleura so neatly." Tom had to teach Cory and Amal what they could expect to see and what might resist vision, guiding their expectations. By teaching Cory and Amal what to expect, Tom was teaching them the "competent deployment" of the practices of professional seeing (Goodwin 1994, 626).

Tom directed Cory to move the instrument to the left. "Let's see if we can expose the esophagus," he said. They lifted the esophagus and cleaned off the remaining attached tissue.

Tom handed the camera to Amal, instructing him to make sure not to rotate it. With his hands free, Tom threaded a piece of drainage tube into the abdomen and wrapped it around the esophagus so it could be gently retracted, revealing more attached tissue. "Now, look at a couple of things," he said. "One is esophageal length. The other is what other stuff is holding us up here. You've got to take all that stuff out." The ability to see the underside of the esophagus was contingent upon moving it aside. Anatomists reveal successively deeper layers of the body typically by removing the preceding layer entirely. For obvious reasons, this is impossible in surgery, and many surgical techniques help make pathologies available for action on living flesh without doing harm. Retracting the esophagus made perception and action possible.

Tom pointed to a structure that looked like a gray slug: "See the spleen up there? See the spleen?" The spleen may look very different in a living patient whose belly is full of carbon dioxide than in a preserved cadaver. And minimally invasive surgery provides an inside-out view of anatomy that differs from open surgery and cadaver dissection. This kind of in vivo anatomy lesson, which was common in minimally invasive teaching surgeries I observed, continually reinforces the knowledge of anatomy in living patients for all present.

More purply tissue came into view. "That's all posterior sac: that's got to go," Tom said. "You have to be really careful in excising the sac that you don't get any stomach. But you start slowly; see where you want to go." If we take this last, cautionary phrase in isolation, "But you start slowly; see where you want to go," we might take it as confirmation of the uncomplicated and linear nature of seeing then acting in this space. Cory had to see where she was working so she would not do any damage, but seeing where to go began with excising the posterior sac: seeing was impossible without action.

I have argued against the notion that surgeons construct a representation in the patient's flesh resembling an anatomical illustration. If there was a representation created at this moment in the surgery, it was Tom's oral mapping of the abdominal space as he pointed out anatomical structures of interest. This social act had at least two pedagogical purposes: identifying the spleen or the vagus nerve showed Amal, who had very little experience in the operating room, what the anatomy looked like when magnified by the laparoscopic camera. For Cory, however, Tom's mapping made the landscape she was working in larger than the point she was working on, encouraging her to broaden her horizon. Broadening the visual horizon at the operative site is an important operating skill. Experienced surgeons remain vigilant for anatomical variations and larger clinical problems the patient may have. Tom's mapping also helped make the two-dimensional image on the monitor into a three-dimensional space. Whenever he identified an anatomical feature, he typically described its location—anterior, deep, left, right—giving these features locations in three-dimensional space, rather than on a grid, using his embodied sense of the abdominal space to help Cory and Amal navigate.

Pink tissue came into view. Translucent tissue surrounded it.

Cory asked, "Is this the stomach?"

"Yes, right there." Tom grabbed a bit of tissue and tugged on it, telling Cory to cut through it. She double-checked his instruction. "Yep." Tom was much less tentative about grabbing and tugging than Cory, who was a fully qualified surgeon but had many fewer years of experience. Pulling the tissue taut resembled guiding a resident's hands with a pointer as described in the previous chapter. Tom showed Cory the line she would follow to separate the attached tissue without damaging the stomach. By showing her the line without oral instructions, Tom allowed her to work seemingly autonomously while shaping the result.

Once Cory pulled the stomach out of the chest, and removed the excess tissue from around the stomach and esophagus, she had completed the most difficult parts of the operation. The team began the work of removing instruments from the patient's abdomen and closing the holes made in it.

Annemarie Mol urges theorists to examine practices that bring an object into being by acting upon it. "Instead of the observers' eyes, the practitioners' hands become the focus point of theorizing," she writes (2002, 152). Mol wants to move away from philosophical problems that make knowledge into a mental representation of some reality in the world. This binary has produced endless debates about the accuracy of the representation and the nature of the real. By describing practices—what practitioners do with hands—Mol shows how practices bring the objects of knowledge into being. Further, she explores the diversity of practices that give a single disease multiple ways of being. Reading this important methodological statement somewhat differently yields insights for surgical knowing. Several observers of anatomical dissection and surgical work have emphasized the visual qualities of these related medical disciplines, focusing either on the visual nature of anatomy teaching or on the construction of anatomical representations in the body undergoing surgery (Good 1994; Hirschauer 1991; Moreira 2004). These writers are themselves observers and they pick up on the aspect of the practitioner's embodiment that they themselves share: sight. What they find are the eyes of the observer who converts seeing into representations (Bourdieu 1977). Arguing for medicine's visuality is correct, but it is partial.

Continuing to the second part of Mol's phrase, focusing on the practitioner's hands promises to eliminate the observer's difficulty separating practice from representation. In the case of the esophageal hernia, focusing on practice allows analysts to rethink the surgery's purpose, which is neither to create an anatomical representation nor exclusively to allow the surgeon to see the patient's anatomy, but to repair the hernia and ease the patient's discomfort. Because this was a teaching surgery, repairing the hernia and teaching Cory how to repair hernias went together: Cory was developing her own embodied skills while she was developing the operative site. Here, Cory's sight was crafted from her own surgical skills joined with a large number of interactions in the operating room, from actions whose purpose appeared to have nothing to do with seeing, such as anesthetizing the patient and filling the abdomen with carbon dioxide, to actions intended to help her see and act, such as pulling tissues taut. Tom, the senior surgeon, also lent his embodied skills and Amal's labor to further the work of perception and action. Thus, focusing on the practitioners' hands shifts attention to the broad purpose of surgical action and to ways surgical action affects practitioners' embodiment and patients' bodies.

Inhabiting Minimally Invasive Space

In the first ethnographic section of this chapter, hands, gestures, and language played a critical role during two phases of a difficult surgery. In the second section, a surgery fellow's ability to perceive and to act was crafted from embodied experiences and sociotechnical interventions in the patient's body. In this section, the perceptual skills needed to work in minimally invasive space differ from those required during open surgery, leading to a new form of virtual embodiment that emerges from the relationships of hands and eyes in surgery.

The experiences of Amal, the surgical resident who held the liver retractor during the esophageal hernia repair, reveal the differences in embodied skills of beginners, competent practitioners, and experts. Amal was just beginning his second month of residency. He had spent a few hours practicing with simulators, which gave him a basic feel for the instruments involved. While the team scrubbed for a second operation, a gallbladder removal, Tom asked Amal if he would like to hold the camera. He eagerly said yes. Once the team had anesthetized and prepped the patient, Cory incised ports in the patient's abdomen. She inserted the camera and handed it to Amal, saying, "You keep the buttons up." The camera is a rigid stalk with a lens on one end that is inserted into the patient's body. At the other end is an easily gripped handle that allows surgeons to zoom in. The camera attaches to a large video monitor and recording deck. Because laparoscopic cameras often are angled, holding the buttons up provides important orienting information to surgeons, though it was unclear whether Amal understood this. Thus, Cory oriented the camera relative to the technology, not relative to the patient's body.

Cory told Amal how to direct the camera so she could see the abdomen from the inside and place several more ports. The "inside" view helped her ensure that she would not place a hole too close to a blood vessel or organ. She began to dissect the gallbladder's connective tissues. She told Amal several times to rotate the camera or pull it back to keep steam and material loosened by the harmonic scalpel from clogging the lens. After half an hour of silently following directions, Amal said, "So 'up' is looking down?" "Yes," Cory said. Tom added, "From the top down. That's what it means." Amal's phrase is revealing: "up" meant moving the camera's base upward, so the camera tip inside the patient's body pointed downward. Seeing down required a counterintuitive movement of hands and instrument. Amal was just becoming aware of how the fulcrum effect applied to the camera.

Cory's repeated urging to pull the camera back to avoid clogging the lens indicated that Amal was not yet aware that he was working in a three-dimensional space. Clearly, he did not know up from down, or close from far, or the most basic rudiments of how to navigate in the three-dimensional abdominal space depicted on the two-dimensional monitor. He had no feel for how the camera related to the inside of the patient's body. As will become clear from the examples that follow, experienced surgeons do more than look at the image on a monitor. They treat these bodyscapes as the three-dimensional spaces they work in, rather than as pictures they look at.

"Operating on Images"

Dr. Harry Beauregard, the gynecologist, started working with minimally invasive technology late in his career. He began doing laparoscopic abdominal surgeries while looking through a microscopic eyepiece, an earlier generation of minimally invasive visualization. He found the transition to the monitor alienating. During an interview, Harry said,

> It was the focus change from the patient to the monitor. That's where the action was, and it was something I had to take into account. I mean I had to go there to do the work that the camera illustrated, allowed me to visualize. And so I would go there to work on the monitor. And so I was leaving the patient and looking up to a monitor where there I could do stuff. And with the tools of the minimal access, if I looked at the patient, I

couldn't do anything. You see how absolute it was? And I could look at the handles, but couldn't see on the inside. It was totally useless. I had to go to the monitor to operate. And that's why I started saying I was operating on images, not on patients.

Harry described the operative site as though it moved to the monitor, which, in terms of vision and action, it did. The position of his hands did not change much from the microscopic system. But he talked as though his entire body moved with his eyes. He experienced himself as no longer working on patients, but on images. Vision and action came together on the screen. His hands were outside the patient and the operative site was hidden inside. To see what he was doing, Harry had to look at the monitor.

To better understand the relationship between surgeons and remote technology, I asked Dr. Anna Wilson, the hand surgeon, to watch videotapes of a shoulder arthroscopy she had performed months earlier and to explain to me what she was doing. Unlike Harry, Anna had performed minimally invasive surgeries since residency. The tapes depicted the scope's view, the view from inside the patient's body. The patient had torn his biceps tendon years before. The destabilizing effect of the tear made his shoulder joint move improperly, wearing down protective cartilage and encouraging arthritic bone growth. The scope magnified the operative site by twenty-five or thirty times, and the scope had a wide-angle lens and an angled shaft that allowed Anna to cover more ground as she rotated the camera. Unlike the view of the abdomen through the scope, the view of the joint's interior was entirely unlike any anatomical view I have seen: the body looked incredibly abstract, like looking through a porthole at a red and white undersea floor with white tendrils undulating in the current. The view made me mildly seasick.

As the camera advanced into the shoulder, Anna said, "This is somebody with a terrible shoulder, a terrible shoulder." She described how she was running fluid through the joint, hence the sea-floor effect.

ANNA: That's the outflow. It's also the cannula for instrumentation in the front. This is not a good first one for you to look at. This is his humeral head and there's just a lot of arthritis, a lot of fibrillation.

RP: So arthritis, it's not like a neat bone growth, it's this messy crap?

ANNA: It's messy crap. It's just bare, bare bone. So I'm coming from behind him and the glenoid is on our left and the big ball is on our right.

So the camera is with me. It's kind of my view from chest level. So here I'm probing. I'm proving that he's got an arthritic shoulder. This is the remnant of his biceps tendon. This will definitely make you dizzy.

RP: You feel that, or you see that?

ANNA: I put through the cannula in front. I take the probe. That's my finger extender.

As this dialogue indicates, Anna had several ways of opening the operative site. The first was navigational. As the video advanced, she named anatomical structures, such as the ball of the humerus and the glenoid, or shoulder socket, as they came into view. One reason to share what she sees while operating, Anna said, is to establish common ground with the surgical team. Verbal navigation can be particularly important with minimally invasive surgery because the two-dimensional view can be deceptive and requires skill to read. Navigating a patient's anatomy this way was not something Anna did only while watching a video with an anthropologist. She also did this in the operating room with residents and fellows. Every surgeon I have watched does this with minimally invasive procedures. But I have never seen surgeons do as much narration during an open surgery.

The second method of establishing the operative site was through probing. Anna said the probe extended her finger. I often heard her tell medical students that instruments are extensions of her body. She sometimes struggled to describe in words exactly how she typically holds an instrument because, for her, the instrument becomes part of her body. Anna did not think about the probe. Rather, she used it as an extension of her finger that was directed toward the arthritis. Probing the arthritis was the important action, not holding the probe. Merleau-Ponty uses the example of a blind man's cane to show how we use instruments to extend our senses—that is, our bodies and ourselves—toward objects in the world (2002, 165).[2] He argues that the cane extends the blind man's consciousness into space. What remains unstated is that, like a surgeon, the blind man, too, needs years of practice to navigate in his world. Further, tapping does not resemble navigating by sight or by unmediated touch. Both cane and probe have structuring effects on their respective users' embodiment.

Anna said something that suggests the broader embodiment at work. She said the image was her view "from chest level." This was an odd statement. We do not have eyes in our chests and, thus, have no view from chest level. But Anna located her body in relation to the patient's body. "The camera is with me," she said. She was standing behind the patient's right shoulder. Shoulder and scope were level with her chest. The technology gave a view from chest level. Just as the probe became her finger extender, the scope became her eye extender. Anna extended this technological eye from her body's position in space to the patient's body. Action began with her body and extended from there. It became a view from chest level. This was clearly not yet the case for Amal, the new resident. He could not quite connect what he saw with his eyes with what he did with the hands holding the camera. I tried to get more detail about what Anna was doing: "So then you feel the arthritis, or you see it?" I asked. "Yeah, both," Anna replied. "It's very much a proprioceptive thing."

Anna proved that the man had an arthritic shoulder by sight and by feel. She verified the arthritis by probing the tissue's hardness. She said her identification of the arthritis was proprioceptive. Proprioception is our sense of our body in space, the sense that allows most of us to know, for example, where our left foot is without looking at it. Anna's statement that the visual and tactile confirmation of arthritis was proprioceptive appears to conflate vision with proprioception and, in a strict, objective definition, would be an incorrect use of the word. But I believe something subtler was at work. Anna oriented her body and instruments so she could best see and operate on the patient's body. The connection between sight and action was so tight that proprioception and vision merged. Anna saw and probed the arthritis through her body. She extended herself—her senses and her being—to the operative site to make the diagnosis.

On the video screen, another right shoulder appeared. Anna used a probe to gently flick a small knob of flesh on the shoulder. She described this as "physical doodling." In other words, she was thinking about what she could do with this injury.

> Actually what I'm doing also is, I'm externally rotating the shoulder to see the tension of the muscle [she points]. That's the middle glenohumeral ligament. You can see the glenoid here. And you can see the humeral head over here. This is also a right shoulder. There's a lot of fibrillation coming down and actually this is probably going to be some of the rotator cuff falling in our face. The fibrillation is that gunky stuff. This is the rotator cuff tear.

Anna located us in relation to the anatomy and diagnosed the injury. She identified messy white tissue descending into the image frame as the rotator cuff tear. She described the tissue as "falling in our face." This odd grammatical construction suggests several aspects of the embodiment at work. Tissue waving against the camera lens showed up on the monitor as tissue blocking our view. Anna, who sat next to me in a computer lab, placed our faces at the meeting place of tissue with camera, oddly merging both of our faces with the technological interface. This suggests that the apparatus of camera and monitor structured her perception: the monitor has just one "face," the camera lens inside the joint. Multiple people can peer through it, however, so it became "our face." In other words, Anna located our faces at the interface of the camera with the interior of the patient's shoulder joint. I have heard Anna make statements like this several times, but only while doing arthroscopy, never while doing open surgery. Unlike Harry, the gynecologist, Anna did not experience this as alienating. She tells her residents that she becomes part of a joint when she does arthroscopy, using an analogy to Heisenberg's Uncertainty Principle to argue that her very presence in the joint causes significant changes. Instead of separating the operative site from the patient, Anna's body merged with the scope as it moved around inside the patient's body. The apparatus became part of her body. It also exerted its own agency in shaping her perception by allowing more than one person to be located in the space created by camera and monitor. Anna located our faces inside the patient's body and on the same scale as the magnified view of the shoulder's interior. As with her view from chest level, Anna located herself where the technology was. Eyes and instruments merged at the operative site.[3]

Anna's experience of inhabiting the patient's body while doing minimally invasive surgery echoed that of other surgeons. I discussed a similar relationship with Dr. Ramesh Chanda, another hand surgeon, who also trained using both open and minimally invasive techniques. What he said is worth quoting at length:

> You have an image on the monitor. You have this thing in front of you, which is the actual patient, the patient's joint or whatever. In addition to this, there is also a third image, and that's the image, which is in your head. And it's a combination of the two, the patient's image that you see and the stuff you see on the monitor, but also takes into consideration some cog-

nitive aspects, some other issues, the haptic feedback you are getting from your hands. It's a mental model or image or whatever and what I have felt as I have gone through my training is that I have tended to use that third image more and more, which in some ways draws upon what I am seeing on the screen, draws upon what I am faced with in front of me and am touching and holding and manipulating. So I am almost like, I almost imagine myself, almost routinely if I am doing an arthroscopy, sitting inside the joint. And I say, oh, OK, I am looking up and I see the scaphoid or whatever, if I am in the wrist joint, for example. And of course the images on the screen are very important [for] guiding, in fact probably the most important. You certainly cannot do without that. But there are other pieces of information and that, in the end, becomes a guide.

Ramesh says he creates a composite bodily understanding of the patient's joint that unites the on-screen visual and the kinesthetic and tactile information coming from instruments and a patient's body with his surgical experience and anatomical knowledge. Anna and Ramesh both stumbled a bit verbally when trying to describe what they experience. Anna said, "It's kind of my view from chest level." Ramesh said, "It's a mental model or image or whatever." Both surgeons are unusually articulate people, and these moments of imprecision reveal how perplexing some of these perceptual relations are. The two surgeons wrestled to describe experiences they have with their bodies. Was Harry's "mental model" necessarily an image in his mind, or did it reside elsewhere in his body? Where was Anna's sight really located? Could it be located at chest level? Anna's body merged with the scope; Ramesh dispensed with the technology and its limitations altogether. He inhabited the patient's body when he operated. He said he did not have this experience when doing open surgery.

I encouraged Ramesh to say more:

RP: It resonates very strongly with something [Anna] said, which is that when she is operating on the shoulder, she is part of the shoulder.

RAMESH: Yes, that's exactly how I feel.

RP: If you're thinking of yourself as inside the joint, do you actually position yourself, like my eyes are sitting on this piece of anatomy looking at whatever?

RAMESH: Yeah, and actually I would say I am sitting on that piece of anatomy, or rather that you are floating around, swimming around in the synovial fluid, so you can move around, look up, look down, look right, left. And actually the other thing is that you can also, in that mental model, come out of the joint. You can go in and out very easily, so you can visualize it from the outside. You can visualize it from the inside.

Ramesh located his whole body inside the patient's body. One could think of this as the disembodied gaze promised by writers about virtual reality (Balsamo 1996; Gibson 1986). But examining what Ramesh does while swimming in the joint suggests that this formulation is misleading. He looks at a monitor and, often, rotates the joint from the outside while using a probe to examine the internal effects of rotating. He said he experiences himself as sitting or floating inside the joint. Further, he draws upon a history of anatomical and surgical interventions into joints. Ramesh's actions condition his ability to be in synovial space. He described this as a synthesis of the view on the monitor with other sensory information, especially kinesthetic information. The perceptual synthesis that Ramesh described also gave him imaginary abilities that are technologically unavailable, such as the ability to move out of and back into the joint at unusual angles. Intriguingly, the mental tools he gave himself are exactly the kinds of technologies that he and other simulation and medical imaging experts wanted to develop. These technologies would allow a physician to glide through the patient's body, across membranes and through tissues, as though through water. His imaginary navigation of the body was also an imaginary of technology.

Multiple sensations are in play during a surgery conducted using minimally invasive tools, including what the surgeon sees on the monitor, the tactile and kinesthetic sensations transmitted from the instruments to the surgeon's hands, and the surgeon's proprioceptive sense of his or her body in space. These sensations come together with the embodied skills a surgeon develops during years of practice, as well as with knowledge of human anatomy and surgical procedure. Harry, perhaps because he did not begin his training using minimally invasive technology, experienced the patient as split in two: the image on the monitor and the actual patient's body. He repeatedly stated that he had to leave the patient's body to work on images. Anna and Ramesh, in contrast, did not consider the monitor as such. The scale of their bodies was radically reduced, focused at the meeting place of scope and joint, swimming in the joint.

During a discussion over coffee, I asked the three surgeons together to speculate about the differences. Harry gave two possibilities. The first related to when during their careers—at the beginning or in the middle—they began working with a monitor. He started late in his professional life, whereas Anna and Ramesh started during residency. Thus, one difference related to training. Harry also suggested that this difference could relate to the size of joints versus abdomens. He said the abdomen is like a large room with darkened corners. It does not feel confined. Anna picked up his metaphor and began to play with it. "A shoulder is like a closet," she said. "Only it's like a California closet where everything should be neatly tucked away." Injuries make things spill out. The joint-as-closet analogy creates a strong sense of the joint's confined spaces and the disorder pathology creates. The patient's body itself contributes to these perceptual effects. Ramesh agreed with Harry and Anna and added that surgeons who work in the abdomen do not manipulate the body from the outside while viewing it from the inside. That is, they manipulate instruments, but do not rotate limbs to see what changes inside the way orthopedists do. This suggests that arthroscopy—minimally invasive surgery in joints—more tightly links the surgeon's body and the patient's body.

Much later, after he read an early draft of this chapter, Harry found another explanation for the differences. He said he is a man whose medical specialty involved treating women's bodies. The intimacy the orthopedists experienced would have felt inappropriate, he said. As a gynecologist, he spent his career with hands, instruments, and eyes in intimate contact with women's bodies. But somehow, inhabiting a woman's body would have felt transgressive, suggesting a difference between putting parts of his body into the patient and putting himself into the patient's body. This suggests that these perceptual relationships also are shaped by gender and cultural experiences. In other words, he tactically objectified his own body as it came into intimate contact with the patient's body.

Csordas (1990) argues that cultural experiences and habits shape perceptions, making a strong case for the historical and cultural forces at work in constructing what counts as an object. All surgeons become habituated to seeking pathological objects in patient bodies. But that does not mean that all surgeons' experiences of patient bodies are identical (see Sacks 2003). Technologies help shape a surgeon's work space. Also, cultural concerns about how one relates to patient bodies can habituate the surgeon to experience particular kinds of relations with patient bodies. Similarly, the amount of time a surgeon has practiced in minimally invasive space can shape these experiences, as can the constraints of working in particular anatomical regions.

Inhabiting Surgical Space

What do we make of these seemingly bizarre perceptual relationships? If Harry experienced his work site as the image, is the image "just" a representation? If Amal had to ask whether up is down, how would he learn to navigate in this space? If Anna experienced the interface of camera and body as an interface of her face and the patient's body, where was the technology? If Ramesh imagined himself swimming in the patient's joint and able to navigate into and out of the joint capsule, where did image end and patient body begin? Was this a complete departure from the bodily relations of open surgery?

To explain the changes in surgeons' location and scale that take place during minimally invasive surgeries, I consider the development of surgical embodiment as entailing a broad perceptual synthesis crafted from years of surgical interactions with patient bodies in the operating room. As Harry said, surgical seeing and acting are inextricable. Csordas's (1990) synthesis of Merleau-Ponty and Bourdieu can help explain sensory experiences as they are distributed by remote technologies. Csordas argues that embodiment is the existential ground of culture. He uses Merleau-Ponty's term "pre-objective" to show how cultural formation can shape perceptions before those perceptions coalesce into objects. By this logic, surgeons' perceptions—their eyes, in Haraway's shorthand—are crafted within a surgical environment (1990, 192). Our culturally informed bodies shape perceptions before they turn into ideas, concepts, representations, and other abstract objects.

The first lessons in the operating room—including scrubbing, maintaining sterility, and obeying staff—defamiliarize trainees with their own bodies, encouraging them to build a surgical stance toward patients and fellow practitioners. Repeated practice of the small actions of surgery, such as retracting and stitching, aggregate and condense to become bodily habits. Years of cultivation of surgical habits leads to surgical skill, a term surgeons use unflatteringly when qualified as technical proficiency alone, but which becomes high praise when incorporated with judgment and knowledge. According to

Merleau-Ponty, "habit" is a "rearrangement and renewal of the body image" through which the body becomes "mediator of a world" (2002, 164). "Skill" connotes the effects of intentional training in ways "habit" does not and can be defined as purposeful habituation that leads to change in body image. Building from this "craft" becomes "skill, presence of mind and habit combined" (Mauss 2007, 58). The skilled body thus becomes the body habituated to particular kinds of intentional action through practice.

The accumulation of craft practices makes the body into a temporal joint that articulates past practices and present conditions. "Our body comprises as it were two distinct layers, the habit-body and that of the body at this moment" (Merleau-Ponty 2002, 95). Thus, the habit-body develops a generalizable capacity, the ability to do something or, more abstractly, the notion that one can do something (see also Dreyfus 1992). Drawing on the experience of amputees, Merleau-Ponty illustrates this with the example of a phantom limb, which joins a body habituated to having a limb to a present marked by loss. In contrast, the habit-body that develops through practice in surgery becomes joined to a present in which variations in the milieu, such as new tools, unusual anatomy or pathology, or changes in team composition, generate improvisations that draw upon the general abilities of the surgeon's habit-body. The crafting of the surgeon's body also has a moral component: skill, judgment, and accumulated procedural techniques all qualify the surgeon to undertake this high-stakes activity.

Merleau-Ponty's habit-body corresponds roughly to Bourdieu's description of how bodily habits can reflect and create culturally conditioned dispositions to act in particular ways (see Csordas 1990, 1995). But Bourdieu's (1977) *habitus* is a more recognizably social concept: dispositions develop through practice in situations in which symbolic, spatial, and social structures instill particular ways of perceiving and acting. Bourdieu does not address how the dispositions of the habitus adapt and change as worlds evolve. Saba Mahmood (2005) makes a stronger case for practice as the embodying force, arguing that practices instill dispositions to act and believe in particular ways. Treating the body as joining condensed social and physical practice with improvised action in the present allows us to consider continuity and change in embodiment. Changes in surgeons' institutional and technical worlds that become absorbed into the larger stream of surgical practice may impact their craft profoundly as they become incorporated into surgeons' embodied repertoires of skills.

Surgeons cultivate specific habits of perception and thought during years of training. Obviously, surgeons' visual and tactile perceptions are highly trained. They must learn to identify anatomy in indistinct flesh. They must also distinguish normal from pathological tissues. And, unlike anatomists, they must learn to repair the patient's body while doing as little extraneous damage as possible. While surgeons learn their craft, the symbolic, spatial, and social structures of the operating room instill particular ways of perceiving and practicing upon the patient's body. New residents mince around the operating room and shrink away from the patient's body, afraid to touch anything. Residents rapidly gain confidence, but even fellows, who are fully qualified surgeons, have much to learn from more experienced surgeons. The differences in confidence, economy of motion, and skill among surgeons with different levels of experience became very obvious to me after a observing just a few surgeries. When Amal first held the camera, he had no idea what to do with his body in the operating room or in relation to the patient. Cory, despite years of surgical training during residency, was uncertain about whether she was seeing the vagus nerve. After twenty years of practice, Tom could rapidly and confidently grasp a bit of tissue in the abdomen without fear that he would grab hold of the stomach. Further, Tom guided and structured Amal's and Cory's experiences so they would learn surgery without harming the patient. In durably embodied ways, trainees learn to do surgery and to be surgeons.

Surgeons learn the body even as they create the body they want to learn. That is, a surgeon learns by repeatedly exposing a patient's anatomy to sight and action. The practitioner's body and the patient's body mutually articulate each other. When blood, tissue, anatomy, or technological failure disrupt sight, the surgeon uses other senses. When technology distributes the patient's body, the equally distributed surgeon's body reunites it through the circuit of his or her own body. These surgeons demonstrate this. Nick showed how hands can be tools for seeing. The entire operating-room staff performed embodied actions that allowed Cory to see. Harry's hands followed his eyes to the monitor. Anna talked about arthritis falling in our collective face. And Ramesh described himself swimming in the joint. These surgeons' entire bodies were focused on the operative site, where seeing and acting come together.

So why do these surgeons describe such strange changes of location and scale of their bodies when doing minimally invasive surgery? The body's sense of space is brought into being through action. This is not a spatiality of position; it is a "spatiality of situation" (Merleau-Ponty 2002, 115). When spatial perception is radically altered by technology, such as an apparatus that distorts vision, making a hugely magnified world appear at a 45-degree angle, the body creates a perceptually altered "virtual body" that "ousts the real one to such an extent that the subject no longer has the feeling of being in the world where he actually is . . . he inhabits the spectacle" (Merleau-Ponty 2002, 291). The virtual body allows the subject to undertake any necessary task. The situation of surgery is to see and to act at the operative site. From an external, objective point of view, the surgeons' perceptions of themselves operating on images, or waving arthritic tissues out of their faces, or swimming inside the joint appear bizarre. And the surgeons themselves, if asked about the actual positions of their bodies in the operating room, would not describe their locations this way. Instead, they would objectify their actions, describing themselves as an observer would.

These statements become clearer if we imagine surgical embodiment as developing from lengthy residence in a surgical culture dedicated to the art of seeing to intervene and intervening to see. The distributed bodies, instruments, sensations, and knowledges all focus on a single event: opening the operative site so the surgeon can work there. The surgeon's body unites sight, action, and technology. Cory had the benefit of extraordinary technological and expert interventions to help her craft the operative site while she crafted her own sight. Harry located himself at the monitor so he could see enough to work. But he experienced his attention as divided between patient and monitor. Anna and Ramesh took a more radical step. They located their bodies in the one place where a person could see and operate without being divided: at the actual operative site, inside the joint.

six

ENTERPRISING BODIES IN THE LABORATORY

There always seems to be more to reality than you
can fit on your computer.
RHEINGOLD 1992, 35

Several actors prominent in the field of virtual reality in medicine described
the field's "Holy Grail" to me. They envisioned an assemblage of graphic,
virtual, and haptic technologies that would allow them to create an interactive, three-dimensional model of a patient's image data that could be incorporated into a simulator. Surgeons could use the simulator to practice a
procedure on a patient's unique anatomy as many times as necessary to
perfect each step. Designers have modeled this type of virtual medical practice, known as "surgical rehearsal," on the military concept of "mission
rehearsal" (Satava 2008, 142). But the vision goes further. A computer would
record each surgical step during the rehearsal. Once perfected, the surgeon
could turn the operation and the recorded actions over to a robot to perform the surgery on the actual patient. The simulator-robot would allow
the surgeon to practice to perfection and to utilize the robot's precise,
unflagging movements to minimize human errors. Though no total system
such as this one exists, this imagined technology reveals how industrial,
military, and medical ideals merge in a transformational vision for future
medical practice.

   This chapter explores the technologization of bodies and practices for
training and profit that is taking place in medical technology design. Many
aspects of medical practice, such as the feel of an ovary or the sense of
the body's three-dimensional structures, are naturalized as embodied technique and appear inaccessible to modeling. Yet multidisciplinary research-

ers working on technology development for medical education want to open even those areas of clinical work that appear most inextricably bound up in practitioners' bodies. Their work entails the disaggregation of the complex relations of patient bodies, practitioner bodies, and instruments as part of the construction of objects and algorithms that articulate the relations of practitioners, medical instruments, and patient bodies in new ways. The process of disassembling embodied practices and recombining them in digital technologies begins from a move seemingly so basic that its significance is easily overlooked: practices that physicians cultivate through years of clinical work become parsed into discrete "skills," which technology designers identify, describe mathematically, and make into digital objects that can be developed into stand-alone technologies or embedded in more complex digital tools (see Strathern 2000, 9). Put another way, clinical relations of bodies to one another, to tools, and to medical knowledges are rapidly becoming fragmented and reconstructed in technological forms. Once extracted from bodies, these objects become available for new kinds of research and for capitalization.

This process of extraction and construction of objects fits what Marilyn Strathern has called the "enterprising up" of natural phenomena (1992, 35). The term originates with the concept of "enterprise culture," the growing trend toward promotion of entrepreneurial values dedicated to capitalization of new or underdeveloped areas of the market (Gray 2007). In some accounts, "enterprising up" also deliberately invokes the transporters used in the television series *Star Trek* to technologically disassemble bodies and reassemble them in new locations (Haraway 1997).[1] Both meanings of the term come into play with the development of teaching technologies for medical education: these technologies do indeed reconstitute bodies and practices in new sociotechnical matrices, making these bodies—or fragments of bodies, knowledges, and practices—available for training, research, and business ventures well beyond their original context. The methods of technologization that I discuss here originate with forms of rationalization native to military training and industrial production. Such solutions hold promise to make medical training and practice more standardized and consistent. But researchers and promoters often fail to recognize that many medical realities, such as a physician's emotional relationship to a patient, may not "fit" neatly on a computer.

This chapter places the future imaginary of virtual reality in medicine against the engineering realities of a multidisciplinary space of a medical school laboratory that builds teaching technologies. I show how professionals versed in the rationalizing logics common among engineers, computer scientists, and educators work with physicians to reconfigure the bodily relations of medical teaching. A long-standing imaginary of medical practice inspired by military and industrial concepts of efficiency and rationality drives this work. This imaginary is leading to the development of digital, anatomical "body objects" designed to be embedded in computers. Further, these technologies promise to shift practitioner embodiment as new practices coalesce around new technologies. I argue that the emphasis these technologies place on technical achievements shifts the focus of medical education toward the perfection of technique (i.e., toward care of the self as the most significant technique of caring for others).

Imagining Virtual Reality and Medicine

The surgical simulator-robot described above has a strong allegiance to military concepts of practice and control that stem in part from the technology's roots in military research, particularly training technologies for pilots and other high-tech military personnel. Virtual reality is a set of visualization, computation, and sensory-enhancement technologies intended to immerse the user in a complex, multisensory world that can simulate anything from the bottom of the ocean floor to the inside of a protein molecule. Virtual-reality research emerged in the 1960s as designers of military display technologies began working on graphics, modeling, and, later, networking elements of immersive environments. The field began with large infusions of military research money, particularly from the Advanced Research Projects Agency (which later became DARPA), which provided funding for long-range research that industry interests found too speculative for commercial development. Ivan Sutherland, the first researcher to articulate a vision for virtual reality, worked in several academic laboratories, training a cadre of researchers who moved fluidly among military, academic, and entertainment research, creating what Timothy Lenoir (2000), a historian of science, has called the "military-entertainment complex."

Early virtual-reality designers envisioned medicine as a logical area in which to apply their research, but hardware and software development for medicine got started in earnest in the late 1970s as researchers adapted medical imaging to computational technologies and techniques developed in military, scientific (mostly biological), and digital entertainment fields (Rheingold 1992). This nexus of research interests continues to affect medical virtual reality in the United States. Federal medical and military sources, including the National Library of Medicine, the Defense Advanced Research Projects Agency, and the Army's Telemedicine and Advanced Technology Research Center, fund much of the research. Companies engaged in military contracting, including Lockheed Martin Corporation, and in game development, including Immersion Corporation, have built medical simulators and simulator components (Satava 2008, 144). Computer experts who began their careers in videogame design have brought programming techniques, including methods for graphic modeling, memory optimization, and collision detection, into medical simulation design. Designers of virtual-reality tools in medicine explicitly credit flight simulation for pilot training as their inspiration for virtual hardware systems and for training and practice technologies, such as checklists, that externalize and make systematic safety checks and procedural steps (Gaba 2000, 2004; Kohn et al. 2000; Satava 2008).[2] This branch of research into medical training technologies thus draws on virtual military training and flight simulation (for commercial and military pilot training) for technological inspiration and for logics of training and practice (Fletcher 2009).

Dr. Richard Satava worked as an Army surgeon for almost two decades before moving to DARPA in the early 1990s, where he helped jump-start the field by channeling funds into research projects.[3] He has published and presented his futuristic technological visions at conferences, such as Medicine Meets Virtual Reality and the American Telemedicine Association, which are important for researchers developing virtual reality, telemedicine, and simulation technologies for civilian and military medical applications. I focus my discussion of the future imaginary of the field on Satava's writing because, as a visionary and funder in the field, Satava has positioned himself to shape how this future vision gets converted into actual projects.

Satava has argued that electronic mediation will lead to a "total revolution of medicine" built around a cluster of technologies for constructing three-dimensional images of the patient, processing and making them manipulable, and disseminating them over computer networks (1997). Although Satava's vision centers on new technology development, he also has described nothing less than a major overhaul of surgical training and practice, building on a vision for medical education that draws as heavily on ideas from military and industrial sources as it does from medical traditions (Kohn et al. 2000; Satava 2008). The training methods Satava argues for are essentially disciplinary, teaching the physical actions of surgery (see Foucault 1977). But Satava and others expect such training to slot into more encompassing medical training regimes, which entail a larger vision of training that works at the service of medicine's most complex clinical and moral dramas.

In a 1995 paper, Satava offered a vision for how virtual technologies would augment practitioners' abilities. He argued that the tools developed using combined imaging, data crunching, robotics, and networking technologies would lead to surgical robots that physicians could operate remotely, possibly also by using augmented reality technologies that would allow them to lay images over the patient's actual body:

> In taking this approach, we are able to "dissolve time and space," the physician can "be" at a distant place at the same time as another person without needing to travel there. But of utmost importance is the fact that the physician can simultaneously bring in many different digital images, such as the patient's CT or MRI scan, and fuse them with real time video images, giving the surgeon "x-ray vision." (334)

Satava wanted to decouple the physical connection between doctor and patient through the use of virtual tools that allow physicians to work over networks in remote or dangerous areas, such as rural communities, battlefields, and outer space. The telemedicine system for remote interaction would be coupled with augmented virtual reality.

These visualization, modeling, and virtual-reality technologies would enable the surgeon to "enhance his skills beyond the frail limitations of the human body" (Satava 2008, 20). Satava's idealized image of the future surgeon resembles a superhero who can defeat time and space and whose X-ray vision allows him to peer through walls (see also Rheingold 1992, 26). This surgeon-as-superhero metaphor should not be underestimated: The kinds of technologies Satava envisions clearly would augment surgeons' control over their practices and the individual bodies they treat. Surgical control has been a powerful motivation for the design and implementation of operating rooms, overhead lighting, and surgical instruments (Adams and Schlich 2006; Schlich 2007). As I discussed in chapter 4, control also is the focus of surgical training, including the development of techniques of the body intended to steady hands and avoid errors. Satava's vision of the mediated surgeon goes much further, however, as he envisions a technologically enhanced practitioner, able to defeat time, space, and the body's opacity (its resistance to vision) through the wonders of technology.

One foundation for the simulator-robot technology described above could be a form of digital patient record that Satava calls a "Holomer," which stands for "holographic medical electronic representation" (Prentice 2002; Satava 2006). The Holomer would be an electronic medical record, resembling systems that many health-care policy specialists have argued are needed to make U.S. health care more efficient and cost-effective. The Holomer would contain much more imaging data and functionality. The Holomer would collect a patient's medical record and several kinds of body scans, including three-dimensional models. Physicians could use the stored images and medical records as baseline studies. Or if the patient needed surgery, the surgeon could practice the procedure on a model made from the patient's Holomer data.

In a 2002 presentation at the Medicine Meets Virtual Reality conference, Satava suggested that patients could donate or sell their Holomer data for pharmaceutical and other kinds of research.[4] Like the simulator robot, the Holomer reveals one of the future narratives that these researchers engage in: the promise of individualized medicine.[5] When critics argue that existing tools for practice, such as simulators based on cadavers, do not reveal the extent of human variation, these researchers counter that future technologies will use individual patient data drawn from such technologies as the Holomer. The Holomer clearly could become a form of "enterprised" patient, a data representation of a patient's body that easily could be transported, aggregated with other patients' data, and made available for research and capitalization.

Satava's research agenda takes inspiration from industrial and military models of training and efficiency. Industry and science (particularly laboratory science) have provided technical and organizational models for surgical training, operating-room organization, and hospital management since reforms of medical education and hospital practice took place during the first two decades of the twentieth century. At that time, efforts focused on making medical practice more scientific, including standardizing education and hospital organization and creating records systems that allow physicians to aggregate patient information (Howell 1995; Stevens 1999). Early twentieth-century rationalization efforts in medicine followed F. W. Taylor's push for "scientific management" (Stevens 1999, 55). But most reform efforts were designed to gain physician acceptance by avoiding measures that might threaten their autonomy in practice and decision making (Samuel et al. 2005, 251). Present-day reform efforts incorporate methods drawn from post–World War II research into technologically complex, tightly integrated systems, such as pilot training (Gaba 2000, 2004; Gawande 2009). They are specifically designed to standardize practice by guiding physicians' decision making.

In talks and papers, Satava has argued that surgical teaching and operating-room care are less effective than industrial methods of reducing errors and enhancing precision and cleanliness. For example, he advocates the adoption of robotic parts changers that would hand the surgeon instruments while simultaneously tracking inventory and managing billing. The parts changer would replace the operating-room scrub nurse. A supply dispenser would replace the circulating nurse and perform some accounting functions in real time that typically take place after the procedure is finished. Satava argues that the system would be faster and more accurate and would remove several vectors for infection (humans) from the operating room. His vision for technological changes clearly is inspired by industrial techniques that move products through factories and keep track of costs: "This is the epitome of efficiency," he wrote, "using robotics, just in time inventory, and supply chain management processes" (n.d.).

Satava argues that surgeons should adopt modeling and prototyping practices that are common among scientists and industrial designers, giving them the ability to model and simulate the effects of various actions. "Scientists and engineers all have a computer (or information) representation of their product (in healthcare the 'product' is the patient)," Satava wrote in a paper supporting research into surgical rehearsal technologies (2006, 3). The reliance on concepts from science and industry is clear, but the language of patient-as-product also is significant to the shifts Satava proposes in four ways. First, it is a reminder of the capitalization of biomedicine, particularly the focus on profits generated in part by cost measures and patient "throughput" (Ludmerer 1999, 350; see also Stevens 1999). Second, it explicitly links medical labor to industrial labor, tying Satava's goal of reworking the medical apprenticeship system to historical shifts from craft to factory labor that have accompanied two centuries of industrialization

(Braverman 1998; Marx 1992; Zuboff 1984). Third, the digital instrument systems for representing and reproducing patient bodies and physician skills that Satava proposes can be "enterprised up," that is, brought into capitalist systems of commodity relations far more easily than skills that remain lodged in practitioners and clinics (see also Strathern 1992). Fourth, though objectification of patients is common in biomedicine, the language of patient-as-product erases the patient as a human person with agency. Satava may be a compassionate physician, but his writings, which tend to promote technological and bureaucratic solutions to medical problems, contain little evidence that he expects patient agency or autonomy to play a role in his revised system of surgical care, nor that he sees patient agency as important for good surgical outcomes. Satava's position toward patients is not unique in this world of medical research.

Satava and others are using simulator development to foster new forms of surgical education by encouraging the development of systematic criteria for assessing apprenticeship training. Satava argues that research into simulator design and into the teaching methods needed to incorporate simulation into medical curricula will lead to the "evolution" of surgical apprenticeships through "objective assessment of surgical skills and converting training from the apprenticeship model to one of criterion-based training" (2008, 141; see also Fried and Feldman 2008). If adopted, outcome measures and other performance criteria that Satava calls for would shift performance assessments from the trained judgment of the senior expert to more bureaucratized metrics for evaluation. Several surgeons I observed resisted such formalized performance measures, arguing that their years of training and experience qualified them to evaluate trainees. Performance criteria potentially threaten this individual and professional approach to training, making trainee performance accountable to a much wider group of evaluators, including hospital managers and professional associations. Though professional and specialist organizations have long maintained training and practice guidelines (Timmermans 2003), training metrics tied to performance criteria could move bureaucratic forms of control deeper into surgical practices and training relationships than in the past. Satava's vision is essentially disciplinary and bureaucratic, entailing the construction of technologies and standards that would ensure the production of surgeons with quantifiable skills. Yet his surgeon-as-superhero image suggests that he sees these changes in surgical technologies and training as empowering.

Social scientists who have examined the turn to virtual reality in medicine have wondered whether these technological developments might have more ambiguous effects on surgical power than Satava imagines, including the possibility that, by distributing knowing across many surgical technologies, the surgeons of the past will become diminished in autonomy and decision-making power. Michael M. J. Fischer suggests that the surgeon may be "reduced from the center of control, judgment, and action to being a technician within a system governed by protocols of best practices, decision trees, cost concerns, and other inputs established elsewhere in the system" (2003, 322). Similarly, Timothy Lenoir argues that the surgeon-hero of the past was the center of perception and action, bringing experience, training, and judgment together to effect a cure (2002, 42). Lenoir says the surgeon who will emerge with these systems will be technologically knowledgeable and adept but possibly will lose autonomy to the bits of knowledge embedded in machines. Further, both patients and practitioners may lose autonomy because these technologies can be designed to record procedures, possibly keeping records of errors for later lawsuits or helping medical bureaucracies deny payment for disallowed procedures (2002, 41). Fischer and Lenoir suggest a diminished role for the perceptions, skills, and judgments that surgeons embody through years of practice, arguing that surgeons will lose some ability to act autonomously as they become increasingly embedded in technologically mediated structures of decision making, cost control, and risk management. Both scholars suggest that surgeons using these systems will come to resemble carefully honed components of a larger technosocial machine.

The difference in perspective between Satava's vision and that of Fischer and Lenoir rests with whether one imagines the surgeon to be the central agent controlling these technologies or the object of control by outside forces. One's view of the potential of these technologies for augmenting surgeons' power or diminishing their autonomy depends largely on one's view of who will oversee the system and what form it will take. More utopian views tend to come from those who imagine themselves as in control of the technology (Turkle 2004).[6] Satava's vision for a technologically augmented supersurgeon keeps the surgeon at the center of agency and action, maintaining the surgeon's traditional professional role. Satava argues that surgical technologies and new training methods will extend and enhance the surgeon's bodily abilities well beyond the confines of the operating room. This vision may help persuade surgeons and other stakeholders to adopt these technologies, rather than furthering concerns about loss of surgeon agency.

Who will use such information gathered by automated systems? Will surgeons and researchers use the data to improve medical practice, or will insurers or hospital managers use them to control costs and reduce risks? Both views likely are partial. The institutional, social, and political milieux of future technology design and medical care will determine whether these technologies augment or decrease surgical power. They may do both: augmenting surgeons' power to see and repair pathologies while simultaneously embedding them in a techno-bureaucratic system that affects their options for treatment. Regardless of whether one sees these technologies as empowering or bureaucratizing surgical work, they will distribute bodies, knowledges, and practices in new assemblages of actors and technologies. They also will shift surgical training toward a model that focuses on an individual's acquisition of specific, measurable competencies, rather than upon the development of larger, less quantifiable clinical abilities. Further, these views of technological surgery systems imagine the patient's body as a dataset that can be accessed, divided, and recombined in new ways, rather than as a person to be treated.

One Laboratory

Satava and others looking at the future imagine that simulators and other medical teaching technologies will be embedded within a reconfigured surgical world of retooled practices, practitioners, and milieux. The work of disassembling bodies, practices, and relations leads researchers to continuously generate new objects, fields, and questions. Developing these tools requires collaboration from practitioners in medicine, engineering, computing, and education. The rise of the "cybersciences" in medicine, biology, and genetics has required new kinds of scientists who have training enough in the field of inquiry to follow research developments, and whose computational skills are good enough to make basic discoveries in informatics (Fujimura and Fortun 1996, 167). I have argued that the logics behind Satava's vision for virtual reality in medicine results in part from Satava's position at the intersection of surgical practice, military medicine, and medical technology design. A closer look at technology design as it has taken place in one laboratory reveals how constructions of bodies and practices from engineering and computer science get incorporated into these technologies.

The Coastal Information and Medical Technologies laboratory (a pseudonym) has been a leader in the development of technologies for simulating patients and medical environments and is fairly typical of the several dozen university-based laboratories around the world where this kind of research takes place. In 2001 and 2002, when I was in residence at Coastal, the research group occupied half a floor of a stucco office building at the far northwest corner of a cluster of medical research buildings on the Coastal campus. The laboratory began in the early 1990s as part of the medical school's Anatomy Division. The group developed out of one anatomist's project to build a digital teaching system based on stereographic photographs of human anatomy. When the project ended, the laboratory began building other tools for teaching anatomy but rapidly branched into other areas of medicine, including development of support tools for the medical school curriculum. The laboratory's role at the medical school combined computational services, such as design and maintenance of an Internet-based curriculum and content service, with applied research, such as the construction of a simulator for teaching gynecological surgery.

The laboratory resembled a small cubicle farm, containing offices, a computer laboratory, a server room, and a small conference room. Computers and devices occupied desks and shelves in most rooms and offices. A closer look revealed the presence of another major interest: medicine and medical education. In an open hallway and waiting area, copies of the *Journal of the American Medical Association* occupied shelves next to *Internet Week, Syllabus, Academic Medicine*, and, bridging the disciplines of medicine and computing, the *Journal of the American Medical Informatics Association*. In computer rooms and individual offices, atlases of anatomy and histology shared space on bookshelves with handbooks on programming and designing with C++, Perl, and Director. Specially designed interface devices, usually attached to computers, hinted at the presence of a third major discipline in the laboratory: engineering. These objects reflected the heterogeneous disciplines that laboratory researchers brought together to design new medical technologies.

The laboratory was genuinely interdisciplinary, housing researchers from multiple specialties in medicine, engineering, educational technology design, and computation around projects related to educational hardware and software design. Most researchers had received training in medicine, computing, education, or engineering. In 2001 and 2002, the laboratory employed up to fifty people, including a director, seven or eight researchers from multiple fields, web designers, project managers, students, and support staff. The group employed roughly equal numbers of men and women and represented an exceptional diversity of races, ages, and cultural backgrounds of U.S. and non-U.S. origins, reflecting a cultural pattern among residents of high-tech communities that value "dense networks of skilled, mobile, and 'diverse' professional workers" (English-Lueck 2002, 20). Researchers in the laboratory included four surgeons, a half-dozen mechanical and electrical engineers, an educational technologies expert, and a physicist doing cognitive research. The lab was organized by project in groups of four to twelve. Some researchers worked on several projects at once, while others were funded for specific projects. Collaborators, including experts in programming and networking, worked remotely from other laboratories at Coastal and in other universities, connecting with the group via telephone, email, and video-conferencing systems. The group received funding from federal, university, and a few corporate sources. The laboratory also participated in efforts among laboratories throughout the United States to develop "collaboratories," a means of dividing up research tasks, sharing information, and parceling out grant money to avoid duplication and share research and resources (Kouzes et al. 1996).

Information and communication technologies greatly extended and strengthened the group's network of collaborators, making the laboratory itself an example of distributed labor. For example, during my second week at the laboratory, I attended a meeting of the group working on Next Generation Internet research, a federal effort to develop and test a gigabit-speed network for scientific and business purposes. The meeting began with group members speaking with a collaborator in the Midwest via an Internet-based video-conferencing system. Laboratory members described their search for tools to measure how applications run over the Internet and the problems that real-time visual, audio, and textual systems run into during moments of heavy network traffic. Networking jargon—terms like "latency" and "jitter" —flew furiously.

Meanwhile, the laboratory's director, Sonja Vidal, an engineer, spoke on the telephone with a technician in the Midwest, who was helping her set up her laptop as a server. She planned to make the two-way video conference into a three-way conference, bringing a group doing related research at a midwestern university into the conversation. She was scheduled to present the laboratory's research results using her laptop to display images on a wall in the midwestern lab, while she talked from the conference system, creating a virtual slide presentation. Once Sonja and a helper got the two systems up and running, she gave her presentation. As she spoke, those of us sitting in the room watched a video of a dissected hand that was transmitted from the laptop at Coastal to a laptop at the midwestern university, then displayed on a wall in the lab in the Midwest, and transmitted back to Coastal over the video-conferencing system. In the middle of Sonja's presentation, the telephone rang: she had a call from a family member in Africa. Sonja clasped her head between her hands and said, to much laughter, "This is too much sometimes, huh? We are all very connected."

Group members take this level of technological connectedness mostly for granted, displaying exceptional ease with mediated communications and virtual interactions. Scientific and funding agencies increasingly are promoting interdisciplinary collaboration across laboratories, even among competing grant applicants. The development of these "collaboratories" stems from recognition that many fruitful problems in science and technology research defy clear-cut disciplinary boundaries (Kouzes et al. 1996). This approach also limits overlapping research and makes laboratories accountable to each other. Laboratories have an enormous amount of scientific and technical knowledge and practice sedimented in their machines and routines (Latour 1987; Latour and Woolgar 1979). In theory, collaboratories should tighten connections among laboratories, reducing overlapping research projects and encouraging investigators to tackle interlocking pieces of technoscientific problems, making them resemble nodes in a network of knowledge production more than scientific enclosures. In practice, from the laboratory work I have observed, true collaborations existed only when specifically written into grants. Larger collaborative efforts mostly involved information-sharing just slightly deeper than might be found at a conference or workshop. But the imaginary of the distributed laboratory intriguingly mirrors that of the reconfigured surgeon. Ideally, wired laboratories can leverage more knowledge developed in more places, transcending the limitations of time and space by taking advantage of new electronic communication tools. This certainly was true of the far-flung network of researchers working with the group at Coastal. Although the laboratory's researchers benefited from extending their networks, they also faced the possibility that their practices would be more closely scrutinized and held accountable to bureaucratic forces located elsewhere. Laboratories, like operating rooms, traditionally have been environments of enclosure, spaces of concentrated productive forces, whose effect is "greater than the sum of [their] component forces" (Deleuze 1992, 1). As with practices in the operating room, many functions of laboratories are being disassembled and redistributed.

Merging Disciplines, Emerging Technologies

Designing surgical simulators and other digital teaching tools requires, at a minimum, software writing and computer modeling skills, mechanical and electrical engineering, knowledge of anatomy, and surgical skill. In my experience, researchers in this multidisciplinary setting were unusually curious about practices and knowledges from other fields. In the laboratory at Coastal, researchers fell into one of two groups that can be loosely described using terms borrowed from information theory. The physicians and educators, "content" people, developed the pedagogical contents of applications and ensured their accuracy and validity as teaching tools. The "information" researchers, mostly programmers and engineers, studied ways to transmit those contents to users, doing networking research, device building, and programming.

Though medicine, computing, and engineering are culturally distinct, a danger exists in describing laboratory members as rigidly bound to medicine or technology design. The physicians and others I have described as occupying the content side of Coastal's research work were highly computer literate. They had learned mechanical concepts and terms from the group's engineers, and all participated in "a computer culture that in one way or another touches us all" (Turkle 1984, 18). Three of four surgeons working in the group had studied programming, hardware wiring, or web design, and the fourth had done extensive work with digitized medical images and models. These surgeons already demonstrated some skills of the technologically adept future surgeon that Lenoir describes (2002). Conversely, most of Coastal's engineers and programmers, whom I describe as information people, had spent years creating medical devices and applications. Most lab members received advanced degrees in either medicine or technology design. Several of them had spent extended time observing practices in operating rooms, anatomy laboratories, and other clinical spaces. Very few researchers were capable of creating contents and the information structures to deliver them to users. Those who were adept at creating content and information structures typically received degrees in medicine, then developed an interest in computing. That "doubly literate" people tended to be physicians, not computer experts or engineers, reflects the development and training histories of medicine and computing work: medicine has high educational and institutional barriers to entry, whereas computer experts take pride in their origins as tinkerers and in their field's (often exaggerated) egalitarian promise.

Coastal's projects often brought researchers' diverse knowledges together in interactions around objects: hardware, software, terminology. These are "object worlds," communities formed around material or conceptual objects (Bucciarelli 1994, 62). Objects become focal points for negotiations about bodies and machines, medical and engineering practices, and their relations. For example, during the network project meeting I described above, an engineer arrived to deliver a new interface device for a virtual-reality laparoscopic simulator. A commercial videogame interface maker that was entering the medical interface market designed and built the device as part of a public-private cooperative agreement that allowed the company to use federal funds and specifications provided by the laboratory's engineers and physicians. The device, thus, had virtual reality's history of relations among industries (including the entertainment industry), universities, and governments built into it.

Dr. Harry Beauregard, a retired gynecologist turned simulation researcher, examined the device together with several members of the lab, including the remotely linked collaborators in the Midwest. Protruding from a black box, the device's handles mimicked the look and feel of handles used in laparoscopic procedures. Harry fiddled with the device for a few minutes, feeling its handles, their weight and movement.

This is a significant advance. It's lighter weight and it doesn't feel so resistant in your hand. . . . These [handles] are lighter weight. They feel less metallic. They are less metallic because they're plastic, and it gives a better sensation. They're still wide. They're still heavier, but they've got to accommodate a lot of stuff. And the rotation works smoothly, just the way it ought to.

Later, Harry introduced the device to one of the remote collaborators. He called it the "Number three interface for the surgery workbench," noting its "five degrees of freedom and force feedback." When Harry described the interface's widely spaced handles and their weight relative to actual surgical instruments, he spoke from his experiences as a surgeon. When he used the word "interface" and related the device's degrees of freedom and force feedback capability, he used engineering terms. The moment reveals the blending of knowledge that occurs in this world. Harry did not write code or develop algorithms, but his fluency with engineering and computing languages enabled him to communicate his experiences and interests in language that engineers could understand.

Coastal's technologies were products of negotiations among physicians, engineers, and computer programmers, who had to develop some proficiency in technical fields outside their own—physicians learned some programming, programmers learned some medicine—to create these objects. The fields represented in the laboratory—surgery, engineering, computer science, and education—are merging in this new disciplinary space not because researchers have worked in shared spaces but because they have worked together to build these technologies. Researchers' shared knowledges can be primarily conceptual—knowing that, rather than knowing how—or they can be more durably embodied as techniques they could use with ease. The "trading zones" (see Galison 1997, 46) for interdisciplinary knowledges at Coastal entailed discursive and material negotiations over individual technologies, making these trading zones specific to projects or technologies. This work of negotiation and construction has fostered development of the field of virtual reality in medicine and has enabled construction of distinctive objects that have become the field's "signatures" (Traweek 1988, 49). In this new research arena, interdisciplinary merging occurred not only in language, but also within the technologies themselves.

Making the varied concepts and languages in this field comprehensible required a sensitivity to potentially awkward and misleading constructions. For example, on my first day visiting the laboratory, during a project meeting, Harry and Dr. Ramesh Chanda discussed their work building surgical simulators. They described their goal of creating a "thriller app," or computer application. "We've made a semantic change from 'killer app' to 'thriller app,'" Harry said. Ramesh clarified, "Somehow 'killer app' doesn't sound quite right in surgical simulation." A "killer app" is a common term in the world of computing for a highly successful application, one that dominates the market, killing the competition. But describing a simulator for teaching medical skill as a "killer" could seem inappropriate. The two surgeons renamed their application, but retained a resonance with entertainment that evoked the field's link to videogaming and commercial software development. Examples of these kinds of word games abounded at the laboratory, revealing how knowledges and sensibilities from the worlds of computing and medicine come together. The shift from "killer app" to "thriller app" reflected the physicians' attentiveness to medicine's humanistic values, as well as the interest in potential commercialization that is ubiquitous in this research field.

Interdisciplinary Biographies and Technologies

When laboratories and research projects become opened to new connections and new worlds, researchers, too, must make connections to new knowledges and practices. Karin Knorr Cetina (2000) argues that laboratories reconfigure both natural objects and scientists. Her observation certainly applied to the Coastal Information and Medical Technologies laboratory. The technologies developed in the laboratory also reconfigured, or had the potential to reconfigure, medical practices. The logics of this reconfiguration did not necessarily follow the bureaucratic system of protocols and systems-level constraints that Fischer and Lenoir feared, though one characteristic of information technologies is that they can easily be adapted to this type of information retrieval and surveillance (Zuboff 1984, 317). Most technologies that were in development at Coastal while I was there followed the logic of engineers, who imagined bodies as dynamic systems, with motions and interactions that could be quantified and replicated. In this section, I recount two examples of technologies that have the potential to alter medical practices that typically have been based on extended sensory training.

A young surgeon's description of her research career captures in microcosm the intersection of medicine, medical education, technology design, and entrepreneurial aspirations that are common in this research field. The surgeon and designer, Dr. Tanya Burrows, has an advanced degree in education. Tanya told me that a love of anatomy, cemented during her first year of medical school, led her to surgery, where she discovered that she had what she called "the surgical eye." "It relates to a visual gift—being able to see things in three dimensions—that I knew I had." With the discovery came a desire to teach. While doing her graduate coursework, Tanya's interest in the sensory aspects of medical technique continued to develop during a course on sensors, during which she began working on a simulator to teach pelvic exams. She taught herself the programming language C++ and wired a plastic and rubber training mannequin with sensors embedded in a model ovary. These sensors calculate the pressure of a trainee's hand as it squeezes the mannequin's ovary. The simulator represents hand pressure as a sliding-bar graph on a computer screen (as pressure increases, the bar goes up). Tanya later worked with private-sector partners to build and market the simulators commercially.

Pelvic exams are difficult to teach, Tanya said, both because the instructor cannot see the trainee's hands and because trainees and trainers alike struggle to communicate sensory experience:

> When I'm teaching this, how can I describe it? There's no uniform language for teaching how a prostate feels or how a cervix feels. . . . It's also very difficult to do the three-dimensional visualizing of the vaginal vault and cervix.

In the absence of an easily imagined anatomical structure and a transparent relationship between tactile sensation and language, Tanya decided to bypass language, creating a visual representation of the pressure a hand applies during palpation. Typically, practitioners embody the sensations of ovary palpation through repetition and practice. In contrast, the simulator augments tactile learning with visual feedback. To create an object that the trainee and instructor would have in common, Tanya constructed a symbolic representation of the relationship of examining body to examined body. The simulator, like other information technologies, "abstracts thought from action" (Zuboff 1984, 75). The skill required to interpret an ovary's status by squeezing with a hand differs significantly from the skill required to read a graph. Reading a graph depicting the pressures of a hand squeezing a model ovary is an example of "intellective skill," the ability to connect symbolic representations, such as the bar graph, to activities occurring in the physical world (Zuboff 1984, 76). Shoshana Zuboff (1989) described a shift from work that required "action-centered" skills, which are inextricably tied to physical and sensory practice, to work that required intellective skills as a significant part of the processes of industrial automation that she documented in the 1980s. The pelvic simulator, however, mixes the two skills, assuming that the user (typically a medical resident) already has intellective skills that can be used to acquire the action-centered skill of palpation. The pelvic simulator alters the trainee's relationship to both instructor and patient by moving the focus from what the hand feels to what the eyes see. Further, the simulator leaves behind those aspects of tactile sense that numbers cannot convey.

Though the pelvic simulator appears to be a straightforward means of teaching the pelvic exam ex vivo, it subtly reconfigures the embodied relations of teachers and trainees, tissues and senses, languages and representations, clinical time and teaching space.[7] Teaching the pelvic exam by traditional means has entailed the efforts of two humans to communicate, however imperfectly, the sensations they experience when their hands are in intimate contact with a third person's reproductive organs. Sometimes the third person—the patient—participates in this communication.[8] By replacing the patient with a model, and by making the model speak to both teacher and student by means of a sliding bar on a screen, the interaction appears to make the embodied relation more precise and to clarify ambiguities in the communication—pressure becomes a numerical value, and its sufficiency instantly can be read off a screen. But the simulator also shifts the nature of the teaching moment. The simulator makes the sliding-bar graph—not hand or ovary—the focal point of the teacher-student interaction.

Tanya's studies of simulator users have shown that students using the simulator rely less on expert supervision for instruction because trainees feel comfortable using the simulator on their own. The simulator cannot easily capture the complexities of linguistic and physical relations between trainee and trainer, and between patient and practitioner, so they are replaced with a visually represented number on a graph. The simulator may improve trainees' palpation skills and, consequently, their abilities to detect clinical anomalies, but it also reduces the clinical relationship to the pressure of a physician's hand on a patient's ovary. This makes the interaction mathematical and, therefore, quantifiable, but it leaves out other aspects of the interaction, such as the tactile "feel" of the ovary, communication with the patient, and some of the teaching interaction with the instructor. Further, the simulator promotes a normative version of the pelvic exam, a form of standardization that may not be desirable if designers expect the simulator to be incorporated into medical programs with varied local practices (see Timmermans 2003, 21).[9] When asked about the limitations of the analogy between simulated bodies and living bodies, Tanya, like many other technology designers, deferred to the future: the simulator helps prepare students for their first living patients. She argued that most parties—trainees, clinical instructors, and patients—would prefer a trainee who had some simulated practice to one with no practice at all. Trainees would learn the subtleties of interpersonal relations during this intimate exam in later clinical encounters. Thus, cultivation of individual physical skills becomes extracted from a larger clinical situation in which trainees must interact with patients. Care of self in this model comes to precede care of others.

Tanya designed the simulator to help trainees better embody palpation skills so they could more effectively apply them to patients. The simulator changes the way trainees embody palpation skill, but it also maintains the physician's body at the center of medical work. In contrast, a technology developed by Sonja, the group director, who is an electrical engineer, privileged mathematical precision and predictive models over the embodiment of skill. In the early 1990s, Sonja developed a computer model that could predict the effects of reconstructive hand surgeries, calculating mathematically the effects of various types of orthopedic interventions, such as reattaching a tendon at a particular location. In an interview, she described how she gathered quantitative anatomical data and what this type of modeling could bring to medicine, particularly surgery:

SONJA: When I first got into this reconstruction of the wrist, I would find all these pictures of the bones and even what looked like three-dimensional drawings, but nowhere could I find something that told me what the actual size of it was in millimeters. So I couldn't find, for example, the moment arm of the tendon that's gliding over these bones and, in the end, I had to slice. I had to work with [a hand surgeon] to slice bones and reconstruct it to get that geometrical information. . . .

RP: Is medicine ready for a more mathematically oriented anatomy?

SONJA: Most people don't need it, I don't think. The people who are forced to need it, they learn it. It can actually do things. For example, for surgeons, it can predict the effect of variations in certain surgeries. You move the tendon five millimeters this way, what's it going to do? The surgeons work that out through their own knowledge and intuition, but you could tell them mathematically that it's going to move the finger in this direction that you don't really want, and you can actually quantitatively tell them.

Sonja described how the anatomical and medical literature she consulted lacked mathematical calculations of relative sizes and angles of bones, ligaments, and tendons in the wrist. Developing models for the motion of tendons over wrist bones demanded precise mathematical measurements of the dimensions and geometric relations of structures. From these data, Sonja could calculate the effects on wrist movement of various locations for tendon reattachment. Existing images of wrist bones, even three-dimensional drawings, did not provide the information that Sonja needed to model wrist motion. Engineers learn early in their training to resolve complex motion into equations, but the idea that a mathematical model of wrist mechanics could predict the outcome of particular surgical actions was new in anatomy at the time. For Sonja, mathematical modeling could help create predictive models of the effects of surgical actions, effects that surgeons typically gauge using carefully crafted perceptual skill and detailed anatomical knowledge. As an engineer, Sonja values creating a quantitative, predictive model over modeling based on surgical intuition. Since this early work, many engineers and anatomists interested in graphic modeling have begun to argue for a more quantitative approach to human anatomy and motion.

Sonja and other engineers I encountered in this field worked to define bodily motion mathematically, resolving movements into force vectors that could be displayed visually using arrows, so users could understand the relative sizes and directions of the forces involved. The dynamic forces of human motion are not easily demonstrated with cadavers. The push by engineers for the development of quantitative anatomical information displays an epistemological preference for quantification: the engineers I encountered wanted to make the enormously complex systems of human bodies comprehensible by representing them in terms of their dynamic properties. The reduction of complex systems to dynamic properties is a basic tenet of engineering education that becomes a taken-for-granted aspect of the engineer's habitus through years of practice (Berg 1997; Bourdieu 1977; Forsythe 2001). But this is not a method native to most areas of biomedical practice.

Whereas the pelvic simulator was intended to help practitioners embody a new skill, Sonja's predictive models worked from the assumption that surgeons could perform better with technological assistance that could offer a precision unachievable by the most dexterous and experienced surgeons. The pelvic model builds upon the assumption that improving medical care can be achieved by improving the self. The predictive model builds upon the assumption that improving care can be achieved by augmenting the self.

Body Objects

Dynamic modeling of bodily movement or function often first involves creation of a static model. Heterogeneous groups of researchers engineer representations of human bodies, such as the mathematical model of hand motion, to inhabit computers. These body objects are teaching tools, diagrams, and models that reflect Coastal's character as a computer research laboratory that develops medical teaching tools. A crumbling cardboard model of a child's skull, an artifact from an early project, sits on a shelf in Sonja's office. Researchers constructed the model by programming a computer to calculate geometry of the skull from the outlines depicted on a series of cross-sectional images created using computerized tomography. Those calculated curves then became outlines of cross sections of skull, which were cut out of cardboard and stacked sequentially to build the skull. The skull was an early proof-of-concept of graphic models built from cross sections of human anatomy. Since the early 1990s, this type of graphic modeling from cross sections has become common for anatomical modeling in many clinical and research applications.

In Harry's office, he had pinned a small pink and white foam model of a uterus to a bulletin board. The uterus served as the basis for a computer-aided design model, part of an early attempt to build a virtual-reality surgical simulator. Harry began the simulator project as a commercial venture in the early 1990s. The project never got off the ground, largely because the field chose to pursue cross-sectional models built from actual patient data instead of computer-aided design models. Among the remnants of Harry's project were the foam model on the bulletin board and its digital doppelganger on a hard drive. When Harry emerged from this venture, he began building models that originated from images of real cadavers (Sonja and Harry began to collaborate in part because of her expertise in this area).

For months, a whiteboard in another office displayed a drawing of a finger overlaid with a schematic intended to show the physics of finger motion and what happens mechanically when it fractures. The drawing was a conceptual sketch for a computer animation of a broken finger driven by a mathematical description of its motion. Later, I saw a computer animation built from this initial sketch: the broken finger had a distinctly unnatural "hitch" in it when it straightened out. The finger model reveals how researchers apply physics equations to static models to put them into motion.

Each of these objects was a body part that had been reconfigured in relation to a particular technology: the skull was a cardboard manifestation of computed cross sections, the finger was a set of force vectors that could show dramatic differences in the motion of a normal finger and a broken finger, and the foam uterus had been broken down into its most elementary shapes and reconstituted virtually (see Downey 1998). Regardless of their purpose or success, such objects reveal how the combined engineering, computational, and medical knowledges of the group came together to build body objects and embed them in simulators and other computational systems.

To build training simulators, researchers create body objects that are incorporated in the computer. This requires a crucial epistemic move: the body must become mathematical, described using equations the computer can interpret. Actions and sensations that trainees usually experience physically must be calculated, just as the finger's motion and the skull's curvature must be calculated in the examples cited above. Calculating surgical action, however, requires three layers of mathematicization. First, the curvature of a skull or other body shape must be calculated. Second, the body's motion, such as the deformation of a breaking finger, must be calculated. Third, the interaction of user and model (which Harry has called "tool-tissue interaction") must be calculated. In the world of surgical simulation, a virtual body must interact with both computer and user as a mathematical and a visual-physical entity. Sonja described the mathematics of creating deformable models of bodies that can interact with virtual tools:

> The only way the computer can understand things is, in this case, through geometry. It needs geometry. It needs to know how to compute a sequence of forces with equations, which previously, in a sense, [surgeons] did in their heads. You knew how to predict what was going to happen. You didn't solve an equation to do that, it was just part of the experience. So it's the computer that forces you to put that mathematical construct on.

Surgeons predict the consequences of their actions based on their own embodied experience and others' experience as it becomes distilled in papers, procedural scripts, and apprenticeship-style teaching. Surgeons' sense of what would result from their actions remains lodged in their bodies. In contrast, computers must "understand" bodies and their actions mathematically. The computer requires that each step in a body's motion be modeled as a discrete mathematical state acted upon by the movements—resolved into forces—of tools wielded by the surgeon. The feel of surgery must be parsed, calculated, incorporated into the computer's programming, and ultimately fed back to the human user, who then will experience the sensations of performing a surgical procedure phenomenologically.

Body objects are hybrids: each, in its own way, is a medical and a computational or engineering object. They are models and representations of bodies, all originating in medicine, that have become intertwined, visually and semiotically, with knowledges culled from engineering and computer science and, physically, with sensors, wires, and processors. Body objects also are narrow because a simulator requires specific mathematical descriptions to calculate a line or determine a trajectory. They cannot be loosely described in ways humans understand intuitively. In this, they differ from the boundary objects that Star and Griesemer (1989) described because boundary objects, such as natural history museum collections, are useful to many types of researchers precisely because they retain a certain looseness in their construction. Body objects serve only two kinds of "users": computers and human users of computers. Body objects are representations of bodies articulated mathematically, so computers can convert them into visual and haptic (tactile and kinesthetic) signals that human users can understand. These are bodies that researchers have purposefully reworked to meet technological needs. Further, body objects primarily represent parts of bodies, rarely whole bodies, and never persons. They are designed specifically to interact with users as body parts, often as tools for teaching specific techniques. As such, their proliferation encourages greater focus on technique in medicine.

In the laboratory at Coastal, bodies of patients become informatic models —body objects—that can be mobilized and recombined in new technologies and different fields of research. Many techniques employed by technology designers originated in nonmedical areas of capitalist production, but profit often is not researchers' primary motivation. Instead, these methods can be mobilized as solutions to problems (or perceived problems) of transparency, communicability, standardization, and prediction that bedevil embodied relations. Tanya Hughes's desire to build a simulator to teach what she could see and feel while closing an incision or palpating an ovary was not motivated solely by the simulator's potential profits. Tanya also wanted to be a better teacher, one capable of articulating her embodied knowledge through the medium of a machine. Similarly, Sonja's work to determine the force vectors related to wrist motion reflected a desire to improve upon physicians' intuitive understanding of motion, which typically develops through years of practice (and can never replicate the precision of a computer). Thus, to render instrumental logics as purely about a mechanistic worldview or purely about capitalization would miss the ways that instrumental techniques, though originating in and often working at the service of capitalist logics, define engineering and computer science approaches that also can be applied to the twin medical goals of healing and teaching.

Technologizing Bodies

The vision of the surgical simulator-robot described above has spurred researchers in laboratories around the world to work on its medical imaging, graphic modeling, simulation, interface design, and robotics components since the late 1970s. The simulator would allow the surgeon to use imaging technologies to reconstruct the patient's three-dimensional anatomy to plan and practice the steps of a difficult surgery. The robot then would convert the surgeon's actions into those of an automaton: unaffected by physical strain, by emotion, or by the patient's suffering. This untiring robot could work all day, day after day, increasing hospital "throughput" of patients. In this imaginary of technology, the patient becomes a "product," the objectified outcome of surgical work, whether performed by a human or a robot. Yet there is something uncomfortable about calling a patient a "product." This language represents a radical objectification of the patient that appears to erase any lingering assumptions that medical "care" is about something more than provision of commodified medical services. This discomfort exemplifies Paul Rabinow's statement that older assumptions often permeate new regimes of thought and practice, creating an "unarticulated uneasiness" (1996, 130). The rise of virtual technologies and bureaucratic techniques does not necessarily cause this uneasiness. Rather, the language of patient as product and practitioner as robot suggests that medical care might become an industrially inspired technical achievement, eclipsing the concept of care as a morally virtuous undertaking. In this section, I explore the logics underpinning the ideal of surgeon-as-automaton and patient-as-product.

Classic descriptions of biomedical practice place great importance on values associated with caring. One widely read medical ethics textbook describes the relationship between care and emotion: "Good health care often involves insight into the needs of patients and considerate attentiveness to their circumstances, which often derives more from emotion than reason" (Beauchamp and Childress 2009, 37). This same text continues at some length about the five virtues of medical morality, including compassion, discernment, trustworthiness, integrity, and conscientiousness. Those virtues have been sorely tested by time crunches and managed care schemas that treat "care" as a commodity to be dispensed as discrete actions and treatments. The virtues of medical morality are, by their nature, individual and unquantifiable. They certainly can exist within a rationalized regime of medicine, but their presence is irrelevant to the execution of medicine as constructed within a technological and bureaucratic framework. Beauchamp and Childress rank technical virtuosity lower than the five virtues, but technical ability is much more easily quantified and verified.

The work of designing simulators, robots, and other digital medical technologies relates loosely to larger efforts to rationalize medical work and medical training. Attempts to rationalize medicine have existed at least since the standardization movements of the first decades of the twentieth century (Stevens 1999; Timmermans 2003). What makes simulator research unique is researchers' attempts to encode expert surgeons' physical skills to help trainees acquire their own skills. Bureaucratic governance within highly rationalized milieux mistrusts individual, internal, emotional, and nonverifiable aspects of professional care, favoring that which is externally verifiable and "objective." Some argue that the current complexity of biomedical systems around the world suggest that lodging techniques, ethics, and responsibility exclusively in the bodies of individual doctors may no longer be an adequate means of achieving high-quality medical treatment (see Gawande 2007).

For Max Weber, rationalization is an important organizing principle for highly complex modern systems (1946, 214). "The more complicated and specialized modern culture becomes," he wrote, "the more its external supporting apparatus demands the personally detached and strictly 'objective' *expert*, in lieu of the master of older social structures, who was moved by personal sympathy and favor, by grace and gratitude" (216). The push for expertise as it is embodied in technology and a more bureaucratic system of protocols and checklists reflects mistrust of subjective forms of expertise, including expertise embodied in individual practitioners. The deconstruction of embodied surgical ways of knowing taking place as researchers develop digital technologies for teaching and practice largely follows the logic of technical fields, particularly engineering and computer science, which value quantification and objectification over experience and intuition. These techno-logics either focus on training the physicians' body, as the example of the pelvic simulator does, or provide information that could bring greater precision to physicians' practices, as the wrist motion program does. Researchers working on these technologies use analytic techniques from engineering and computer science to disassemble patients' bodies and physicians' practices and recombine them in formalized, often digital, forms for the purpose of redistributing, technologizing, and capitalizing them in new ways. "Personal sympathy," such as it exists, has become increasingly separated from technical skill and often is considered a desirable but unnecessary addition to the work of medical treatment.

One critical move of technologization is the division of a physician's professional abilities into the knowledges, skills, and physical forces that one applies to other bodies. Originally associated with craft labor, the breaking up of craft into discrete skills is bound up with the history of industrialization and management control over production processes (Braverman 1998; Marx 1992; Noble 1979; Taylor 2009). Integral to its present-day conception is a relation to commodification of workers' abilities that leads workers and employers to treat acquisition of skills as necessary for the continuous development of qualified workers (Urciuoli 2008). What counts as skill often becomes redefined as that which can be quantified or measured, so its acquisition can be measured. The pelvic simulator, for example, defines palpation as the pressure of a hand on an ovary, separating palpation from the larger sociomedical interaction of physician with patient. Skills extracted from professionals and made into objects are visible to others, mobile, and capable of being reembodied in computer technologies. When hidden inside patients' and practitioners' bodies, as well as in relations that take place in operating rooms and clinics, medical practices are difficult to capitalize. But once extracted as body objects that can be embedded in technological systems, they become fair game to be "enterprised up" as research tools and commercial ventures. Satava's Holomer is a perfect example of medical information about a human body that has been beamed onto a disk and thus becomes available for research or capitalization. These engineering logics take medical practices—some of the most physical and intimate forms of relationship of one body to another—and resolve them into their component forces. Few acknowledge that difficult-to-quantify aspects of this relationship, such as the effects of a physician's kind words or gentle stroke on the hand, get written out of the equations.

In Satava's writing, the surgeon is a highly trained, technologically augmented technician who is capable of treating patients with an array of sophisticated resources. Satava wants to base surgical education on quantifiable performance measures, as well as to evaluate and measure such seemingly subjective medical abilities as judgment. Although Satava couches his claims in terms of the surgeon-as-superman, he argues that the changes he proposes will improve physicians' relationship to patients by improving their ability to provide care. "The future is not about technology, it is about human caring" (Satava 1997, 201). Despite this caveat, the meaning of "care" in Satava's writings rests more upon the practitioner's ability to provide care that is the product of a surgeon's level of technical proficiency than upon the physician's ability to provide compassionate treatment. This invokes the split between care as technique and care as caring that Rosemary Stevens attributes to the gendered and professional divisions that existed between physicians and nurses in the first half of the twentieth century (1999, 66). Though many of the sexual divisions of labor that have marked the medical and nursing professions have eroded, the gendered distinctions that make technical work the physician's province and leave caring work to nurses remain. The work of caring often becomes coded as "soft" or as "woman's work" and becomes suspect in the masculinized world of rationalization.

I have often heard patients say they would prefer a doctor who is technically gifted but cold to a doctor who is compassionate but less gifted. These patients thus split physicians' technical accomplishment from patients' affective needs and medicine's moral virtues, often implicitly suggesting that the two cannot coexist, as though the technically gifted surgeon must also be a hyperrational automaton or a surgical robot. Care does not disappear in this calculus. Rather than care for persons, the object of care for physicians becomes technique, or care of self (Deleuze 1988; Foucault 2005). The biomedical care of the self has a moral component. As I described in chapter 4, the ethics of doing no harm make the acquisition of technical proficiency a moral imperative of biomedicine, splitting technique from aspects of care, such as compassion, which focus on the patient as subject. Care of self becomes the means of caring for others.

seven

THE ANATOMY OF A
SURGICAL SIMULATION

During a discussion about virtual-reality simulators, a hand surgeon working on simulator design drew a diagram on a napkin, depicting two poles
connected by a line. He wrote "implicit/apprenticeship" at one pole and
"explicit/VR" at the other. He explained that surgeons learn many of their
skills by imitating their superiors. These skills are rarely broken down into
their component parts. To build a virtual-reality simulator, however, researchers must make those actions explicit. They must disassemble embodied actions into discrete behaviors, translate bodily actions into equations
describing their physics, and recompose them in virtual space. In other
words, bodies and their relations in surgery are reconstructed as forces
interacting according to physical laws that can be computed. Trainees ideally will have a physical experience similar enough to surgery on living
patients that they can learn from the experience. To achieve this, surgical
action must be made explicit for computers, though what gets made explicit
as steps for trainees gets made explicit as equations for computers. Researchers describe this process as the construction of a "patient on demand," which is an object that is available whenever a trainee needs to
practice and can be reset as often as needed for a trainee to perfect a skill.

During years of extended apprenticeship in clinical settings, surgical
trainees acquire a "muscular gestalt" that leads to "the power to respond
with a certain type of solution to situations of a certain general form"
(Dreyfus 1992, 249). According to Hubert Dreyfus, developing a muscular
gestalt is one of the many things a computer cannot do. Yet the simulator
must help trainees develop one. To do this, the computer facilitates a visual
and kinesthetic interaction between the surgeon-user's body and a virtual

patient's body, constructing the user's actions and the model body's reactions as graphic and haptic (tactile and kinesthetic) feedback. Haptically enabled devices provide physical feedback from a virtual object to a user, creating the sensation of interacting with a material object. Adding haptics to a simulator makes a tight link between sensation and action, creating a research challenge for simulator makers.

The construction of simulators involves at least three distinct research areas: graphic modeling, haptic interface design, and research into haptic knowing. Each research area requires surgeons, computer experts, engineers, and others to articulate bodies and actions graphically (for users) and quantitatively (for computers) and to incorporate these articulations into software and interface devices. Studying simulators provides an opportunity to examine the reconstruction of surgical action by showing how researchers doubly articulate—for computers and users—the bodily relations of surgeon and patient. Put another way, the relations of bodies and instruments in surgery must be articulated for the computer so the computer can articulate surgical action for the trainee.

In this chapter, I dissect the research that went into creation of a surgical simulator designed to teach minimally invasive gynecological procedures, such as the removal of an ovary. An interdisciplinary group of researchers at the Coastal Information and Medical Technologies laboratory developed the simulator. Investigating the process of simulator construction shows how technology designers raise new questions about preexisting practices: questions that are relevant for practitioners, designers, and social scientists. The ethnographer Stefan Hirschauer extrapolates from surgeons' sports and war metaphors to argue that surgery can be described in terms of "relations of force" (1991, 282). Simulator designers, who must create bodies and relations for the computer, literally construct the actions of surgery as relations of forces. That is, they must construct surgical actions as forces that can be computed by computers. I call this reciprocal construction of bodies and machines "mutual articulation."

Mutual Articulation and Surgical Simulation

Mutual articulation provides a framework for studying surgery and surgical simulation that focuses attention on what occurs at the interface of a surgeon's hands and a patient's body. "Mutual articulation" follows from Bruno Latour's concept (2004) of "articulation," which describes how bodies come into being through sensory interactions with the world. Latour acknowledges the difficulty of describing what a body is. He argues that the body is most usefully imagined as an interface that becomes increasingly describable as it engages with more elements. Bodies and body parts come into being through the articulation of differences. Following this approach, attending to the body means focusing on ways bodies learn to register and distinguish objects. Latour cites the example of a kit the perfume industry employs to teach future perfume makers the art of smelling. Using this kit, students learn how to differentiate extremely dissimilar smells and then to identify progressively more subtle smells. Skilled perfume experts become known as "noses" (2004, 207). The metonym reveals how sniffing skill and body part become synonymous, coming into being together. Latour's theory rests on multiple meanings of the word "articulation" as "a joint," in the sense of a body with joints and of "speaking intelligibly" ("articulate"), making articulation material and linguistic. Viewed from this perspective, much of medical education entails articulating two bodies—the patient's body and the physician's body. According to Latour, scientific and technological instruments extend the senses beyond the unmediated body's capabilities. Coming to know the world, whether through the senses or through the mediation of instruments, becomes a process of articulating differences in the world.

The concept of articulation works well when, as occurs in the case of the perfume kit, the teaching tool is standardized and stable. In surgery, however, a surgeon must create the surgical site, sculpting flesh, with all its variations, into an operative site. In surgery, knowledge of the object is embodied in the surgeon at the same time that the surgeon brings that object into being. Patient and surgeon shape each other through a process of mutual articulation. The physician constructs the operative site from the indistinct tissues of the patient's body (Hirschauer 1991), even as surgical practice defines and reinforces the surgeon's skill. Mutual articulation becomes particularly important when examining relations of bodies and instruments in complex activities, such as surgical training. Bodies affect and are affected by each other in multiple ways that often are only partially determined.

Considering bodies in surgery as mutually articulated allows reexamination of classic ethnographic work on surgery. For example, Hirschauer says physicians acquire two bodies. They learn an "abstract body," which is the body as it is represented in anatomy texts and plastic models. They also acquire their own bodies as experienced practitioners. He describes anatomical knowledge and surgical experience as being engaged in a "permanent cross-fading of experience and representation" (1991, 310). Hirschauer argues that surgeons reproduce the abstract body depicted by anatomical atlases in the patient's body. Knowledge and skill develop together, combining "the anatomical *knowing that* of the visible, and the anatomical *knowing how* of making something visible" (310, emphasis in original). And he says anatomical images reflect the physical means—usually dissection—of their production. But, although Hirschauer connects abstract anatomical knowledge as contained in atlases to the skills needed to produce those images, he says, "the body of the anatomic atlas, with its clearcut divisions, different colors, numbered and labeled structures, is present in the surgeon's mind" (310). Hirschauer creates a separation between the skilled work of hands and the visual knowledge of the atlas, which he says resides in the mind. A surgeon's anatomical knowledge, according to this view, exists separately from anatomical skill.

Hirschauer's notion of abstract anatomical knowledge and the surgeon's ability to sculpt the body to resemble an anatomical model suggests that a representation of human anatomy becomes housed somewhere inside the surgeon (typically imagined as inside his or her mind). The idea of anatomy as a static textbook representation contained in the mind creates sharp distinctions among knowledge, body, and world. According to this view, the surgeon's body simply follows the orders of an executive consciousness to act upon passive objects. This view creates several problems. It renders the body as a mechanical prosthesis of mind. It reduces all that is external to passive recipients of the mind's orders. And it creates the problem of ensuring that the picture in the mind accurately reflects reality in the world, creating an aporia between mind and world that is impossible to bridge. Considering the creation of anatomical knowledge as the development of physical skill that comes with years of practice allows one to consider not the accuracy of an internal mental or visual model, such as may or may not exist, but simply the surgeon's ability to sculpt the operative site in the patient's body to effect desired changes without doing harm. Thus, surgical knowledge can be thought of at the interface between a surgeon's hands and a patient's body, as it exists in practice. Whether taught by a simulator or by another surgeon, the surgeon crafts his or her ability to construct an anatomical model from highly variable patient bodies. Simulation reveals that the patient's body plays a role in that shaping.

Examining anatomical knowing as it is practiced in the act of operating upon a living body—studying practice at the interface of a surgeon's hands and a patient's body—eliminates worries about the completeness or accuracy of mental models and about the surgeon's ability to translate mental knowledge into physical action. Hands, eyes, and mind are no longer considered separately. Practicing on patient bodies teaches young doctors how to make the fine visual and visceral distinctions among tissues that they will need as surgeons. Surgeons in teaching hospitals use real bodies, and the contrasts between them, to teach trainees to see and to feel differences among tissues. Medical residents learn these distinctions through the process of practicing upon bodies. The abstract anatomical body depicted in atlases and models does not exist in the flesh until it is created by an anatomist. The anatomical body comes into being through practice. Surgeons typically do much less delineating and differentiating among tissues than anatomists because surgeons must limit the time they spend dissecting and the damage they do to living bodies. In both cases, practitioner and body mutually articulate each other as trainees learn to create the anatomical body or operative site from an undifferentiated, unarticulated cadaver or patient body.

The objectification and instrumentalization of the relationship of hands, instruments, and anatomies that occurs when designers build surgical simulators breaks the process of surgery into many components, forcing surgeons and programmers to make explicit elements of the tactile experience of surgery, such as the elasticity of a uterus or the delicacy of an ovary, that often remain tacit. The process of construction of a surgical simulator reveals how surgical skill must be articulated for the computer and, ultimately, for its users. This, too, is a process of mutual articulation. Engineers and programmers build new relationships between hands and machines by decomposing the action of hands into two components: action and sensation. Hands learn while they do. Eyes and other sensory organs also learn while they do, but the connection is much less direct. Studying simulator research thus opens up new questions for observational studies of surgery, particularly about such areas as haptic knowledge and the social aspects of surgery that cannot be taught with a simulator (Collins et al. 1997). Simulator researchers articulate the physical connection between hands and model for the computer, working to understand how learning occurs in the passage from hands to object and back.

Materializing the Virtual Patient

Traditional methods of practicing surgical technique outside the operating room include suturing bananas and other natural objects, practicing on rubber and plastic mannequins, and performing procedures on cadavers. All are used in practice, but they have limitations. Bananas bear some tactile resemblance to skin, but the analogy to surgery ends there. Mannequins are expensive and wear out quickly. Cadavers require the presence of an anatomy laboratory and staff, who must maintain a willed-body donation program, an expense many medical school administrators want to reduce.[1] A procedure can only be performed on a cadaver or a rubber model a few times before it falls apart.

Medical technology researchers are building two types of computerized simulators: physical simulators, in which a mannequin with sensors represents a human patient's body, and virtual-reality simulators, in which a graphic creation existing entirely in the computer models the patient's body.[2] Virtual-reality simulators, which are the focus of this chapter, hold promise for teaching skills, such as cutting, that would rapidly destroy a mannequin.[3] Researchers cite several reasons for adopting such simulators. Unlike dissection, simulation is reversible—the computer can be reset—so students can practice as often as needed to acquire a skill. The computer also can track student progress and, ideally, suggest corrective measures, which may help students master good technique. Designers also argue that the adoption of simulators will allow beginning trainees to learn some basic skills before working on patients in the operating room, ideally reducing operating-room errors.[4] Further, medical education reformers want to use simulators to ensure that surgical trainees get more systematic practice with many procedures (Satava 2008, 147). An influential Institute of Medicine report recommended the widespread adoption of simulation as a means of teaching practices that can reduce medical errors (Kohn et al. 2000). Simulator makers also are discussing their technologies with specialty certification boards, which could add a skills test on a simulator into existing qualifying exams. Extending the networks of simulation supporters to specialty boards might ensure simulators' adoption by medical schools, their use by trainees and, ultimately, their success (see Latour 1987, 1990).

Most virtual-reality simulators are designed to teach minimally invasive surgical procedures. There are three reasons for this. First, the navigation of an operative site via the mediation of a monitor that takes place with minimally invasive surgery is the inspiration and motivation for building virtual-reality simulators. Second, minimally invasive procedures require surgeons to work over a fulcrum (just as the oars of a rowboat are used over the fulcrum created by the oarlock) in a three-dimensional space that is represented in two dimensions. Because of these perceptual shifts, minimally invasive procedures require more practice to learn than open procedures. Third, open surgical procedures are more difficult to simulate, and students and residents can practice many skills of open surgery on ordinary objects. Many virtual-reality simulators are prototypes and, though some commercial systems exist, their adoption by medical schools has been slow. The expense and technological challenges of simulators make their future uncertain.[5] Simulator designers themselves often say their creations do not "feel right," but the more important questions are whether simulators provide good enough feedback to help trainees develop the muscular gestalt of surgical action and whether clinical curricula can be revised to incorporate them in training programs.

Because minimally invasive surgical action already takes place on the monitor, the move to simulate these procedures is easier than with open surgery. Although efforts exist to simulate open surgery, surgeons often use their hands directly inside the body when doing open surgery, which would be more difficult to simulate than surgery with instruments. And minimally invasive surgery involves more kinesthetic than tactile sense, making the provision of haptic feedback easier. Simulating surgery also takes advantage of a feature of all surgeries: the operating field is separated from the rest of the patient's body, which usually remains covered with sterile drapes (Hirschauer 1991, 299). A simulated patient represented as a fragmented body part on a computer monitor resembles the surgeon's visual experience of the operating field more than one might imagine.

The virtual-reality system requires a user, graphic models of patient body and surgical tools, an interactive device designed to look and act like the surgeon's end of an instrument, and two computers, one to manage the haptic device, and another to run the simulation. Making the system work requires definition of how these components work together. Materializing tools and bodies in cyberspace requires what are, in effect, three feedback loops that make up the interaction between user and model. The first—or virtual—feedback loop defines the interaction between instrument tips and model body as the model responds to the instruments and, in turn, provides haptic feedback to the user. This is the domain of computer modeling. Researchers—programmers and surgeons—wrestle with this question: How can we create a graphic and physical model to interact with the instrument? The second—or mechanical—loop describes the interaction between the user's hands and the instruments as the instruments respond to user and model. This is the domain of mechanical engineering research, which aims to answer another question: How can we ensure that our device works properly—feeding correct haptic information to the virtual world and back to the user's hands? The third—or embodied—loop connects the user's intentions to the user's hands, while hands and device interact. The embodied loop represents the domain of haptics research, and this question predominates: How do bodies learn, and how do tactile and kinesthetic actions lead to craft skills?

Each of the feedback loops that describe the interactions of user and simulation represents a research area among simulation experts. Each research area requires a mathematical description of the virtual patient's and the material user's bodies as they interact with the simulation. Though I describe these loops as independent entities and though, at Coastal, they represent somewhat independent research projects, the goal is to build a simulator from this complex assemblage of hardware, software, and expertise that can provide a visual and physical experience similar enough to performing surgery to help the student learn. Each of the simulator's components defines the relationship between model and user slightly differently, but together they should give the user a seamless experience of surgery.

Modeling: Constructing the Model Patient's Body

The laboratory's laparoscopic simulator contains a model of the female pelvis built from ninety-five photographs of cross sections of a female pelvis. The sections came from a thirty-two-year-old woman who donated her body to the university before she died. Anatomists froze the woman's pelvis and shaved sections off the frozen block at two-millimeter intervals. As they exposed each section, they took photographs that eventually were digitized and made available to other researchers for use. Anatomists have used these kinds of techniques to cross-section anatomical specimens since the mid-nineteenth century. Though initially developed for embryological specimens too small for traditional dissection methods (Hopwood 1999), cross-sectional anatomy later became a means of correlating anatomy with radiological images. More recently, anatomists have used these techniques to develop image databases (like the female pelvis) suitable for graphic modeling. The adoption of century-old techniques for computational purposes begins to reveal the number and complexity of techniques and technologies enfolded in simulators.

Dr. Harry Beauregard used the collection of cross-section photographs as the foundation for Coastal's virtual-reality simulator. He spent more than a year examining each digital cross section, which he calls a "slice," then tracing the structures he wanted to model into files using an early version of PhotoShop, a commercial image-manipulation application: each file contained one cross-sectional image. He described this process, known as "segmentation," simply as "drawing circles" around each structure he wanted to model and saving the contents of each "circle" as a "mask" with its own computer file.

> I would make a mask, and I would put it in the muscle file. And I'd make a mask and I'd put it in the bone file. And then I'd go to the next slice, put the bone in the bone file. Next slice. And so I ended up with all of these files that had individual masks, and then we took the software . . . and made models from those masks.

Harry initially segmented only the reproductive system, leaving the six pelvic bones and many muscles as undifferentiated aggregates labeled "bone" and "muscle," respectively. Subsequent iterations differentiated pelvic bones and muscles and added less critical features, such as fat. Later, Dr. Ramesh Chanda segmented the bones and muscles. They produced twenty-two hundred masks from the ninety-five cross-section slices encompassing the female reproductive system and the surrounding musculoskeletal system. Segmentation includes several of the "transformative practices" that Michael Lynch identifies in relation to model making, including "upgrading" the images by making strong borders between tissue types and "defining" the images by sharpening contrasts (Lynch 1988, 160–61). Modelers do not segment cross sections to make them legible to human eyes. Rather, anatomists segment cross-sectional images to create outlines that can be integrated into computer-modeling programs, that is, to articulate cross sections for computers.

The division of labor between Harry and Ramesh occurred because each physician had a different area of anatomical expertise. Ramesh compared the difference between Harry's anatomical expertise as a gynecologist and his own as a hand surgeon to geographical knowledge of highways and interstates in the San Francisco Bay Area:

> I think it is a question of with what granularity you look at [the body], with what amount of detail. To try to give an analogy, it's like . . . a map. If you look at a map, say you're looking at the map of the Bay Area, and it's an overall map, and you say, there's [U.S.] 880 and there's [U.S.] 101, and you have a fair idea of the map, and that's your basic anatomy. But now if you want to know about Palo Alto, then you need to zoom down. Oh, there's El Camino, and there's this, and there's this. So now you know a little bit more detail there. It hasn't changed your 880 and 101 knowledge, which is over the Bay Area. . . . So, if you're talking about the radial nerve, if someone doesn't have to deal with the radial nerve surgically, they have an idea, OK, the radial nerve comes from there and goes there. But the finer bends and curves only somebody who is dealing with it would know.

Surgeons and anatomists often analogize human anatomy to a map, for example, by describing anatomical features that help them navigate as "landmarks." But the analogy misses several complexities inherent in anatomical segmentation. First, cross-sectional images of the body have no labels to guide the surgeons as they segment. Second, though some radiological images, notably computerized tomography, are cross sections, surgeons rarely see actual bodies in cross section, so interpreting cross-sectional images requires extrapolating from a two-dimensional section to the three-dimensional body: the equivalent, perhaps, of reading a map of the Bay Area from a diagram of its geological strata.[6] The level of anatomical knowledge required to segment one female pelvis also speaks to the specialization of surgical-anatomical knowledges and to the difficulty of producing a comprehensive model body.[7] The anatomical body, even in a partial area, such as the pelvis, required digital articulation by specialists from two surgical disciplines. This is an example of Annemarie Mol's "body multiple" (2002): the female pelvis is a single, albeit complex, anatomical region that, in surgical practice, can be a gynecological pelvis, an orthopedic pelvis, a vascular pelvis, and more. Anatomical terms and structures are a fundamental medical epistemology, knowledge that, at a general level, all biomedical physicians can assume they share. But human bodies have far more structures, systems, bends, and folds than even senior anatomists can master in a lifetime. A multiplicity of practices brings different areas of an anatomical region into being.

Up to this point, medical experts—the two surgeons—did the work of delineating body parts. The next steps multiplied the body in another realm of practice: the world of computer modeling, a subspecialty of medical informatics. A computer-modeling student took the segmented masks and computationally stacked them to create models of organs, muscles, bones, and other features (just as stacked slices of bread create a loaf). To connect cross sections into a surface model, the student transformed stacked outlines into a "mesh," a digital, mathematically generated net that mapped the model's surface. A digital mesh resembles a nylon stocking that has been stretched over a body part. Modeling using this technique takes advantage of a digital photograph's resolution into pixels. Once the two surgeons outlined the structures to be modeled on the two-dimensional cross sections, the student wrote computer algorithms to connect the outlined pixels across adjacent cross sections, articulating physiological geometries for the computer. These connected pixels formed a mesh conforming to each structure's surface. Because this model is made of both graphic pixels and the mathematical mesh, the model body is simultaneously a graphic and a mathematical construction of a body—a model that a human user can manipulate in ways the computer can calculate. These graphic models are "silicon second natures," digital artifacts that reproduce natural objects, but also offer to replace them as resources for learning and research (Helmreich 1998, 11–12).

Harry, who spent eighteen months doing the first segmentation of the female pelvis, described the first time he saw the reconstructed uterus made from the masks he drew:

> The thing that blew me away was not what I expected to see, but what I hadn't expected to see, and that is where the utero-sacral ligaments attach to the cervix and support the uterus in the pelvis. There are a couple of little bumps, little sharp points there where those take off that I could see [on the model]. And, of course, that relates a lot to my surgery, which is on those ligaments where endometriosis occurs. So many laparoscopies I did finding endometriosis on those ligaments and in the region of the pelvis that I was so drawn to the image. There they are. And I could see them.

Harry described the process of drawing outlines of structures on cross-section photos as a process of abstracting the human body's complexity and specificity into circles (outlines of structures) placed in computer files. But when the model came together, the resemblance of the model uterus in the computer to an actual uterus surprised him; all those tedious months of drawing circles had produced a model that looked like a uterus. The utero-sacral ligaments depicted on the model looked like ligaments he had operated upon.

By drawing outlines of anatomical structure that could then be computationally stacked, Harry and Ramesh were able to reassemble the pelvis in the computer. Modeling transformed the photographic cross sections into a neat, three-dimensional model uterus that had already had fat dissected away, in other words, a graphic model that resembled a pelvis that an anatomist had already sculpted into a pelvis suitable for anatomical imaging. Harry and Ramesh planned to later segment fat and other missing tissue to more accurately reflect the body a surgeon encounters. Using a computerized drawing pen instead of a scalpel, Harry articulated a model body that inhabited the computer. The model body then affirmed for Harry that this computational procedure represented his experience and produced a tool he considered adequate for teaching surgical practices to simulation users.

The digital pelvis is a laboratory object, a model of the original object (in this case, a human body), detached from its natural environment, and no longer beholden to the original's temporality (Knorr Cetina 2000, 27). Unlike a living or dead human body, the model body can travel through a computer network, can be pulled apart and put back together, and can be modified to reflect pathologies, all without causing it harm. The model body resembled a Latourian "immutable mobile," in its "mobility, stability, and combinability," but it relied upon a computer for its existence (Latour 1986, 7). Though highly mobile, it could only exist inside its computational environment. The body becomes a body object, a digital reconstruction of the original, designed so humans and computers can work with it. Though mobile, educators could only use the model in this state for teaching anatomical structures.[8] It was visual, but it could not yet interact with the user as a material body would. It was not yet a patient, and it was not yet prepared for surgery—even virtual surgery—because surgery, at its most basic physical level, involves interactions of bodies and instruments.

Before the model pelvis could become a "patient-on-demand," it had to become responsive to surgical action. In Latourian terms, it had to become articulate, or able to be "moved, put into motion by other entities, humans or non-humans" (2004). To put the model pelvis into motion, a programmer named Patrick Flynn added algorithms to the model to describe how tissues would stretch, separate, or come together—that is, how tissue would deform —when pulled, cut, or sutured. Patrick began with the mesh structure of the surface model and defined the lines connecting points on the mesh as springs. Pulling on any point of the virtual mesh would cause the surrounding virtual springs to stretch, "deforming" the model according to well-defined physics equations that describe the resistance of springs. Spring-based deformations effectively reproduce the small, relatively slow movements of tissue that are common in surgery (more dynamic action requires different equations). Stiffer springs lead to tougher-feeling tissues. Patrick articulated the body's ability to be moved by surgical instruments as the movements of springs, making these movements calculable by the computer. The physical forces a surgeon applies when prodding or pulling a body part were articulated as the forces of pushing on springs. Flesh became mechanical.

To set values for spring stiffness, Harry and Patrick approximated the feel of pelvic tissues, trying to encode Harry's physical memories, which he called "haptic memories," of the feel of performing surgery on various tissues. Harry expressed his haptic memories in terms of his sense of differences among tissues and his sense of the feel of a particular tissue.[9] To develop the haptic program, Harry and Patrick created algorithms that attempted to represent Harry's physical experience in a form the computer could use. To do this, Patrick had to learn something about surgery. He learned the physical differences between structures in a woman's reproductive system. He also learned some terminology of anatomy and surgery. Once he had developed an algorithm to describe differences in how tissues feel, Patrick also had to describe Harry's actions. He said he created a description of "how the world works" at a deeper level than typical surgical instructions to cut, clamp, or suture by putting data-capture gloves on Harry's hands while he worked and then letting the computer map his motions as a continuous stream of forces acting on the model. In effect, the computer made equations to describe the movements behind each surgical action.

Articulating digital bodies for the computer also can lead to fascinating verbal articulations. During a demonstration, Harry ran into a technical glitch. He could not feel any resistance coming from the virtual tissues. Patrick tried to describe to Harry how the uterus should feel:

> Hey, do you want me to reset your uterus there? . . . Do you want me to bump up the stiffness so it behaves like muscle? Now it's behaving like a thin skin. I think that's something I learned from you: that the uterus is basically like a tough muscle. Now it's behaving like a thin skin.

The idea of "resetting" comes from computer science and shows how the conceptual vocabulary from that discipline contributes—sometimes awkwardly—to defining the body in the world of virtual anatomical modeling and surgical simulation. Patrick described what he had learned from Harry about how tissues feel. Mathematically, he attempted to approximate Harry's bodily experience, which usually remains tacit, into spring equations.

Traditionally, surgeons understand the toughness or delicacy of tissues in their bodies and might communicate the feel of a particular tissue to a student as a general warning about the potential to harm delicate tissue, such as a warning that damaging or cutting a nerve during surgery could be a "million-dollar [malpractice] injury." Harry's understanding of tissue feel came from years of practice. Constructing a quantitative model of a patient body's physical response to surgery only becomes necessary when the knowledge moves from body to computer. To prepare the model body for surgery, Patrick had to make it capable of responding to surgical action by making it deformable. This is the type of "mathematical construct" that Sonja Vidal, the group director, referred to when she said that knowledge that once was primarily experiential must become mathematical when translated into a computational idiom. Patrick and Harry articulated the feel of the model body's movements in relation to Harry's bodily experience by translating it into algorithms. In turn, they expected the differences in tissue feel incorporated into the model to make trainees' bodies articulate; the encoded differences were designed to help students learn the feel of model bodies, feel that ideally would later allow trainees to move easily from simulated to material bodies.

How tissues feel when manipulated by a gloved hand can be described in words, but only using relative terms, such as "delicate" and "tough" (Pinch et al. 1996). Students can use these descriptions to guide them while they develop a "muscular gestalt," a feel for the effects of their actions on bodies. But the computer requires muscular knowledge of difference to be articulated as explicit mathematical values. Harry constructed differential values from his experience, and Patrick translated these into mathematical descriptions of tissue feel. The model's deformability does not, cannot, exist apart from the thing with which it interacts, in this case, the surgeon's body as mediated by instruments. Deformability is a quality of model bodies defined exclusively at their interface with other bodies. Values of tissue feel used in deformable models are products of the mutual articulation of bodies.

Interacting: Characterizing the User's Body

By making the virtual model deformable, programmers built the possibility of movement into the model body, but the model could not yet be put into motion by a user. The next key step in making the surgical simulator was to create a mechanical device to act upon the body. Because the user activates the device, which then acts upon the model body, the device becomes, in effect, a bridge from a body in the real world to a model body in the virtual world.[10] A bridge can take the form of several types of device, but ones I have seen share this feature: they all exist both on and off the screen. This existence in both worlds resembles many gaming devices, but medical researchers pay more attention to giving users a realistic feel for surgical interaction. The coupling of haptic action and reaction is tighter and more rigorously defined and is itself a unique research area. Coastal's gynecology simulator uses a two-handed, or "bimanual," device designed to mimic the feel and motion of instruments used in laparoscopic surgeries. The laboratory developed the device jointly with a commercial manufacturer of medical and videogaming devices. The device is a heavy metal box with two protruding handles. Each handle has a scissorlike mechanism at the end that allows the user to manipulate virtual instrument tips.

When a user turns the instrument on, graphic representations of surgical instrument tips—the patient ends—appear on the computer screen in the same space as the body model. A multiprocessor graphics computer runs the simulation. The computer uses a method known as "collision detection," which tells the instrument tips and model body to react when they enter each others' coordinate space (that is, when they touch). Collision detection is its own mathematical art form, becoming especially tricky when objects interacting in virtual worlds must deform, like tissues, rather than collide, like hard objects. Patrick told me that the simulator's first collision-detection algorithm tended to make the model body explode on contact, a less-than-desirable response from a simulator designed to teach surgical skill. Later iterations allowed slow-moving instruments to pass right through the model uterus (also undesirable). Exploding ovaries and ghost uteri reveal the precision with which the interactions of bodies must be defined. In videogame design, unintended effects often simply become incorporated into the fantasy world. But the pedagogical goals of surgical simulation require more mathematical elaboration.

Outside the computer, the surgeon's ends of the instruments resemble surgical instruments whose virtual tips move as the user moves the handles, giving the illusion that real handles and virtual tips are continuous. Closing the metal, scissorlike handle in the real world clamps the virtual instrument tips in the virtual world. When the user pulls the handle, the virtual tip and tissue move with it. The device acts in two directions. The bimanual device allows the user to perform actions on the handles that translate into action at the tips, which, in turn, act on the model body. The device also provides haptic feedback to the user's hands.[11] When users clamp the instrument onto a virtual ovary, for example, they feel a distinct snap as the instrument locks onto the ovary and resistance when they pull the virtual tissues. In reality, users are pulling on the physical interface handle; on the screen, the instrument tip retracts, pulling the ovary with it. Harry calls these actions "tool-tissue interactions," a phrase that redefines surgery from the actions of one person upon another to the interactions of tool and tissue.

Within the context of the mechanical feedback loop, the user's body emerged in relation to the haptic device as engineers designed the device and began to study how it operates in practice. Louis Gibson, a senior mechanical engineer, said that engineers and surgeons had lengthy conversations during the design process to resolve such details as distance between the handles and the range of movement the device should have:

> There was considerable debate from engineers like me who wanted to simplify things by removing some degrees of freedom, but surgeons argued you needed it.

Louis's comment captures in mechanical detail one of the most significant differences between engineering and medical ways of interacting with the world. Engineers favor simplifications that make calculation easier, whereas physicians insist that details matter. Each new capability makes the device more difficult to manage mechanically and computationally, but surgeons demand fidelity to surgical experience. Realism required that the device attempt to mimic not only the feedback of interacting with patients' bodies, a software design challenge, but also the spatial and tactile feel of instruments themselves, a hardware design challenge. Designing a device that could correctly interpret the signals received from the human user, execute the signaled actions, then feed the haptic response back to the user, gave rise to a fascinating problem: characterizing the human user's effect on the system. During an eight-hour meeting of laboratory researchers with Fred Phillips, an external reviewer and an expert in educational technologies, Louis and Sonja Vidal, the lab director, tackled the question of how to consider the user's body as it interacts with the device:

> LOUIS: We will have to do a study that accounts for variability among subjects.
> SONJA: When [our collaborator in Texas] uses [the device maker's] stuff, she's always complaining that she's not getting the kind of frequency response they claim it should have.
> LOUIS: The dynamic response slows if a human hand is holding the device.
> SONJA: It's like having a sloppy, wet mass holding the thing.

Human bodies, viewed here as research objects, create several challenges for investigators. Bodies are variable, that is, not all bodies affect the device the same way. In terms of this system, a hand, what Sonja calls a "sloppy, wet mass," is heavier than a device handle and exerts uneven forces on it. But the hand is "sloppy," meaning those forces cannot precisely or consistently be resolved into vectors, and "wet," meaning that simple physics equations describing the effects of forces of one object on another are confounded by the squishy nature of flesh, whose movements should be defined using equations for deformable objects, becoming altogether more difficult. In other words, users' bodies slow the device down in unpredictable ways, compromising its ability to faithfully transmit the sensations of interacting with the model. The collaborator in Texas articulated the device's response by performing repeated trials that characterized how it acted under many precisely controlled conditions. The research question became how to manage the effects of this "sloppy, wet mass" (or many, varied sloppy, wet masses) on the device's response.

In surgery, the surgeon's hands and tools, when they're performing well, are the unproblematic agents of surgical action. This is the essence of medical embodiment: with years of practice, surgeons learn to use tools as extensions of their bodies that can interact with the world in ways they could not do unassisted. But the effect of the surgeon's—or user's—body on the bimanual device and on the virtual simulation must be characterized mechanically and compensated for by the simulator, so that the interaction of cyberbody and material body feels like an interaction between two material bodies. The user's and the model body's ability to mutually articulate each other depends, first, on the engineers' ability to account for the resistance of hands to physical characterization. Bodies become a messy set of forces that trouble programmers', surgeons', and device makers' abilities to re-create a good enough feel of performing surgery on a live body. This requires articulating the user's body for the instrument and for the programs that control the device. Researchers must account for the sloppiness and variabilities of user's bodies so the user can properly articulate the model body and receive useful physical feedback. The user's body must be articulated for the device, so it can articulate the feel of doing surgery for the user.

Embodied Knowing: Integrating and Translating Skill

The embodied feedback loop—the work of perception and interpretation that occurs in the user's body—takes up the question of what we learn through our bodies and how sensations transmitted to the body are interpreted and learned. Sarah Hartmann, a physicist turned cognitive scientist, spent several years doing haptics research at Coastal. She conducted a series of experiments intended to elucidate poorly understood haptic concepts, such as the delineation of edges, which we use to understand our world through tactile and kinesthetic sense. She also investigated how many times a particular pattern in space must be repeated before the body learns the pattern. She wanted to better understand the role of physical learning in surgery. Improved understanding of haptic learning could help designers and engineers develop more effective devices, including surgical simulators. She summed up the research project as the attempt to characterize "somato-conceptual" intelligence:

> Haptic sensations are personal. I cannot tell you exactly what I feel. It's personal. It's felt by the touching person only. It's determined by the

touching forces. Each person exerts different forces. There's a different coefficient of forces for muscle, so we experience different things.

According to Sarah's definition of haptic cognition, material bodies become bodies that exert forces on objects and receive forces from those objects, an articulation of the body similar to the body articulated for the computer. This is no accident: scientists measure sensations as forces sent and received when bodies and objects interact. The conceptual definition of haptics reflects haptics as they are measured, that is, as the play of forces. According to this concept of haptic learning, physical experience becomes reduced to a set of forces exerted upon and received by muscle, so muscular forces interacting with an object determine experience and learning. Sarah's definition of haptic learning brackets the contributions of other types of experience—of affect, of cognitive and haptic memories, of procedural scripts, and of explicit instruction. These kinds of effects are difficult or impossible to quantify.

Studying the path from physical force to learning presents enormous problems for researchers. The problem gets redefined in terms of the forces transmitted to hands and the user's interpretation of those forces. During the same external review cited above, researchers tackled the problem of how to understand what happens inside the user's body:

SARAH: How do you make it so everybody feels the same thing?

FRED: It gets metaphysical very quickly. If we all touch the table, do we all feel the same thing?

SARAH: It's a bad question because you can't answer it.

FRED: It's a good question; it just shows you're not a philosopher.

SARAH: Yes, but as a physicist, I understand the question.

FRED: That's because physics and philosophy are close together.

Sarah's question begins from an assumption that simulator users should have roughly the same physical experience when they use the simulator. The question founders, however, on classical philosophical problems of representation: if builders assume that the simulator's job is to create a faithful representation of the feel of surgery in the user's mind, then the correspondence between how the simulator represents the feel of surgery and whether the user takes away an "accurate" feel of surgery become meaningful, and impossible, questions (Bergson 1998; Latour 2004; Mol 2002). Fred's comment about metaphysics shows that the possibility of shared physical experience rests on indeterminacies of bodily knowing that are resistant to investigation by scientific means. The physical forces of touching certainly can be examined scientifically, but how a user experiences these forces, and how the forces of touching get bound up with the user's previous experiences and other confounding factors make determining whether everyone *actually* feels the same things nearly impossible to answer. If the question about the relationship of haptic feel to user experience gets defined in terms of experience, then it becomes metaphysical, outside the scope of scientific investigation, because it gets deeply into the nature of mind, perception, and the individual interpretation of experience.

The group works neatly around the impossible metaphysics of touch, by finding that the problem, when redefined in terms of the interactions of device and user (the forces of touch), becomes available to analysis:

RAMESH: What is felt by the user? What is the force? What is the interpretation of force by the user? Is it possible to measure?

SARAH: Different surgeons would make the same interpretation when they feel the same lump.

FRED: That's as far as you can go. If everybody says it's a ring, you're in good shape.

LOUIS: Or 85 percent of them.

FRED: But if you want to get to their subjective experience, then it's the metaphysical problem. . . . You could frame it as a signal to noise problem. You can't guarantee the same experience for everybody. But if you can build enough signal into it so most people give you the same interpretation. . . .

SONJA: There may be various sources of signal. How do you know what they're telling you?

RAMESH: What in the brain it is, you can't measure it.

FRED: You know right where they are [as they interact with the simulator] and you know what they're interpreting.

This conversation reveals how the researchers constructed the surgeon-user's body so they could manage it. The user's body came into being in relation to the device when the researchers defined experience as a relationship of signal sent by simulator to behavior enacted by user. The group recognized that if it tried to answer the question in terms of subjective

experience, the result would be inaccessible to medical, cognitive, or engineering research. We can image brains, but not minds or experiences. What
a user senses through his or her body—the connection between forces on
muscles and descriptions of experience—resists scientific research. If haptic
knowledge consists of forces exerted on users' bodies and the interpretation
of those forces, then studying the connection between force and interpretation becomes very difficult.

To work around the interpretive problem, the researchers reformulated
the user's subjective experience as a question of consistency of interpretation or, in more scientific terms, reproducible results. They realized they
could not know what bodies experience directly or whether two people
experience the same sensations when touching the same object. They could
not know whether many users' internal experiences of touching an object,
such as a lump, are identical, but they knew that many surgeons would give
the same interpretation of that object. As Fred suggested, shifting the definition of haptic experience away from metaphysical questions about internal
experience—away from the body's physical and subjective insides—and toward the body's interaction with an object might allow researchers to elicit
consistent interpretations of that experience.

Defined as a body that palpates and interprets a lump, researchers can
study what a user's body knows. As engineers, however, they could go one
step further. They could augment the signal from the object to encourage
more consistency among interpretations. By defining haptic cognition as a
relation of signal to noise, they could ensure that the device would send a
strong enough message to the user's body that most users would give the
same response. By observing how the user interacts with the model, they
could begin to understand which signals are strong enough to provide a
consistent interpretation. This is the computational equivalent of building a
perfume kit. By making smells undiluted and highly differentiated, perfume
makers can teach beginning students to distinguish them (Latour 2004).
Similarly, by making a lump or a ring highly distinct from the tissues
surrounding it, simulator makers could ensure that most users would recognize it.[12] Doing so, however, would require understanding what kinds of
signals a user might respond to (what sensations tell users whether they are
touching, say, a kitten or a fish). This problem leads to new questions for
haptics research and new articulations of bodies as they interact with the
world through touch.

During this conversation, the pathway between the user's body and the ability to provide a consistent interpretation became, in effect, black boxed. It could not be mathematicized like a model patient's body or characterized like a device might be. Rather, haptics researchers constructed the user's body in relation to the signal the rest of the system sends to the user's body and the fidelity with which the user interprets the signal. The question is no longer what the body is, but how the body interprets action; the ontological body becomes the interpreting body. The challenge shifts from trying to characterize what happens inside the user's body toward understanding how to create a model body that surgeons are sensitive to in identical—or mostly identical—ways. Augmenting the model's signal could make the interpretations of experience more consistently articulate.

Vision, Touch, Embodiment

The simulator is an assemblage of hardware and software, shaped by researchers from multiple disciplines. Simulator research falls into three areas—modeling and deformation, interactive device making, and studies of haptic knowing. Research into each of these areas requires definitions of the model patient's body, the user's body, and their surgical relations. Within each research area, designers encode the physical connection between user and model as the play of forces on objects. Simulator makers make mathematical models of surgical actions that usually remain tacit, such as the movements a surgeon makes when clamping, cutting, or suturing, and the response of tissues to those movements. I have laid out how each of the three research areas articulates the user's body in relation to the simulated model body and vice versa. What remains to be done in this section is to consider some implications of mutual articulation in surgical simulator design.

At each stage of this research, designers articulate the user's body for the simulation system. The representation of Harry's physical experience that gets incorporated into the model shapes how the model reacts to users' actions.[13] Patrick defined the model body's resistance to surgical instruments in relation to Harry's embodied memories. Patrick and Harry designed the resulting algorithms describing the model's resistance using spring equations to shape future users' bodies. Engineers worked to tweak the haptic interface so it could compensate for the fleshiness of the user's body well enough that the mutual shaping of model and user could provide a meaningful learning experience for beginning surgeons. To do this, researchers studied many bodies so that they could incorporate a model of their variations into the device. And haptics researchers wanted to define what parts of physical interaction would be meaningful for learning by studying what happens at the interface of body and model. They reasoned that they could vary the signals the model would send to the user to elicit particular interpretations. The model's ability to articulate the user's body would be measured in terms of users' interpretations. At each stage of this research, the user's body was articulated in relation to the simulation system and vice versa.

The design of haptically enabled interfaces that feed sensory information to the user's hands makes the mutual articulation of the user's and the model's bodies apparent because the connection between hands and model must be carefully constructed. Technologically and physiologically, the link between the object's effects on the user and the resulting action is much tighter with touch than vision. Haptics researchers describe how touch differs from other senses: "Touch and force sensations convey information about the environment by that enabling action. Successful bodily acting requires 'touch and feel' information from the environment simply because, unlike any other sense, haptics (touch and kinesthetics) is not only a sensory channel to receive information, but also a channel for expressiveness through actions. The hands are both sensors and actuators, using sensory information to control their acts" (Reiner n.d., 2). The dual nature of hands—they are sensors and actuators—connects an actor to an object much more directly than does vision, smell, or hearing. Hands simultaneously perceive an object and act directly upon it. The effects of touch can be measured as effects on the object. Simulator researchers at Coastal wanted to design a model of tissue feel that could provide the muscular gestalt, or generalized embodied feel, which Dreyfus describes (1992, 249). To do so, they considered boosting the simulator's signal strength to make interpretation more consistent among users. With a simulated model body, researchers could study directly what forces users exert when cutting, clamping, or suturing tissues. Researchers also knew that they could observe exactly what part of the model would react to the body's actions, making the study of the connection between signal and interpretation more direct. Because hands themselves contain the means of both sensation and action, they embody mutual articulation in a way that forces researchers to place tight constraints on the connection between sensing and acting. Fred made the critical point about touch and cognition: "You know right where they are, and you know what they're interpreting." The hand, as a perceptual instrument that senses while it acts can make studying the interpretations that result from these perceptions and actions easier to study than other senses.

Simulator researchers, if they can make haptically enabled simulators work properly, can guide and enhance the student's tactile learning. Embodying surgical ability requires the expert guidance of senior surgeons. The intertwining of sensation, action, and interpretation can be constructed at an interface with an object as the ability of the user to articulate the model body through dissection and the ability of the model to articulate the user's body in terms of surgical skill.

The concept of mutual articulation for understanding surgical simulation addresses a problem that arises when discussing simulation. Latour's concept of articulation (2004) specifically attempts to avoid a world of subjects and objects in which a subject houses an internal representation of an object whose accuracy must be verified. In this chapter, I have avoided calling the simulation's visual and haptic signals "representations" because the language of representation would mean that the simulator would house a technological representation of surgery intended to help users create an embodied representation of surgery. This "second-order" representation would be impossible to verify as "accurate" because it would produce exactly the problem that Sarah, the haptics researcher, raised in the reviewer discussion: verifying users' experiences. Thus, the language of representation leads to metaphysical questions about reality and fidelity that are impossible to answer. Mutual articulation leads to a more productive solution by allowing one to consider the kinds of bodies that simulation research articulates and the questions about bodies and practice that unfold from those articulations. Though researchers argue about fidelity at every level of the process of simulator construction, they ultimately come to a similar conclusion by choosing to worry about what the user does with the simulator rather than what the researcher experiences. Thus researchers, too, avoid questions about what the user knows in favor of questions about what the user does.

With a simulated "patient-on-demand," students may have many more opportunities to practice surgical procedures when they want, as often as they want, and on as many types of pathologies as can be programmed.

Haptics changes the nature of the interaction from viewing and perhaps acting upon the body with a mouse to *feeling* the cyberbody react. The incarnation of cyberbodies that can provide haptic feedback will make these interactions bodily in ways unlike earlier computer technologies, undoubtedly with implications for other fields in which haptic interactions are important. Haptics research, as a field that studies how hands learn, can reveal how bodies mutually shape each other. Additionally, information gathered from research into modeling, deformation, mechanical haptic interfaces, and physicians' embodied practices contributes not only to simulator research, but also to the development of future medical and surgical technologies, such as radiological modeling, surgical planning, remote surgery, and surgical robotics.

At each point in the creation of the surgical simulator described here, researchers pooled various disciplinary knowledges of anatomy, surgery, computation, education, cognition, and engineering to develop objects (models, software programs, devices) that have carefully defined relationships to the user's body. Researchers also created interpretations of what human bodies are in relation to these objects; they articulated the body in new ways. These technological practices for reconstructing human bodies and interacting with them are multiple but not unconstrained. The simulation must be relevant for the medical student. It must work as a teaching tool. To succeed, simulators must not only articulate patients' and users' bodies as they relate in surgery, they must also help incorporate knowledge of those relations—surgical skill—into the student's body.

Conclusion

Ted Porter (1992) argues that the highly formalized languages of mathematics are more mobile than other kinds of languages but that humanists are widely suspicious of them. Humanists' suspicions often reflect the difficulties that formal languages have of capturing what is situated and contingent—and therefore unquantifiable—about human activity, including values, ethics, affects, as well as unexpected phenomena that emerge from new interactions (see Suchman 1987). For simulators, patient bodies are pixels, surgeons' bodies are forces, and surgery is the play of forces on pixels. The interplay of forces erases what is social, contingent, and affective from the labor of surgery. The erasure of social context in surgical simulation may not pose many difficulties for medical educators: supporters suggest that simulators could speed up trainees' learning, allowing them to arrive in the operating room better prepared to start practicing. They like to argue that patients probably would prefer to be treated by trainees who had received some simulated practice rather than those with no practice at all. Trainees would thus get a head start by developing some technical skills using a simulator. The relational and contingent aspects of surgery would come later.

One aspect of the shift to simulators bears further exploration: simulators change the nature of practice. One form of practice, the dominant form of practice in medical education, entails engaging in one's profession or exercising one's skills in the pursuit of that profession. This is practice within a milieu, learning the technical and social requirements of working as a professional. This kind of practice is precisely what the simulator cannot encode. The second, and different, definition of "practice" is to exercise oneself, pursuing a skill to require or maintain proficiency. This definition of the word puts the emphasis on mastering the skill rather than on working within a sociotechnical context. These are not hard distinctions: learning to practice a profession, especially in medicine, requires mastery of many skills that, as I argued earlier in this book, accumulate and aggregate within the cultural context of medical work to become part of the embodied professional known as a physician. Simulators place more emphasis on skill-building aspects of surgical learning. This may be appropriate. Pianists, for example, practice scales, compositions, and difficult passages for hundreds or thousands of hours before performing. But the focus on technical practice begs for further explication of those aspects of surgical performance that cannot be encoded in a simulator.

CONCLUSION

New technologies can change the nature of practice, perception, and experience, but their effects depend on how they become incorporated into a social milieu. Since the turn of the twentieth century, physicians have received training by doing clinical work in teaching hospitals, acquiring skills and values from those with more training and experience, gradually embodying the perception, affect, ethics, and judgments of physicians. Administrators, insurers, and practitioners have argued for decades that this system of situated medical learning is inefficient, requiring time, labor, and resources that harried hospital staff increasingly lack. Further, they argue, trainee development can be highly contingent upon the skill and interest of individual physicians or clinical groups.

In response, curriculum reformers and technology developers want to retool clinical apprenticeships by making training more systematic and more standard in the hope that all practitioners will receive the education they need to provide adequate care. They are working to build new training systems around simulators that can act as "patients on demand," artificial bodies that trainees can practice upon whenever they want and as often as they need to hone their skills. Simulators thus promise to become essential components in teaching programs that require trainees to develop competence with specific tasks, filling in gaps left in clinical education. Yet the concept of the patient-on-demand and the new training regimes proposed for it often neglect ways in which medical embodiment forms part of a larger acculturation that takes place within a highly structured milieu and entails lessons that go far beyond the technical skills a simulator can teach.

Surgical trainees have long honed basic skills, such as knot-tying, by practicing on objects such as bedposts and drawer handles. But the embodied lessons, such as maintaining control to limit harm, which surgeons repeatedly reinforced in clinical activities that I observed, reflect a situated and culturally specific form of education that differs from the drill-and-assess methods promoted by simulation proponents. Here, I recount one example from my own experience to show the lessons that situated training can provide. The laboratory at Coastal University where I spent much of my time doing research for this book had an active haptics research program, investigating tactile and kinesthetic sensation as bodily experience and as an engineering challenge for designers trying to virtually reproduce the haptic sensations of interacting with physical objects. I had taken an anatomy class, but, uncertain of my role as participant-observer, I had declined opportunities to dissect. Once I started researching haptics, however, I realized that I would have to experience the sensations of actual dissection to better understand attempts at digital representation of sensation.

The day finally came after Dr. Ramesh Chanda had given a demonstration of hand anatomy to a mechanical engineering class. Ramesh is a surgeon and anatomist who worked on simulator design and other technology projects at Coastal. During the demonstration, Ramesh and another surgeon had dissected a cadaver arm procured for the purpose of identifying hand and arm structures for the gathered group of students. After everyone else had left, Ramesh asked me if I would like to dissect. We had recently observed another surgeon do an ulnar nerve transposition, a procedure to move the ulnar nerve from its normal position in the elbow to relieve the pain of a pinched nerve. Ramesh was eager to try the procedure.

Technicians had placed the fleshy arm, which had been severed at the shoulder, on a dissecting table and shrouded its upper half in wraps intended to keep it moist. We unwrapped the arm, revealing a tattoo in faded ink. It said, "Vivien Leigh, 1944." Later that day, I wrote these notes:

> I ask if this would be a good time to cut. [Ramesh] says yes. . . . The arm is
> fleshy, fat even, and severed at the shoulder. Tattooed on the arm in blue
> ink with no embellishment is a name, "Vivien Leigh," and a date, 1944. I
> wonder at this date. Is this when the man whose arm this was had the
> tattoo made? Is it when he first saw Vivien Leigh? Is this a tattoo [that he
> got while doing military service]? Did he have a wife? What did she think
> when she saw this tattoo? I knock on the head of the humerus, which
> looks like the top of a white mushroom, but is hard and a little bumpy.

In the laboratory, I set aside my questions about the tattoo and focused on Ramesh's instructions. He showed me where to start the incision and how to proceed. I began to cut, and he promptly stopped me. I had begun to cut with the knife at the wrong angle to the skin: I should hold the knife at 90 degrees to the skin, he said, or the skin would tear more than necessary. I began again. The skin felt fibrous under the knife. The first cut was too shallow to penetrate the skin, so I cut again. Beneath the skin were several inches of yellow fat, which Ramesh instructed me to cut through. I gingerly sliced through the fat, which was greasy and unpleasant, but the knife sliced downward easily.

Evidently, I was moving too slowly because Ramesh took the knife from me and rapidly descended through the fat to expose the elbow. He kept dissecting and, finally, opened the joint and began to explore its interior. At his instruction, I reached into the incision, feeling the bony groove of the elbow joint. My gloved fingers touched something broad and flat that might have been the nerve. I remembered another surgeon's observation that large nerves feel like linguine. I ran a finger along the nerve's smooth surface. Ramesh then opened the incision further and moved the ulnar nerve out of its normal groove in the elbow. We were done.

The ulnar nerve transposition done in the anatomy laboratory is a good example of the kind of action a simulator might reconstruct: each action, from the angle of the knife to the pressure required to cut the skin to the sensations of skin and fat under the knife, is typical of a sensation that simulator researchers want to encode. One of Ramesh's colleagues coined the phrase "tool-tissue interactions" for various surgical actions, including dissection, an attempt to rework surgical language to more easily communicate surgical actions to engineers. But the phrase brackets many aspects of the interaction, aspects that I argue are vitally important for analysis of medical education.

First, what I learned during this experience went far beyond the haptics of cutting and the immediate visual perception of the elbow's structure. The tattoo opened up the social life of the man whose arm I was dissecting, even if it evoked more than it explained. The tattoo reminded me that this arm had belonged to a living, breathing person, someone who had lived a long life and who had, at one time, cared enough about a movie star to put her name on his arm. Repeatedly, I observed anatomy students finding evidence from a life engraved upon or hidden inside their cadavers. The discovery of an artificial hip joint or a pair of breast implants, for example, often led to questions similar to mine: Who was the person who inhabited this body? How did this person live? These moments, more powerful because they are surprising, connect body parts to human lives. Thus, they "activate the person," shifting the human body's ontological status from object to person (Strathern 2004, 8). The cadaver is no longer a living person who has animation and agency, nor is it an object that has never lived (Johnson 2010, 2). The cadaver is neither person nor thing. It is both and neither. The cadaver's ontological indeterminacy leads to extraordinary reflections by medical students on life, death, and medical work. Ideally, over the course of medical training, such reflections evolve into a nuanced stance toward cadavers (and, later, patients) that acknowledges their dual nature as persons and things. The too-common failure among physicians to develop a nuanced stance toward patients, their bodies, and their ailments reveals the difficulty of making these ontological distinctions and contributes to patient complaints that their physicians treat them as objects, numbers, cases, or body parts, but not as persons.

Second, after speculating about the man's life, I shifted to the mushroom-like quality of the humeral head. The passage reveals this as a movement from activating the person who had been tattooed to objectifying the arm by considering the hardness of the joint's bony surface. As I have discussed, objectification can be a means of creating distance from personhood. This distance can be an important tactic for patients and practitioners (see Lyon and Barbalet 1994; Thompson 2005). I was about to cut into this man's arm and felt some trepidation about the act I was about to undertake. But unlike a tattoo, a humeral head, though undeniably human, is part of a person that nonsurgeons almost never encounter and that likely evokes personal responses in very few people. It certainly did not for me. Scrutinizing the humeral head distanced me from the arm's personhood, just as the tattoo activated it. Like the surgeon who compared the tactile feel of nerves to pasta, I further distanced myself from the arm's humanity by likening it to a mushroom. I became curious about the humeral head as an object, not least because it was wider and flatter than I had imagined. This is an example of ontological choreography, the improvisational shifting from person to thing that is so common in medicine (Thompson 2005, 189). I created emotional distance by likening a body part to an object, a mushroom, whose thingness is unproblematic.

In the anatomy laboratory, medical students begin to embody an affective stance toward bodies by interacting with cadavers. Many anatomy programs use the cadaver's ontological duality—its nature as person and thing—to encourage students to objectify the body or activate the person as needed. The situated milieu plays a role in these tactical uses of objectification. The cadaver is objectlike when it is shaved, embalmed, and prepared for dissection as a laboratory object. Yet remainders of the person the cadaver once was, the tan line from a wedding ring or a missing appendix, bring the cadaver's former personhood into view. Further, the status of most cadavers as bodies that individuals choose to donate mark them as former persons with agency to decide their body's fate after death. The ability to objectify the body or activate the person can be emotionally adaptive when doing clinical work: practitioners and patients alike benefit at times from thinking of the body as an object. At other times, activation of the patient's personhood is essential when giving good or bad news to a patient, for example, or when speaking with the patient's family.

Even within the most sterile of anatomy laboratory environs, the life, death, and family of the former patient are never far away. Once, while unwrapping another arm intended for dissection, anatomists found a gold wedding band that hospital staff should have removed. They immediately stopped work. They then soaped the finger so they could gently slide the ring off, vowing to return it to the family. The group of anatomists and surgeons working on the arm exhibited a kind of sober concern that the ring be returned to its rightful owners and that the social order (which separates the cadaver-as-laboratory-object from its former life) be restored. Medical schools want to encourage this kind of concern among new students. Whereas the clinical environment and the need for emotional distance might encourage objectification (or even the black humor made famous by fictional accounts, such as Samuel Shem's *House of God*), important bodily markers of individuality, such as the ring, and memorial services for medical school cadavers reinforce the activation of the person.

The third significant component of the arm dissection was sensory: the visual, auditory, and tactile qualities of the interaction shaped my memories in ways unlike most instructional experiences I have had. Years later, I can still feel the sensations of the steel knife in my hand and the sensory differences between cutting skin and cutting fat, as well as the tactile differences among fat, bone, muscle, and nerve as they came into contact with my gloved fingers. These sensations are durably embodied, even though they have not been repeated, reinforced, or made routine as they would be for a medical student. Affect, too, plays a role in these memories. I can call up the sensations of, say, cutting chicken to prepare a meal, but the haptic memories are not as powerful, nor is the situation (the occasion, the room, its inhabitants) etched as indelibly in my memories. Further, cutting into human bodies is sanctioned and supervised in anatomy laboratories.

During this interaction, I wanted to properly dissect the arm, out of respect for Ramesh as a teacher and colleague and out of respect for the tattooed man who donated his body so others could learn. Anatomy students and teachers alike testify to the power dissection has to evoke strong emotions and extraordinary philosophical reflections. For me, the experience cemented my conviction that dissection is a powerful, multisensory means of introducing students to biomedicine's technical, affective, and relational demands. For medical students, dissection represents an intense first immersion in medicine's language, culture, and techniques of the body. Like dissection, biomedical practice contains both human relations and scientific understanding.

While cadaver dissection grounds medical students' early encounters with biomedical epistemology, surgeons build on sensations of examining and touching body parts to develop a perceptual syntax that allows them to read a body's structures and symptoms. This perceptual syntax builds from the assumption basic to biomedicine that disease results from biologically based pathology. Technologies like minimally invasive surgical instruments, cameras, and monitors maintain biomedicine's underlying biological assumptions, but they also have changed the perceptual relationship among bodies in surgery.

Minimally invasive tools depict the surgery on a two-dimensional monitor, flattening the body's spaces, but surgeons can maintain a relationship to the patient's body that resembles the relationships of open surgery by orally constructing the space in three dimensions, navigating body structures that come into view as the camera moves. Further, the camera's magnification of the body's structures changes the relationships of scale of surgeon and instrument to patient. The mediating effects of minimally invasive technology lead some surgeons to experience genuinely new perceptions, such as the feeling that their eyes are coextensive with a tiny camera threaded deep into a joint. By "placing" their perceptions inside the patient's body—where the action is—surgeons doing minimally invasive surgery reconstruct the relationships of hand to eye that occur in open surgeries. Virtual-reality simulators can help teach the physical skills, including working over a fulcrum, necessary to navigate a body depicted on a monitor. They might also help trainees experience the perceptual shifts that minimally invasive surgery can induce. But learning to navigate may be more difficult without verbal construction of the three-dimensional space of the sort I always observed among teaching surgeons.

In addition to experiencing the emotional effects of activating the person and objectifying the body, as well as the sensory effects of cutting into human skin, I also observed Ramesh's teaching, which provided the fourth lesson of the elbow dissection. Ramesh allowed me to make a mistake, then corrected me. Because this was a cadaver, not a living arm, I could not have harmed it. But Ramesh had long since embodied the ethical imperative to do no harm and he imparted it in every training interaction I have observed in which he played a role. I even saw him place a guiding hand on the hand of an inexperienced simulator user to show him how to properly dissect virtual tissues. Whether they were in an operating room, an anatomy laboratory, or a simulation center, Ramesh and other surgeons I observed taught trainees to limit damage when dissecting living, dead, or virtual tissues. Ramesh was neither harsh nor judgmental, but whether because I had begun with a mistake or because the stakes of cutting a human body seem high, the moment stands out in my memory more than other, more abstract teaching moments. Anatomists and surgeons alike, particularly those who are critical of reduction or elimination of medical school dissections or of turning to simulation, argue that the emotional charge of making a mistake while working with actual human tissue gives the learning experience more power.

I have often observed teaching by error correction take place during teaching rounds in the hospital and in operating rooms. For example, I began this book with an account of a slip of the knife toward the hepatic artery that could have endangered a patient's life. After Dr. Nick Perrotta, the attending surgeon, guided his trainee past the danger, he made a joke that revealed the professional stakes for the surgical fellow if he had severed the patient's artery. Surgeons often teach by letting the trainee stray just a bit. They then issue a timely warning and, when the danger is past, make a joke about the consequences of straying. By making trainees work at their limits, then by reviewing their mistakes, surgeons encourage trainees to embody techniques intended to prevent slips, techniques that range from continual repetition of anatomical architecture to bracing one's wrist to prevent the hand's natural tremor from interfering with one's work. This kind of teaching gives trainees the illusion of working autonomously. As trainees advance, the illusion of autonomy comes closer to reality. Technical skill thus becomes a critical component of the ethical imperative to do no harm.

Heavily supervised practices impress upon residents that they must continuously hone their skills to maintain bodily control and avoid doing harm to patients. Over time, skills become durably lodged in practitioners' bodies, developing into generalized dispositions to perceive, to feel, and to behave. In the operating room, close supervision by senior surgeons helps trainees develop control over their surgical actions. By working narrowly within a frame of perception and action that the surgeon constructs, the trainee can work at the edge of his or her ability to learn new skills. This closely supervised work includes continual verbal reinforcement of the values of control, as exemplified by Ramesh's instruction to cut the skin at a 90-degree angle to make the incision cleaner. Physical feedback and continual reminders—through corrections, jokes, and stories—about the need for tightly controlled action help the trainee embody an ethic of doing no harm.

Medical embodiment begins with the accumulation and aggregation of skills, especially as they combine with vast quantities of information medical students eventually must bring to bear upon clinical problems. By placing embodiment at the center of medical knowing, I have shown how actions and interactions with patients, supervisors, and technologies contribute to the construction of medical perceptions, affects, judgments, and ethics. I have shown the many ways that a biomedical *habitus* develops during the grueling years of medical school, residency, and beyond.

From the first cut in the anatomy laboratory, physicians learn their craft by imitating those more skilled and, eventually, by doing years of supervised practice in hospitals. They develop an affective stance toward patients by imitating supervisors, dissecting cadavers, and later, treating patients within situated milieux that teach them how to objectify bodies and address persons. Residents juggling long lists of daily tasks in the clinic steep themselves in the lessons of the hidden curriculum, positive and negative tacit messages about comportment, treatment of patients, ethical practices, and emotions that their supervisors might themselves struggle to articulate (Hafferty and Franks 1994; Ludmerer 1999).

The cadaver's former personhood, which gets repeatedly activated over the course of a dissection, makes it an emotionally and pedagogically powerful experience for medical students. Though cadaver dissection is a form of simulated clinical activity, the cadaver's former personhood continually reminds trainees that medicine involves interacting with and treating human beings. In contrast, a simulator can evoke the human body, but it cannot activate a personhood that never existed. Of course, activating personhood is not a simulator's intended purpose. Instead, it exists to provide an object to practice upon that can be reset when an error occurs and can be practiced upon until a trainee achieves technical mastery. In some cases, simulators also exist to activate the medical situation, such as a rapidly deteriorating emergency in the operating room. But the stakes of both uses differ from the stakes of dissection. Dissection activates the person both to help medical students come to grips with medicine's moral and emotional dramas and to teach trainees that keeping patients' personhood in play matters. Thus, dissection can help students develop multiple aspects of clinical practice, including mastery of dissection technique and anatomical structure, diagnosis of cause of death, and emotional grappling with death and with taboos against cutting into a human body.

As Dr. Ernan Tomaso, a physician and anatomist, told me:

> One important thing people forget is that, in the field of medicine, you deal with human beings. You deal with treating human beings. You're dealing with life and death. If all you're dealing with are cold holograms or plastic models, you lose that respect. If you're dealing with a cadaver, you're dealing with a real human body. That can translate later on, when you're treating real people. It helps you deal with human beings as human beings, rather than as objects.

Ernan argues strongly for cadaver dissection as a significant component in the development of medical compassion and a nuanced emotional stance toward patients. In contrast, the stakes of simulated practice involve the embodiment of medical techniques using teaching methods that are more easily standardized and assessed according to uniform criteria than traditional teaching in clinics, which relies more heavily upon assessments by individual teaching physicians. Further, teaching with simulators could fill in gaps left by clinical work that are more or less complete depending upon the contingencies of the patient population's needs at any given moment. In contrast to dissection, medicine's moral and emotional dramas remain far from this bureaucratized model of teaching.

The differing stakes of clinical training and simulated practice can lead to pedagogical confusions that reveal what is at stake in a transition from situated clinical teaching under the supervision of a master surgeon to a system involving simulated practice and bureaucratic assessment measures. Some lessons contained in clinical teaching have no simple analogue in simulated teaching. The second vignette with which I opened this book described a question that I asked three surgeons who also are simulator designers, "Is it OK to let your students kill the virtual patient?" Dr. Anna Wilson answered, "Of course. They're going to do it anyway." The response made Ramesh and Dr. Harry Beauregard uncomfortable. All three surgeons were accustomed to teaching in the anatomy laboratory and operating room, spaces where respect for bodies is paramount and instructors reinforce the imperative to "do no harm" at every opportunity. Killing the virtual patient posed an ethical dilemma for Harry and Ramesh, even though "killing" it could not harm it. One could simply reset. Indeed, proponents of virtual anatomical and surgical training cite this as a benefit of simulators because a trainee can practice until he or she perfects the technique. And the benefits of repetitive practice should not be underestimated. The technical and ethical guiding that teaching surgeons do was missing. This lack made my two surgeon friends uncomfortable. Harry, Ramesh, and Anna, despite their technology work, remained strong advocates for surgical teaching and supervision in the operating room. These surgeons' roles as teachers of surgery compelled them to teach not only the technical skills of surgical practice, but also the social and ethical behaviors appropriate for a surgeon. The discomfort Harry and Ramesh described makes perfect sense if the virtual patient is a stand-in for the living patient, as the cadaver often is treated, and if the virtual world stands in for the operating room. But Anna's comment, "They're going to do it anyway," contains more possibilities.

When Harry and Ramesh worried about letting trainees kill the virtual patient, they viewed the simulated body as a surrogate that could stand in for the patient. They argued that, as teachers, they would expect their trainees to treat the virtual patient as they would a cadaver, as a surrogate for the patient that demanded respect. According to their logic, both cadavers and virtual patients should be treated with a respect that could translate into respect for patients. Further, they argued for their role as teachers who help trainees embody the imperative to do no harm. Their role was to teach trainees the skills necessary to act on behalf of a patient's interests.

Anna, however, viewed the virtual patient as a practical tool for embodying technique that could be detached from its symbolic connections to the patient. Following this usage, the simulator becomes a training tool that could be utilized like other practice tools, such as bananas, which can be used to practice suturing. In this register, her answer becomes quite interesting. "They're going to do it anyway" has two meanings. First, trainees are likely to kill the virtual patient because they do not yet know what they are doing. The simulator would forgive beginners' "fatal" mistakes by allowing them to reset. In actual surgery, resetting is not an option; surgeons must carefully structure a trainee's actions to ensure the surgery's ultimate success.

The second meaning of Anna's statement is that trainees turned loose on a machine for which killing is a low-stakes activity might take it as an opportunity to experiment. Instead of killing the patient they are "killing" a virtual patient, a patient that can be reset for another try. Since such play can be treated as the manipulation of images largely detached from personhood, these activities become a form of exploration. According to this view, virtual patients are designed to teach surgical techniques, such as cutting, stitching, manipulation of tools in a three-dimensional space as depicted in two dimensions on a monitor. Thus, despite their constructed evocation of the patient's body, the simulators can teach technique in the absence of the social matrix of the operating room. Unlike cadavers, virtual-reality simulators do not act as surrogates for patients.

But Harry and Ramesh clearly wanted to treat the virtual patient as if it were a surrogate for the patient. I have watched them demonstrate their simulator, and they replicate their style of teaching in the operating room, even putting their hands over a user's hands to guide them to the right actions. Harry's and Ramesh's discomfort at Anna's response emerges from their belief that they must teach technical skills and ethical behavior to trainees. Allowing trainees to kill even a virtual patient would be an abrogation of that duty. For Harry and Ramesh, the question was whether the virtual patient as surrogate for the living patient would encourage enough attentiveness to the norms of surgical behavior that it could stand in for the patient to teach not only the techniques of surgery, but also the meanings and values of surgery. This is the form of teaching that surgeons master and practice. Anna argued that simulators might effectively teach surgical technique. At one point, she expressed hope that simulation would "speed the learning curve" in the operating room, saving precious moments under anesthesia for the patient and work time for the surgeon. But she imagined that trainees would treat it as an object for practice with much less connection to the patient than a cadaver: the simulator would create a space where they could explore what it would be like to kill the virtual patient without repercussions or recriminations. It is another form of exploration, one that has immense power, but it is not the form taken by traditional medical teaching.

The balance of medical interest seems to favor treating the virtual patients as surrogates for living patients. This approach drives research into instruments and, especially, into graphic modeling that seeks to ever more faithfully represent the patient. This search for computational fidelity seems to be driven by physician concerns about developing patient models and tools for interaction that might distance them too much from actual patients. Yet most plans for teaching with simulators suggest the second approach to training. Simulators tend to be located in spaces away from operating rooms. Trainees receive instruction in their use, but supervision typically is not the close oversight by surgeons that trainees receive in the operating room. In these simulator laboratories, trainees can practice techniques with little of the careful technical and normative guidance that teaching surgeons provide. Opportunities for killing the virtual patient are rife.

Pragmatically, I wonder whether clarifying the work that the simulator is expected to do—whether it provides a full-blown surrogate for operating-room training or provides a place to practice technique—might not make simulators more useful. Anthropologically, though, I am intrigued by the ways in which designers of medical training simulators seek to ground their flight into the world of images and models in the carefully constructed norms and behaviors of traditional medical practice, while simultaneously making it easier to extract technical practice from those same norms and behaviors. Concerns about whether trainees using simulators could stray too far from standard practices are expressed primarily as concerns about simulators' visual and haptic fidelity, but some part of these discussions reflects practitioners' worries that medical training might stray too far into the world of image manipulation and away from training to do no harm.

Technology designers have argued that virtual patients offer options to reset, reverse, and keep trying that neither cadavers nor living patients offer. If the virtual patient is solely a surrogate for the living patient, then an instructor's duty would be to strongly discourage the trainee from killing it on the grounds that "do no harm" is a moral imperative that cannot be transgressed even in the virtual clinic. If, however, the instructor takes the virtual world as a place where trainees can explore the meaning of a patient's death, including a death at their hands, then new possibilities open for instructors to explore the meaning of "do no harm" with their charges.

The development of virtual teaching technologies requires the articulation of relationships among bodies in surgery and among digital elements in the simulator. This requires the creation of objects, such as models of body parts and algorithms describing their motion. These objects then become replicable and mobile. They also can be made available for capitalization. This deconstruction of bodies, relations, and actions reveals the mutual articulation of the patient's and the practitioner's bodies in surgery, as patient bodies become crafted for surgical action while practitioners deepen their embodied knowledge of patient bodies.

Yet moves to extract medical teaching from the clinic shift the notion of practice from practice within a profession to practice of specific skills isolated from the larger milieu of clinical work, reified as significant components of a physician's skill set and privileged over other aspects of medical professionalism that are more difficult to isolate, such as the ability to provide compassionate care. While constant practice is important within medical apprenticeships, the repetition occurs within the structuring milieu of the clinic accompanied by the social, ethical, and affective lessons of caring for real patients. Disciplinary and bureaucratic styles of medical teaching, such as using simulators to isolate and drill skills or following evaluation criteria detached from the oversight of a specific surgeon, encourage trainees to practice procedures as often as necessary and with as many variations as necessary to develop an embodied mastery of its steps. Mastery of technical skill becomes its own goal, whereas most surgeons argue that it is only a small portion of a surgeon's abilities. The positive and negative moral lessons of the hidden curriculum become lessons to be learned elsewhere.

Clinical teaching as disciplined drilling and as situated practice are inter-mixed in many medical training programs. And each type of learning has its strengths. But when they come into competition, as they have in debates over dissection, the two sides tend to disagree about whether medical edu-cation should be exclusively about constructing technically adept practi-tioners or whether medical teaching also should encourage the develop-ment of humanistic values, such as compassion. These types of debates raise questions at the heart of what constitutes good medical care in the twenty-first century, such as whether compassion is vital to the healing arts or whether it is a desirable but ultimately unnecessary adjunct to technical expertise.

In places where virtual-reality simulators have entered surgical curricula, beginning trainees say they appreciate getting "a feel" for the instruments of minimally invasive surgery before they are called upon to use them in the operating room. But they also acknowledge that such practice gives only a modest boost to a beginner's skills. Simulated teaching could become incor-porated into situated teaching regimes, or it could become a core technol-ogy in a reconfigured disciplinary and bureaucratic mode of instruction. Thus simulators may become practice and assessment tools for surgical skills, routing verification of competence away from individual surgeons and into the simulator system. But another possibility exists.

The germ of another method of teaching can be found in Ramesh's and Harry's methods of training with a simulator. When they laid a hand on the user's hand to guide the user to correct practice, they were replicating the type of teaching that takes place in the operating room. It involves many of the relational aspects of traditional teaching, especially close supervision and guidance. Yet the stakes are very different. One wonders whether the imperative to do no harm can be embodied in a situation in which one truly can do no harm. Yet precisely this openness, this sense that old questions can be reopened and new ones can be explored, gives simulation research immense potential for future exploration of care, harm, control, and em-bodiment in biomedicine. The question becomes, then, not how faithfully new technologies replicate what exists now, but how they might open new questions and offer new solutions for medical care.

NOTES

Introduction

1. All first-year residents have already completed their M.D. This book uses pseudonyms for all actors, who I interviewed or observed. Occasionally, it uses real names when the speaker made a public statement, such as a speech or published document. To better preserve my informants' anonymity, I often do not locate them with respect to the hospitals where they worked. The differences between academic medical centers in the United States and Canada were small at this level of practice. I have tried to point out relevant variations where they occur.

2. Classical and modern versions of the Hippocratic Oath can be found at classics.mit .edu/Hippocrates/hippooath.html; members.tripod.com/nktiuro/hippocra.htm; www.indiana.edu/~ancmed/oath.htm; and http://www.pbs.org/wgbh/nova/doc tors/oath_modern.html (accessed August 12, 2008).

3. Embodied learning may be described in terms of cognitive science and mental models in part because of the relative impoverishment of language describing learning by bodily means. Learning by touch, hearing, smell, and other sensory modalities may simply lack vocabulary. However, I would argue that this strengthens my contention that a Euro-American cultural bias privileges sight and cognition.

4. Merleau-Ponty uses the term "perceptual syntax" (2002, 42) to argue that the perceptual field—those conditions that structure perception—must be constituted before they can become accessible to judgment. Similarly, I use the phrase to suggest that cultural assumptions and training structure a physician's perception.

5. Some scholarly work claimed that Joseph Paul Jernigan, the death-row inmate whose body became the Visible Human Male, agreed to the procedure to avoid death in the electric chair. This claim (see Csordas 2001; Van Dijck 2005) is false. Texas has executed prisoners exclusively by lethal injection since 1982. Jernigan's lawyer suggested that, although Jernigan had signed an organ donor card, he had no idea how his body would be used (Kasics 2003).

6. Although funding for medical care in the United States is dramatically different from that in Canada, far fewer differences exist at the level of training. Canadian and American surgeons regularly trade residents and fellows across borders, and important techniques are studied by all. I suspected that Canadian surgeons may

find it easier than their U.S. counterparts to decline to operate on terminally ill patients, though this suspicion would require more research to prove.

One. "A Fascinating Object"

1. I consider personhood from within the anthropological tradition most commonly associated with Marcel Mauss (1985). According to Mauss, the notion that the person equals the self is unique to post-Enlightenment European thought. European philosophers, beginning with Descartes, argued that the individual self is a unique stable entity. These ideas of personhood and individuality are not necessarily universally shared. The European notion of the individual as the paradigmatic example of the person gives meaning to the idea of the mortal human being. These ideas give meaning to European and American ideas about death and the body.
2. Thompson (2005) has said that objectification of one's body is a common phenomenon, but that it is used in particular ways in biomedical settings (Society for the Social Studies of Medicine, 2007 Annual Meeting, Montreal, Canada).
3. Although unclaimed bodies may still be used for teaching in the United States, the 1968 Uniform Anatomical Gift Act made voluntary donation the primary means of procuring bodies.
4. Evidently, the slogan originated with blood donation (Sharp 2006, 13).
5. United States law treats bodies differently from other material and intellectual goods; profiting from sale or exchange of bodies and their parts is illegal. Thus, persons can donate some body parts or donate their whole bodies after death, but neither they nor others can profit from the transaction. Some shady dealers have found their way through legal loopholes that allow recovery of expenses (Cheney 2004).
6. In practice, families have a great deal of influence over the fate of their loved one's body. Donors must sign paperwork signaling their desire to donate their bodies for research, but family members usually can override the wishes of the deceased.
7. Of course, the availability of older cadavers is greater. Younger ones, especially those who die from injury, more often are candidates for organ donation.
8. Frederic Hafferty describes a similarly strange postdissection experience as "passing cars became motorized coffins, piloted not by people, but by soon-to-be-cadavers" (1991, 81). The anatomy laboratory's ability to linger in the mind and senses in such strange ways reveals just how emotionally powerful these moments are.

Two. Cutting Dissection

1. My research primarily involved anatomists who argued for the value of dissection. These anatomists have convinced me that dissection provides students with an experience that includes visual, spatial, structural, and emotional components. As such, I favor the continuation of cadaver dissection in medical schools, but I also believe that digital anatomy teaching can provide its own important lessons.
2. Some anatomy departments have injected new energy into their research programs by becoming more focused on what might be called "applied anatomy,"

that is, anatomy that focuses on the informational needs of medical technology designers and bioengineers.

3. I also have heard biologists, who increasingly rely on computation as an analytical tool, argue that they must return to the "real" biology to open up new questions.

4. Anatomical terms drift a bit from discipline to discipline. For example, an anatomist told me that the apex of the lung is, for anatomists, a particular point at the top of the lung. In contrast, the apex of the lung for radiologists is a larger region in the same location. Nevertheless, even with this drift, the terms are close enough for most medical communication.

5. Death puns are ubiquitous among anatomists and medical students taking anatomy. In this setting, they become jarring.

6. This is the technology behind a number of anatomy exhibits that went by names such as Bodyworlds that toured the world around the turn of the millennium.

7. Ian Hacking describes George Berkeley's eighteenth-century theories of vision as an integration of two-dimensional vision with tactile perception to make vision three dimensional, that is, "we have three-dimensional vision only after learning what it is like to move around the world and intervene in it" (1983, 189). This argument resonates with more recent animal experiments in cognitive science indicating that physical exploration of an environment speeds the acquisition, at least in cats, of perceptual abilities (Varela 1992).

8. The Visible Human Male's body was the body of a thirty-nine-year-old death-row inmate named Joseph Paul Jernigan. Jernigan was missing one testicle and an appendix, among other features that made his body different from truly canonical anatomy. The Visible Human Female's body was that of a fifty-nine-year-old Maryland woman who died of a heart attack. Much has been made of the fact that she was postmenopausal when she died (Cartwright 1998). These details reveal how every individual body, no matter how close to a normalized ideal, reflects individual variations and life circumstances.

Three. Cultivating the Physician's Body

1. I recall a conversation between a senior resident and a resident just starting his third year. The senior resident described the third year as more enjoyable than the first two, not least because third-year residents begin to have more teaching opportunities.

2. Joan Cassell (1998) describes abusive training of female surgeons, especially in the 1980s, when she did her research. Her purpose is to show the gendered experiences of many female surgeons, especially the pioneers. Harsh treatment of surgical trainees has been a hallmark of surgical discipline. Such treatment also reinforced surgery's normative masculinity, not least by singling women out for harsh treatment.

3. Surgical residencies take an average of five years and can include a year or two of fellowship afterward that is designed to polish off a surgeon's skills within a particular subspecialty.

4. I discuss this further in chapter 6.

5. The lessons of the hidden curriculum bear some resemblance to tacit knowledge,

those aspects of practice that cannot be communicated by formal means. Tacit knowledge has an extensive literature in science and technology studies, but tacit knowledge has been most effectively deployed in studies of scientific replicability while attending less to issues of acculturation and embodiment (see Collins 1985, 1987, 1994a).

6. I discuss articulation further in chapter 7.

7. I have seen physicians engage in competitive banter about the differences between internists who "think" and surgeons who "do." I have even seen a veterinarian (another type of biomedical practitioner) defer to a veterinary surgeons' expertise in using his fingertips to palpate a lump, describing himself as a "thinking type" of practitioner. In doing so, he played down his own abilities by deferring to his colleague, while simultaneously taking advantage of Euro-American traditions that privilege those who work with their minds over those who work with their hands.

8. A few U.S. surgeons suggested that some treatment decisions are dictated not by their best judgment of needed tests and treatments but by standards of care dictated by malpractice and insurance issues. These physicians argued that these standards of care sometimes were excessive, leading them to perform unnecessary or unnecessarily invasive procedures because they did not want to be accused of having done something less than the maximum possible.

9. Ramesh is from India and went to medical school in India, then did a residency in the United Kingdom before moving to the United States. The ways biomedicine morphs when it moves outside North American and European settings are complex and beyond the scope of this book, but Ramesh was reflecting biomedicine's European cultural and philosophical traditions by separating emotions from rational thought.

10. Jerome Groopman argues that feelings for a patient—whether positive or negative —can be a factor in physicians' mistakes. He cited a case in which his dislike for a patient led him to tune out her complaints and thereby miss a fatal diagnosis (2008, 24–25).

Four. Techniques and Ethics in the Operating Room

1. Dr. Claire Wendland, personal communication.

2. Thomas Schlich says that anesthesiologists use a similar construction, calling their work "controlled poisoning" (2007, 236).

3. Medical ethicists have used "ethic of care" to mean how practitioners do their work, what motives guide them, and "whether their actions promote or thwart positive relationships" (Beauchamp and Childress 2009, 36). This medical ethical definition resembles the sense in which I use the term, but my focus is on the embodiment of such an ethic rather than its elaboration as an abstract principle.

4. A third type of surgical ethnography documents the effects of surgical interventions, such as organ transplantation, as they relate to sociocultural issues outside the operating room (Cohen 1999; Hogle 1999; Lock 2002; Scheper-Hughes 2000; Sharp 2001, 2006). These ethnographies represent important discussions of the

cultural issues related to life, death, and the prolongation of life for a few privileged individuals, often at the expense of less privileged individuals. My purpose
here is to examine ethics as they are constructed within the context of residency
training. Discussions of broader social and political issues that have surgery at
their center are outside the scope of this chapter.

5. Hirschauer says drapes provide a "situational focus" on the operative site (Hirschauer 1991). I believe this is correct, but I want to extend the focusing effect to
the operating room and its surroundings.

6. For a debate on the relationship of instrument requirements and ritual practice in
the operating room, see Collins 1994a, 1994b; Fox 1994; Hirschauer 1994; and
Lynch 1994.

7. Financial pressures are among the reasons that researchers are developing surgical
simulators. They hope to remove some aspects of surgical training from the
operating room.

8. Control at the end of a surgeon's career may mean the unpleasant acknowledgment that one's faculties are no longer adequate for the rigors of surgical practice.
This aspect of surgical life cycles merits a study of its own.

9. This particular surgeon practiced in a Canadian hospital, which likely means that
the factors he considers when deciding whether or not to operate differ somewhat
from factors affecting decisions by his counterparts in the United States. For
example, concerns about liability and insurance requirements sometimes compel
U.S. surgeons to operate. Canadian surgeons are not similarly constrained.

10. The use of hardware to surgically knit or stabilize bones is known as "osteo-
synthesis." For a history of this orthopedic technology, see Schlich 2002.

11. Carpal tunnel syndrome is a form of repetitive strain injury in which overuse
causes tissues in the tight space where wrist meets hand to swell, irritating nerves
in the same space.

12. Several surgeons I worked with lamented their residents' lack of preparation,
saying their surgical instructors expected them to review anatomy and procedure
before entering the operating room. They attributed the change either to changes
in residents' hours or to larger cultural shifts in trainees' sense of their own
responsibility.

13. "Spare parts" is a term I heard regularly in anatomy laboratories and operating
rooms to designate redundant or vestigial body parts that surgeons use to replace
damaged body parts. The term speaks to the mechanical view of the body common in medicine, particularly surgery (see Fox and Swazey 1992).

14. My thanks to Joseph Dumit for pointing this out.

15. This passage through the abdominal wall, found only in men, explains why many
more men than women get inguinal hernias.

16. Medical students often use sexual mnemonics to help them memorize anatomical
structures. One surgeon I know speculates that sexual mnemonics may be easier
to remember because they locate themselves in the same region of the brain that is
damaged when someone has Tourette's Syndrome, a neuropsychological disorder
that causes physical and verbal tics and, in some cases outbursts of profanity.

While this hypothesis is unlikely to form the basis of future studies, it does reveal the biomedical bias toward localizing phenomena in anatomy.

17. Putting surgery on a screen this way inspired developers to create virtual-reality surgical simulators with the hope that students would develop proficiency with the complex visual-spatial relations of minimally invasive surgery outside the operating room (Satava 1997).

18. My thanks to Joseph "Jofish" Kaye for suggesting that I observe whether surgeons or trainees bob their heads to get a better view while doing minimally invasive surgery.

19. The value of surgical stillness is one driver behind the development of robotic surgery: a robot will always remain perfectly still, will always perform an action in exactly the same way, will never crumple with fatigue, and will never develop a tremor as it ages.

20. While my presence in the operating room might have affected surgeons' displays of temper, their concentration on the problems at hand is such that I suspect that they often forgot I was there.

21. My thanks to Julie Livingston for suggesting I look more closely at the effects of jokes in the operating room.

22. Real-time comparison is one of the most effective teaching methods for revealing subtleties of anatomy and procedure. For example, a surgeon pointed out an arthritic joint to me, but I could not recognize the pathological nature of the joint surface until she showed me a healthy joint a few hours later. The arthritic knuckle was reddened and roughened, whereas the healthy knuckle was pearly white and smooth.

23. Studies showing a positive correlation between videogame play and surgical success have received recent attention in medical and popular literature in the past three years (Rosenberg et al. 2005; Rosser and Lynch 2007).

24. While individual expressions of surgical character vary widely, qualities such as decisiveness, confidence, and attitudes that could be considered "macho" are among the dispositions that surgeons develop, somewhat of necessity, through practice that requires rapid judgments about procedures that could have profound consequences for a patient's life or livelihood.

25. Medical students use "scut," an acronym for "some clinically useful training," to describe tasks that have no clear relevance to medical practice. These may include very low-level tasks.

26. "Control" as value and ethic has had much broader resonance throughout the histories of Europe and North America since industrialization, but this larger history must be localized in particular contexts to be meaningful.

Five. Swimming in the Joint

1. Minimally invasive surgery has not been an economic boon in Canadian hospitals because moving more patients through a single-payer system does not increase a hospital's billing.

2. The blind man's cane has a long history as a philosophical example, originating with Descartes and used by Heidegger, Merleau-Ponty, and Polanyi.

3. For a discussion of experiments demonstrating perceptual changes that occur with technological mediation, see Reeves and Nass 1996.

Six. Enterprising Bodies

1. Strathern does not mention *Star Trek*, but Haraway (1997) makes the connection.
2. The connections between flight simulation and surgical simulation go well beyond inspiration and include some technologies, as well as some logics of training, such as checklists and other training and practice protocols.
3. Although I have used pseudonyms for most actors in this ethnography, Satava is a well-known figure in the world of virtual reality in medicine, and I am drawing upon his public talks and papers, so I have chosen to identify him.
4. The history of uses of patient tissues and information suggests that practitioners are more likely to profit from the sale of data about patient bodies than the patients themselves (see Landecker 2000; Rabinow 1996).
5. Many medical projects built on informatics, including the Human Genome Project, a massive effort to map the human genome, have touted the promise that the development of massive individual and population databases will lead to new medical discoveries and the promise of treatments tailored to individual bodies. To date, the promises greatly exceed the results.
6. Virtual-reality systems designers eschew notions of artificial intelligence in favor of "intelligence augmentation" (Rheingold 1992, 37). For these designers, concerns about who might be in control of surgical systems should be resolved by creating machines that remain firmly under human, not machine, control.
7. Whether these reconfigured practices change women's experiences of pelvic exams is a worthy topic for future research.
8. Many medical schools hire "standardized patients," individuals who volunteer or get paid to undergo physical exams, including pelvic exams, conducted by medical students. Some of these standardized patients receive training in how to communicate with the trainee.
9. For example, a pair of Swedish gynecologists who had done some research with the simulators said the model uterus was too stiff to allow them to turn the uterus over to examine it completely, which is standard practice in Sweden but not in North America.

Seven. Anatomy of a Surgical Simulation

1. Anatomy programs also face competition from cadaver brokers, who provide bodies for various types of continuing medical education seminars. These lesser-known and sometimes questionably legal uses of cadavers have led to charges of illegal body sales against some medical schools and their employees (Cheney 2004).
2. A third type of visualization system, "augmented reality," seeks to put virtual structures and actual hands and tools in the same space, usually through the use of special screens and/or glasses. Augmented reality systems are not part of this discussion. The premise of surgical simulators most closely resembles that of flight simulators, in which students practice physical and cognitive skills, sometimes following simulated scenarios. Other simulations, of economic processes

for example, are primarily mathematical constructs that sometimes represent numbers graphically, but lack physical feedback.

3. The social challenges of incorporating simulators into traditional medical school curricula may be a challenge as great or greater than the technological challenges of building simulators; these social challenges include such questions as how to restructure curricula and students' time to accommodate simulation exercises. Simulation researchers now recognize the need for curricular reform to accompany technology design and have called for a broad overhaul of residency education that would put simulator practice at the center of a more standardized and rigorously assessed surgical education (Fried and Feldman 2008; Satava 2006).

4. Simulator researchers cite a report on errors in medicine by the Institute of Medicine (Kohn et al. 2000) as a strong justification for the repetitive procedural training a simulator can provide. See also Gawande 2002.

5. Since I began fieldwork in 2001, mannequin-based simulators, which are widely available commercially, have become the fastest growing area of the simulation market, though virtual-reality simulators still are in development.

6. One anatomist I encountered teaches students to check their knowledge of anatomy by attempting to label structures on cross sections. He says the ability to mentally "rotate" a two-dimensional image by 90 degrees and then label its structures indicates that the student has begun to understand anatomical terminology and the body's three-dimensional structure.

7. An anatomist who works on computer applications for teaching anatomy told me that research funding practices also stand in the way of creating comprehensive anatomical applications. Funding agencies will pay for new applications, usually limited to one area of the body, but claim that applying new computer technologies to an entire body is production work, not research, and ought to be done by the private sector. However, this anatomist claims, and others confirm, that most companies have found that the labor of creating a comprehensive computer body model is not worth the cost.

8. See http://summit.stanford.edu/ourwork/PROJECTS/LUCY/lucywebsite/infofr .html (accessed March 1, 2003).

9. The model is an ideal body: it does not take into account variations among patient bodies or differences in individual surgeons' tactile sense, though these are additions that simulator makers say they will incorporate into future iterations.

10. I do not use the obvious word "interface" here, though it is technically correct, because it has visual implications that I want to avoid.

11. Some experiments have been done with haptic interaction between two users in remote locations, but technically this creates a problem separating signals that are feeding forward from users' bodies from signals that are simultaneously feeding back to users' bodies. Human nervous systems have no trouble with this kind of "signal processing," but it remains a challenge for machines.

12. "Upgrading" (Knorr Cetina 2000) of a sensory signal is a common pedagogical method in medicine, in which physicians must learn to make fine distinctions among tissues. For example, an artist with whom I took an anatomy course discovered just how impossibly large her anatomical atlas had made tendons in

the wrist to make them legible when she tried to make her own drawings of the wrist. She realized that the tendons depicted in her atlas would not fit in a normal human wrist.

13. The gynecologist plans to incorporate values for haptic feel based on the experiences of many surgeons in a future iteration of the simulator.

REFERENCES

Adams, A., and T. Schlich. 2006. "Design for Control: Surgery, Science, and Space at the Royal Victoria Hospital, Montreal, 1893–1956." *Medical History* 1:73–94.

Balsamo, A. 1996. *Technologies of the Gendered Body: Reading Cyborg Women.* Durham: Duke University Press.

Barden, C. B., M. C. Specht, M. D. McCarter, J. M. Daly, and T. J. Fahey III. 2002. "Effects of Limited Work Hours on Surgical Training." *Journal of the American College of Surgeons* 195:531–38.

Beauchamp, T. L., and J. F. Childress. 2009. *Principles of Biomedical Ethics.* New York: Oxford University Press.

Becker, H. S., B. Geer, E. C. Hughes, and A. L. Strauss. 1961. *Boys in White: Student Culture in Medical School.* New Brunswick, N.J.: Transaction.

Berg, M. 1997. *Rationalizing Medical Work: Decision-Support Techniques and Medical Practices.* Cambridge, Mass.: MIT Press.

Bergson, H. 1998. *Creative Evolution.* Mineola, N.Y.: Dover.

Bosk, C. L. 1979. *Forgive and Remember: Managing Medical Failure.* Chicago: University of Chicago Press.

Bourdieu, P. 1977. *Outline of a Theory of Practice.* Cambridge: Cambridge University Press.

Braverman, H. 1998. *Labor and Monopoly Capital: The Degradation of Work in the Twentieth Century.* New York: Monthly Review Press.

Bucciarelli, L. L. 1994. *Designing Engineers.* Cambridge, Mass.: MIT Press.

Bynum, C. W. 1992. *Fragmentation and Redemption: Essays on Gender and the Human Body in Medieval Religion.* New York: Zone Books.

Carlin, A. M., E. Gasevic, and A. D. Shepard. 2007. "Effect of the Eighty-Hour Work Week on Resident Operative Experience in General Surgery." *American Journal of Surgery* 193:326–30.

Cartwright, L. 1997. "The Visible Man: The Male Criminal Subject as Biomedical Norm." In *Processed Lives: Gender and Technology in Everyday Life,* ed. J. Terry and M. Calvert, 123–37. New York: Routledge.

Cartwright, L. 1998. "A Cultural Anatomy of the Visible Human Project." In *The Visible Woman: Imaging Technologies, Gender, and Science,* ed. P. Treichler, L. Cartwright, and C. Penley, 21–43. New York: Routledge.

Cassell, J. 1991. *Expected Miracles: Surgeons at Work*. Philadelphia: Temple University Press.

Cassell, J. 1998. *The Woman in the Surgeon's Body*. Cambridge, Mass.: Harvard University Press.

Cheney, A. 2004. "The Resurrection Men: Scenes from the Cadaver Trade." *Harper's*, March, 45–54.

Christie, A. 2001. "Integrating Dissection." *The Connective Issue*. http://www.tuftsissue.com (accessed February 1, 2002).

Clarke, A. E., J. K. Shim, L. Mamo, J. R. Fosket, and J. R. Fishman. 2003. "Biomedicalization: Technoscientific Transformations of Health, Illness, and U.S. Biomedicine." *American Sociological Review* 68:161–94.

Cohen, L. 1999. "Where It Hurts: Indian Material for an Ethics of Organ Transplantation." *Daedalus* 128:135.

Collins, H. M. 1985. *Changing Order: Replication and Induction in Scientific Practice*. London: Sage.

Collins, H. M. 1987. "Expert Systems and the Science of Knowledge." In *The Social Construction of Technological Systems*, ed. W. E. Bijker, T. P. Hughes, and T. J. Pinch, 329–48. Cambridge, Mass.: MIT Press.

Collins, H. M. 1994a. "Dissecting Surgery: Forms of Life Depersonalized." *Social Studies of Science* 24:311–33.

Collins, H. M. 1994b. "Scene from Afar." *Social Studies of Science* 24:369–89.

Collins, H. M., G. H. DeVries, and W. E. Bijker. 1997. "Ways of Going On: An Analysis of Skill Applied to Medical Practice." *Science, Technology, & Human Values* 22:267–85.

Collins, T. J., and R. L. Given. 1994. "Status of Gross Anatomy in the U.S. and Canada." *Clinical Anatomy* 7:275–96.

Coy, M. W. 1989. *Apprenticeship: From Theory to Method and Back Again*. SUNY Series in the Anthropology of Work. Albany: State University of New York Press.

Csordas, T. J. 1990. "Embodiment as a Paradigm for Anthropology." *Ethos* 18:5–47.

Csordas, T. J. 1993. "Somatic Modes of Attention." *Cultural Anthropology* 8:135–56.

Csordas, T. J. 1995. *Embodiment and Experience: The Existential Ground of Culture*. New York: Cambridge University Press.

Csordas, T. J. 2001. "Computerized Cadavers: Shades of Representation and Being in Virtual Reality." In *Biotechnology and Culture: Bodies, Anxieties, Ethics*, ed. P. Brodwin, 173–92. Bloomington: Indiana University Press.

Das, V. "Public Good, Ethics, and Everyday Life: Beyond the Boundaries of Bioethics." *Daedalus* 128:99–133.

Daston, L., and P. Galison. 2007. *Objectivity*. New York: Zone Books.

Daston, L., and K. Park. 1998. *Wonders and the Order of Nature*. New York: Zone Books.

Deleuze, G. 1988. *Foucault*. Translated by S. Hand. Minneapolis: University of Minnesota Press.

Deleuze, G. 1992. "Postscript on the Societies of Control." *October* 59:3–7.

DelVecchio Good, M.-J. 1995. *American Medicine: The Quest for Competence*. Berkeley: University of California Press.

Despret, V. 2004a. "The Body We Care for: Figures of Anthropo-zoo-genesis." *Body & Society* 10:111–34.

Despret, V. 2004b. *Our Emotional Makeup.* Translated by M. de Jager. New York: Other Press.

Douglas, M. 1966. *Purity and Danger.* New York: Routledge.

Downey, G. L. 1998. *The Machine in Me: An Anthropologist Sits among Computer Engineers.* New York: Routledge.

Downey, G. L., J. Dumit, and S. Traweek. 1997. "Corridor Talk." In *Cyborgs and Citadels: Anthropological Interventions in Emerging Sciences and Technologies,* ed. G. L. Downey and J. Dumit, 245–63. Santa Fe, N. Mex.: School of American Research Press.

Dreyfus, H. 1992. *What Computers Still Can't Do: A Critique of Artificial Reason.* Cambridge, Mass.: MIT Press.

English-Lueck, J. A. 2002. *Cultures@Silicon Valley.* Stanford, Calif.: Stanford University Press.

Fadiman, A. 1998. *The Spirit Catches You and You Fall Down.* New York: Farrar, Straus and Giroux.

Fiege, M. 2007. "The Atomic Scientists, the Sense of Wonder, and the Bomb." *Environmental History* 12:578–613.

Fischer, M. M. J. 2003. *Emergent Forms of Life and the Anthropological Voice.* Durham: Duke University Press.

Fletcher, J. D. 2009. "Education and Training Technology in the Military." *Science, Technology, & Human Values* 323:72–75.

Forsythe, D. E. 2001. *Studying Those Who Study Us: An Anthropologist in the World of Artificial Intelligence.* Stanford, Calif.: Stanford University Press.

Foucault, M. 1972. *The Archaeology of Knowledge and the Discourse on Language.* Translated by A. M. Sheridan. New York: Pantheon.

Foucault, M. 1973. *The Birth of the Clinic: An Archaeology of Medical Perception.* Translated by A. M. Sheridan. New York: Vintage.

Foucault, M. 1977. *Discipline and Punish: The Birth of the Prison.* Translated by A. M. Sheridan. New York: Vintage.

Foucault, M. 1984. *The Foucault Reader,* ed. P. Rabinow. New York: Pantheon.

Foucault, M. 1986. *The Care of the Self.* Vol. 3 of *History of Sexuality.* Translated by R. Hurley. New York: Pantheon.

Foucault, M. 2005. *The Hermeneutics of the Subject: Lectures at the Collège de France 1981–1982.* Translated by G. Burchell. New York: Picador.

Fox, N. 1994. "Fabricating Surgery: A Response to Collins." *Social Studies of Science* 24:347–54.

Fox, R. C. 1957. "Training for Uncertainty." In *The Student Physician: Introductory Studies in the Sociology of Medical Education,* ed. R. K. Merton, G. G. Reader, and P. L. Kendall, 207–41. Cambridge, Mass.: Harvard University Press.

Fox, R. C. 1988. *Essays in Medical Sociology.* New Brunswick, N.J.: Transaction.

Fox, R. C., and J. P. Swazey. 1992. *Spare Parts: Organ Replacement in American Society.* New York: Oxford University Press.

Fried, G. M., and L. S. Feldman. 2008. "Objective Assessment of Technical Performance." *World Journal of Surgery* 32:156–160.

Fujimura, J., and M. Fortun. 1996. "Constructing Knowledge across Social Worlds: The Case of DNA Sequence Databases in Molecular Biology." In *Naked Science: Anthropological Inquiries into Boundaries, Power, and Knowledge*, ed. L. Nader, 160–73. New York: Routledge.

Gaba, D. M. 2000. "Structural and Organizational Issues in Patient Safety: A Comparison of Health Care to Other High-Hazard Industries." *California Management Review* 43:83–101.

Gaba, D. M. 2004. "A Brief History of Mannequin-Based Simulation and Application." In *Simulators in Critical Care and Beyond*, ed. W. F. Dunn, 7–14. Des Plaines, Ill: Society of Critical Case Medicine.

Galison, P. 1997. *Image and Logic: A Material Culture of Microphysics.* Chicago: University of Chicago Press.

Gawande, A. 2002. *Complications: A Surgeon's Notes on an Imperfect Science.* New York: Henry Holt.

Gawande, A. 2007. "The Checklist: If Something So Simple Can Transform Intensive Care, What Else Can It Do?" *New Yorker.* December 10, 86–101.

Gawande, A. 2009. *The Checklist Manifesto: How to Get Things Right.* New York: Metropolitan.

Geurts, K. 2003. "On Rocks, Walks, and Talks in West Africa: Cultural Categories and an Anthropology of the Senses." *American Anthropological Association* 30:178–98.

Gibson, W. 1986. *Neuromancer.* New York: Ace.

Goffman, E. 1961a. *Asylums.* New York: Anchor.

Goffman, E. 1961b. *Encounters: Two Studies in the Sociology of Interaction.* Indianapolis: Bobbs-Merrill.

Good, B. J. 1994. *Medicine, Rationality, and Experience: An Anthropological Perspective.* Cambridge: Cambridge University Press.

Goodwin, C. "Professional Vision." *American Anthropologist* 96:606–30.

Goody, E. N. 1989. "Learning, Apprenticeship, and the Division of Labor." In *Apprenticeship: From Theory to Method and Back Again*, ed. M. W. Coy, 233–56. Albany: State University of New York Press.

Gray, C. 2007. *Enterprise and Culture.* New York: Routledge.

Groopman, J. 2008. *How Doctors Think.* New York: Mariner.

Gusterson, H. 1996. *Nuclear Rites: A Weapons Laboratory at the End of the Cold War.* Berkeley: University of California Press.

Gusterson, H. 2001. "The Virtual Nuclear Weapons Laboratory in the New World Order." *American Ethnologist* 28:417–37.

Gusterson, H. 2005. "A Pedagogy of Diminishing Returns: Scientific Involution across Three Generations of Nuclear Weapons Science." In *Pedagogy and the Practice of Science*, ed. D. Kaiser, 75–107. Cambridge, Mass.: MIT Press.

Haas, J. 1989. "The Process of Apprenticeship: Ritual Ordeal and the Adoption of a Cloak of Competence." In *Apprenticeship: From Theory to Method and Back Again*, ed. M. W. Coy, 87–114. Albany: State University of New York Press.

Hacking, I. 1983. *Representing and Intervening: Introductory Topics in the Philosophy of Natural Science.* Cambridge: Cambridge University Press.

Hafferty, F. W. 1988. "Cadaver Stories and the Emotional Socialization of Medical Students." *Journal of Health and Social Behavior* 29:344–56.

Hafferty, F. W. 1991. *Into the Valley: Death and the Socialization of Medical Students.* New Haven, Conn.: Yale University Press.

Hafferty, F. W., and R. Franks. 1994. "The Hidden Curriculum, Ethics Teaching, and the Structure of Medical Education." *Academic Medicine* 69:861–71.

Hahn, R. 1983. "Biomedical Practice and Anthropological Theory: Frameworks and Directions." *Annual Review of Anthropology* 12:305–33.

Haraway, D. 1990. *Simians, Cyborgs, and Women: The Reinvention of Nature.* New York: Routledge.

Haraway, D. 1997. *Modest_Witness@Second_Millenium.FemaleMan©_Meets_Onco Mouse™: Feminism and Technoscience.* New York: Routledge.

Heidegger, M. 1996. *Being and Time.* Translated by J. Stamborough. Albany: State University of New York Press.

Heinrichs, W. L., and S. Srivastava. 2001. "The Changing Culture of Surgery." Unpublished working paper. Stanford University School of Medicine.

Helmreich, S. 1998. *Silicon Second Nature: Culturing Artificial Life in a Digital World.* Berkeley: University of California Press.

Herzig, R. 2006. *Suffering for Science: Reason and Sacrifice in Modern America.* New Brunswick, N.J.: Rutgers University Press.

Hirschauer, S. 1991. "The Manufacture of Bodies in Surgery." *Social Studies of Science* 21:279–319.

Hirschauer, S. 1994. "Towards a Methodology of Investigations into the Strangeness of One's Own Culture: A Response to Collins." *Social Studies of Science* 24:335–46.

Hogle, L 1999. *Recovering the Nation's Body: Cultural Memory, Medicine, and the Politics of Redemption.* New Brunswick, N.J.: Rutgers University Press.

Hopwood, N. 1999. "'Giving Body' to Embryos: Modeling, Mechanism, and the Microtome in Late Nineteenth-Century Anatomy." *Isis* 90:462–96.

Howell, J. D. 1995. *Technology in the Hospital.* Baltimore, Md.: Johns Hopkins University Press.

Hutchins, E. 1993. "Learning to Navigate." In *Understanding Practice: Perspectives on Activity and Context,* ed. S. Chaiklin and J. Lave, pp. 35–63. Cambridge: Cambridge University Press.

Johnson, B. 2010. *Persons and Things.* Cambridge, Mass.: Harvard University Press.

Kant, I. 2007. *Critique of Judgement.* Translated by J. C. Meredith. Oxford: Oxford University Press.

Kasics, K. 2003. *America Undercover: The Visible Corpse.* HBO documentary. Air date: January 26.

Katz, P. 1981. "Ritual in the Operating Room." *Ethnology* 20:335–50.

Katz, P. 1999. *The Scalpel's Edge: The Culture of Surgeons.* Boston: Pearson Allyn and Bacon.

Keane, W. 2007. *Christian Moderns: Freedom and Fetish in the Mission Encounter (The Anthropology of Christianity).* Berkeley: University of California Press.

Keller, E. F. 1984. *A Feeling for the Organism, 10th Anniversary Edition: The Life and Work of Barbara McClintock.* New York: Times Books.

Kleinman, A. 1997. *Writing at the Margin: Discourse between Anthropology and Medicine.* Berkeley: University of California Press.

Kleinman, A. 1999. "Moral Experience and Ethical Reflection: Can Ethnography Reconcile Them? A Quandary for 'The New Bioethics.'" *Daedalus* 128:69–97.

Knorr Cetina, K. 2000. *Epistemic Cultures: How the Sciences Make Knowledge.* Cambridge, Mass.: Harvard University Press.

Kohn, L. T., J. M. Corrigan, and M. S. Donaldson. 2000. *To Err Is Human: Building a Safer Health System.* Washington, D.C.: National Academies Press.

Kopytoff, I. 1986. "The Cultural Biography of Things: Commoditization as Process." In *The Social Life of Things: Commodities in Cultural Perspective,* ed. A. Appadurai, 64–91. New York: Cambridge University Press.

Kouzes, R. T., J. D. Myers, and W. A. Wulf. 1996. "Collaboratories: Doing Science on the Internet." *IEEE Computer Magazine* 29:40–46.

Kristeva, J. 1982. *Powers of Horror: An Essay on Abjection.* Translated by L. S. Roudiez. New York: Columbia University Press.

Kuriyama, S. 2002. *The Expressiveness of the Body and the Divergence of Greek and Chinese Medicine.* New York: Zone Books.

Landecker, H. 2000. "Immortality, in Vitro: A History of the HeLa Cell Line." In *Biotechnology and Culture: Bodies, Anxieties, Ethics,* ed. P. P. Brodwin. Bloomington: Indiana University Press.

Langwick, S. 2011. *Bodies, Politics, and African Healing: The Matter of Maladies in Tanzania.* Bloomington: Indiana University Press.

Laqueur, T. 1990. *Making Sex: Body and Gender from the Greeks to Freud.* Cambridge, Mass.: Harvard University Press.

Latour, B. 1986. "Visualization and Cognition: Thinking with Eyes and Hands." In *Knowledge and Society: Studies in the Sociology of Culture Past and Present,* ed. H. Kuklick and E. Long, 1–40. Greenwich, Conn.: Jai Press.

Latour, B. 1987. *Science in Action.* Cambridge, Mass.: Harvard University Press.

Latour, B. 1988. *The Pasteurization of France.* Translated by A. Sheridan and J. Law. Cambridge, Mass.: Harvard University Press.

Latour, B. 2002. "Morality and Technology: The End of the Means." *Theory, Culture, and Society* 19:247–60.

Latour, B. 2004. "How to Talk about the Body? The Normative Dimension of Science Studies." *Body & Society* 10:205–29.

Latour, B., and S. Woolgar. 1979. *Laboratory Life: The Construction of Scientific Facts.* Princeton, N.J.: Princeton University Press.

Lave, J., and E. Wenger. 1991. *Situated Learning: Legitimate Peripheral Participation.* Cambridge: Cambridge University Press.

Lawrence, C. 1998. "Medical Minds, Surgical Bodies: Corporeality and the Doctors." In *Science Incarnate: Historical Embodiments of Natural Knowledge,* ed. C. Lawrence and S. Shapin. Chicago: University of Chicago Press.

Lenoir, T. 2002. "The Virtual Surgeon." In *Semiotic Flesh: Information and the Human Body,* ed. P. Thurtle, 28–51. Seattle: University of Washington Press.

Lévi-Strauss, C. 1973. *Tristes Tropiques.* Translated by J. and D. Weightman. New York: Penguin.

Lock, M. 2002. *Twice Dead: Organ Transplants and the Reinvention of Death.* Berkeley: University of California Press.

Lock, M., and J. Farquhar, eds. 2007. *Beyond the Body Proper: Reading the Anthropology of Material Life*. Durham: Duke University Press.

Ludmerer, K. 1999. *Time to Heal: American Medical Education from the Turn of the Century to the Era of Managed Care*. New York: Oxford University Press.

Luhrmann, T. M. 2000. *Of Two Minds: The Growing Disorder in American Psychiatry*. New York: Knopf.

Lutz, C. 1986. "Emotion, Thought, and Estrangement: Emotion as a Cultural Category." *Cultural Anthropology* 6:1–16.

Lynch, M. 1990. "The Externalized Retina: Selection and Mathematization in the Visual Documentation of Objects in the Life Sciences." In *Representation in Scientific Practice*, ed. M. Lynch and S. Woolgar, 153–86. Cambridge, Mass.: MIT Press.

Lynch, M. 1994. "Collins, Hirschauer, and Winch: Ethnography, Exoticism, Surgery, Antisepsis and Dehorsification." *Social Studies of Science* 24:354–69.

Lyon, M. L., and J. M. Barbalet. 1994. "Society's Body: Emotion and the 'Somatization' of Social Theory." In *Embodiment and Experience*, ed. T. J. Csordas, 48–68. Cambridge: Cambridge University Press.

Mahmood, S. 2005. *The Politics of Piety: The Islamic Revival and the Feminist Subject*. Princeton, N.J.: Princeton University Press.

Martin, E. 2000. "AES Presidential Address: Mind-Body Problems." *American Ethnologist* 27:569–90.

Marx, K. 1992. *A Critique of Political Economy*. Vol. 1 of *Capital*. Translated by B. Fowkes. New York: Penguin.

Mauss, M. 1985. "A Category of the Human Mind: The Notion of Person; the Notion of Self." In *The Category of the Person*, ed. M. Carrithers, S. Collins, and S. Lukes, 1–26. Translated by W. D. Halls. New York: Cambridge University Press.

Mauss, M. 2007. "Techniques of the Body." In *Beyond the Body Proper*, ed. M. Lock and J. Farquhar, 50–68. Translated by B. Brewster. Durham: Duke University Press.

Merleau-Ponty, M. 1964. *The Primacy of Perception: And Other Essays on Phenomenological Psychology, the Philosophy of Art, History and Politics*. Edited by J. M. Edie. Translated by W. Cobb. Evanston, Ill.: Northwestern University Press.

Merleau-Ponty, M. 2002. *Phenomenology of Perception*. Translated by Colin Smith. London: Routledge.

Mol, A. 2002. *The Body Multiple: Ontology in Medical Practice*. Durham: Duke University Press.

Moreira, T. 2004. "Coordination and Embodiment in the Operating Room." *Body & Society* 10:109–29.

Myers, N. 2007. "Modeling Proteins, Making Scientists: An Ethnography of Pedagogy and Visual Cultures in Contemporary Structural Biology." Doctoral dissertation. http://hdl.handle.net/1721.1/40976.

Netter, F. 1997. *Atlas of Human Anatomy*. Teterboro, N.J.: Icon Learning Systems.

Noble, D. F. 1979. "Social Choice in Machine Design: The Case of Automatically Controlled Machine Tools." In *Case Studies on the Labor Process*, ed. A. Zimbalist, 18–50. New York: Monthly Review Press.

Papp, K. K., E. P. Stoller, P. Sage, J. E. Aikens, J. Owens, A. Avidan, B. Phillips, R. Rosen, and K. P. Strohl. 2004. "The Effects of Sleep Loss and Fatigue on Resident-

Physicians: A Multi-Institutional, Mixed-Method Study." *Academic Medicine* 79: 394–406.

Pickering, A. 1995. *The Mangle of Practice: Time, Agency, and Science.* Chicago: University of Chicago Press.

Pinch, T. J., H. M. Collins, and L. Carbone. 1996. "Inside Knowledge: Second Order Measures of Skill." *Sociological Review* 44:163–86.

Plato. 2007. *The Republic.* Translated by D. Lee. New York: Penguin.

Polanyi, M. 1962. *Personal Knowledge: Towards a Post-Critical Philosophy.* Chicago: University of Chicago Press.

Polanyi, M. 1966. *The Tacit Dimension.* Garden City, N.Y.: Doubleday.

Pollock, D. 1996. "Training Tales: U.S. Medical Autobiography." *Cultural Anthropology* 11:339–61.

Porter, T. M. 1992. "Quantification and the Accounting Ideal in Science." *Social Studies of Science* 22:633–51.

Prentice, R. 2002. "Conference Report: MMVR02/10 — Digital Upgrades: Applying Moore's Law to Health." *Medscape TechMed eJournal* 2. http://www.medscape.com/viewarticle/430200 (accessed March 1, 2004).

Prentice, R. 2005. "The Anatomy of a Surgical Simulation: The Mutual Articulation of Bodies in and through the Machine." *Social Studies of Science* 35:837–66.

Prentice, R. 2008. "The Visible Woman." In *The Inner History of Devices,* ed. S. Turkle. Cambridge, Mass.: MIT Press.

Pryde, F. R., and S. M. Black. 2006. "Scottish Anatomy Departments: Adapting to Change." *Scottish Medical Journal* 51:16–20.

Rabinow, P. 1996. *Essays on the Anthropology of Reason.* Princeton, N.J.: Princeton University Press.

Rajchman, J. 1988. "Foucault's Art of Seeing." *October* 44:88–117.

Rapp, R. 1999. *Testing Women, Testing the Fetus.* New York: Routledge.

Reeves, B., and C. Nass. 1996. *The Media Equation: How People Treat Computers, Television, and New Media Like Real People and Places.* Cambridge: Cambridge University Press.

Reiner, M. 2001. "The Role of Haptics in Immersive Telecommunication Environments." Unpublished working paper. Stanford University School of Medicine.

Rheingold, H. 1992. *Virtual Reality.* New York: Simon and Schuster.

Richardson, R. 1987. *Death, Dissection, and the Destitute.* Chicago: University of Chicago Press.

Rorty, R. 1979. *Philosophy and the Mirror of Nature.* Princeton, N.J.: Princeton University Press.

Rosaldo, M. Z. 1984. "Toward an Anthropology of Self and Feeling." In *Culture Theory: Essays on Mind, Self, and Emotion,* ed. R. Shweder and R. Levine, 137–57. Cambridge: Cambridge University Press.

Rosenberg, B. H., D. Landsittel, and T. D. Averch. 2005. "Can Video Games Be Used to Predict or Improve Laparoscopic Skills?" *Journal of Endourology* 19:372–76.

Rosser, J. C., Jr., and P. J. Lynch. 2007. "The Impact of Video Games on Training Surgeons in the Twenty-First Century." *Archives of Surgery* 142:181–86.

Sacks, O. 2003. "The Minds Eye: A Neurologist's Notebook." *New Yorker.* July 28, 48–59.

Samuel, S., M. W. Dirsmith, and B. McElroy. 2005. "Monetized Medicine: From the Physical to the Fiscal." *Accounting, Organizations, and Society* 30:249–78.

Satava, R. M. 1995. "Medicine 2001: The King Is Dead." In *Interactive Technology and the New Paradigm for Healthcare*, ed. R. M. Satava, K. Morgan, and H. B. Sieburg. Amsterdam: IOS Press.

Satava, R. M. 1997. "Virtual Reality for Medical Applications." *Information Technology Applications in Biomedicine.* Unpublished talk prepared for IEEE Engineering in Medicine and Biology Society, Region 8 International Conference. Prague, Czech Republic, September 7–9.

Satava, R. M. 2006. "How the Future of Surgery Is Changing: Robotics, Telesurgery, Surgical Simulators, and Other Advanced Technologies." Unpublished article. http://depts.washington.edu/surg/Future-of-Surgery-0606.pdf (accessed November 10, 2008).

Satava, R. M. 2008. "Historical Review of Surgical Simulation—A Personal Perspective." *World Journal of Surgery* 32:141–48.

Satava, R. M. 2004. "Telemedicine, Virtual Reality, and Other Technologies That Will Transform How Healthcare Is Provided." Unpublished paper prepared for 2nd CREST Symposium on Telemedicine, Tele-immersion, and Tele-existence. University of Tokyo. December. 10. http://depts.washington.edu/biointel/index.html (accessed November 10, 2008).

Scheper-Hughes, N. 2000. "The Global Traffic in Human Organs." *Current Anthropology* 41:191–224.

Scheper-Hughes, N., and M. Lock. 1987. "The Mindful Body: A Prolegomenon to Future Work in Medical Anthropology." *Medical Anthropology Quarterly* 1:6–41.

Schlich, T. 2002. *Surgery, Science, and Industry: A Revolution in Fracture Care, 1950s–1990s.* Houndmills, Basingstoke, England: Palgrave.

Schlich, T. 2007. "The Art and Science of Surgery: Innovation and Concepts of Medical Practice in Operative Fracture Care, 1960s–1970s." *Science, Technology, & Human Values* 32:65–87.

Segal, D. 1988. "A Patient So Dead: American Medical Students and Their Cadavers." *Anthropological Quarterly* 61:17–25.

Sennett, R. 2009. *The Craftsman.* New Haven, Conn.: Yale University Press.

Sharp, L. 2001. "Commodified Kin: Death, Mourning, and Competing Claims on the Bodies of Organ Donors in the United States." *American Anthropologist* 103:112–33.

Sharp, L. 2006. *Strange Harvest: Organ Transplants, Denatured Bodies, and the Transformed Self.* Berkeley: University of California Press.

Shem, S. 2003. *The House of God: The Classic Novel of Life and Death in an American Hospital.* New York: Dell.

Spencer, A. U., and D. H. Teitelbaum. 2005. "Impact of Work-Hour Restrictions on Residents' Operative Volume on a Subspecialty Surgical Service." *Journal of the American College of Surgeons* 200:670–76.

Spitzer, V. 1996. "The Visible Human Male: A Technical Report." *Journal of the American Medical Informatics Association* 3:18–130.

Star, S. L., and J. R. Griesemer. 1989. "Institutional Ecology, 'Translations' and Boundary Objects: Amateurs and Professionals in Berkeley's Museum of Vertebrate Zoology, 1907–39." *Social Studies of Science* 19:387–420.

Stevens, R. 1999. *In Sickness and in Wealth: American Hospitals in the Twentieth Century.* Baltimore, Md.: Johns Hopkins University Press.

Strathern, M. 1992. *Reproducing the Future: Essays on Anthropology, Kinship, and the New Reproductive Technologies.* Manchester, England: Manchester University Press.

Strathern, M. E. 2000. *Audit Cultures.* New York: Routledge.

Strathern, M. E. 2004. "The Whole Person and Its Artifacts." *Annual Review of Anthropology* 33:1–19.

Suchman, L. 1987. *Plans and Situated Actions: The Problem of Human Machine Communication.* Cambridge: Cambridge University Press.

Suchman, L. 2002. "Located Accountabilities in Technology Production." *Scandinavian Journal of Information Systems* 14:91–105.

Taschen, A. 2001. *Encyclopedia Anatomica.* Florence, Italy: Museo La Specola.

Taylor, F. W. 2009. *Principles of Scientific Management.* Ithaca, N.Y.: Cornell University Press.

Thompson, C. 2005. *Making Parents: The Ontological Choreography of Reproductive Technologies.* Cambridge, Mass.: MIT Press.

Timmermans, S. 2003. *The Gold Standard: The Challenge of Evidence-Based Medicine.* Philadelphia: Temple University Press.

Traweek, S. 1988. *Beamtimes and Lifetimes: The World of High Energy Physicists.* Cambridge, Mass.: Harvard University Press.

Turkle, S. 1984. *The Second Self: Computers and the Human Spirit.* New York: Simon and Schuster.

Turkle, S. 1995. *Life on the Screen: Identity in the Age of the Internet.* New York: Simon and Schuster.

Turkle, S. 2004. "'Spinning' Technology: What We Are Not Thinking about When We Are Thinking about Computers." In *Technological Visions*, ed. M. Sturken, D. Thomas, and S. J. Ball-Rokeach. Philadelphia: Temple University Press.

Turner, V. 1967. *The Forest of Symbols: Aspects of Ndembu Ritual.* Ithaca, N.Y.: Cornell University Press.

Urciuoli, B. 2008. "Skills and Selves in the New Workplace." *American Ethnologist* 35:211–28.

Van Dijck, J. 2005. *The Transparent Body: A Cultural Analysis of Medical Imaging.* Seattle: University of Washington Press.

Van Gennep, A. 1908. *The Rites of Passage.* Chicago: University of Chicago Press.

Varela, F. 1992. "The Reenchantment of the Concrete." In *Incorporations*, ed. J. Crary and S. Kwinter, 320–38. New York: Zone Books.

Waldby, C. 2000. *The Visible Human Project: Informatic Bodies and Posthuman Medicine.* New York: Routledge.

Weber, M. 1946. *From Max Weber: Essays in Sociology.* Edited by H. H. Gerth and C. W. Mills. Translated by H. H. Gerth. New York: Oxford University Press.

Young, K. 1997. *Presence in the Flesh: The Body in Medicine.* Cambridge, Mass.: Harvard University Press.

Zare, S. M., J. Galanko, K. E. Behrns, M. J. Koruda, L. M. Boyle, D. R. Farley, S. R. Evans, A. A. Meyer, G. F. Sheldon, and T. M. Farrell. 2004. "Psychological Well-Being of Surgery Residents before the Eighty-Hour Work Week: A Multi-institutional Study." *Journal of the American College of Surgeons* 198:633–40.

Zetka, J. R. 2003. *Surgeons and the Scope.* Ithaca, N.Y.: Cornell University Press.

Zuboff, S. 1984. *In the Age of the Smart Machine: The Future of Work and Power.* New York: Basic Books.

Zuger, A. 2004. "Anatomy Lessons, a Vanishing Rite for Young Doctors." *New York Times.* March 23. http://www.nytimes.com/2004/03/23/health/23CADA.html.

INDEX

Pseudonyms are designated by asterisks.

cognitive model of medical knowing, 12–15, 88, 98

compassion, 127–31, 226, 261, 266

control, 29, 137–69; anatomical knowledge as expression of, 152–55; and bodily discipline, 143; in career life cycle, 167, 271n8; central importance of, 137–38; as ethical practice, 138, 139, 165–68, 169; and imitation of superiors, 165–66; nonverbal guiding as expression of, 156–57; physical expression of, 147–52; preparedness as expression of, 147–52; procedural understanding and confidence as expressions of, 157–65; restraint as expression of, 145–46; role of time in, 143–44; and Satava's technological vision, 203–4; sterility protocols, 140–43; and surgical embodiment, 139–40; and surgical *habitus*, 140; as technique of the body, 138, 139; and training surgical techniques, 165–68; of violence, 137, 167

Corso, Jeremy,* 148–52

Csordas, Thomas, 18, 194, 195

decision making: and emotional management, 130; and experience, 145–46; rules-based decision making, 12; and spatial awareness in surgery, 120; standardization of, 205; technologies for, 72, 205; value of, 118

Defense Advanced Research Projects Agency, 202

De Humani Corporis Fabrica (Vesalius), 41, 73, 76

Despret, Vinciane, 15–16, 131, 133

detachment, 28, 36–38, 52, 66–67, 128–30

Douglas, Mary, 67

Dreyfus, Hubert, 89, 227, 249

electronic medical records, 204

embodiment in surgical learning, 6–9, 9–12, 260

emotions and emotional lessons: and cadaver dissection, 10, 33–38, 40, 41, 47–51, 58–62, 86–87, 258, 259, 261; cultural construction of, 65–67; and detachment, 28, 36–38, 66, 128–30, 257; and errors in clinical practice, 270n10; and judgment, 66, 127–29, 131, 133; management of, 127–31; role of, in medicine, 224; and simulation technologies, 225

English, Jill,* 64–65, 66, 115–16, 134, 173–74

"enterprising up," 200

Epidemics (Hippocrates), 11, 60

errors in clinical practice: and anatomical knowledge, 89–90; and emotions, 270n10; and reforms advocated in medical education, 19, 123, 232; stakes of, 164; Satava's vision for reducing, 205; and simulation technologies, 232, 274n4; as teaching tools, 259; and work hours of residents, 123–25

ethics and moral formation, 49; and cadaver dissection, 35–36, 49, 50–51, 60–61, 259; and control of violence, 137, 167; and decision making, 145–46; Hippocratic Oath and "do no harm," 11, 60, 137, 159, 169, 259–66; and imperative of control, 169 (*see also* control); outside the biomedical frame, 169; role of technical proficiency in, 8, 11, 138, 140, 166–68, 226, 260; of simulation technologies, 2, 262–66; and surgical *habitus*, 140; as techniques of the body, 10, 138; term, 270n3; violence vs. harm in, 60, 137; and virtues of medical morality, 224

evidence-based medicine, 12

exam preparation, 80–81, 97, 232

Farquhar, Judith, 9, 15

fellowships for surgery, 119–21

Fetters, Graeme,* 80, 98

Fischer, Michael M. J., 207, 215

Flynn, Patrick,* 239, 240, 241–42, 248

Foucault, Michel, 8, 140, 159, 175

Fox, Renee, 36–37, 41, 128

Franks, Ronald, 106, 107

"gaze," 175–76, 193. *See also* perception in biomedicine

gender differences, 163–64, 226, 269n82

Goffman, Erving, 65, 141

Gold, Emily,* 125–26, 163–64

Good, Byron, 37, 108, 109

Griesemer, James R., 222

Groopman, Jerome, 103, 270n10

habits and habituation, 107, 140, 195–97

habitus, 8, 14, 67, 140, 196

Hafferty, Frederic W., 51, 106, 107, 109, 268n8

Haraway, Donna, 195

Hartmann, Sarah,* 244–46, 250

Heidegger, Martin, 148

Heinrichs, W. Leroy, 107–8

"Helping Hands Syndrome," 142

hidden curriculum of medical school, 104–10; affective abilities, 123; embodiment of, 135; management of emotions, 127; and simulation technologies, 265; and tacit knowledge, 269n5

hierarchy in medical education, 113, 135, 139–42, 150, 165

Hippocratic Oath, 11, 60, 137, 159, 169, 267n2

Hirschauer, Stefan, 70, 180, 228, 229–30, 271n3

Holomers (holographic medical electronic representations), 204, 225

Hunt, Richard,* 34, 75–76, 82–84, 90–91, 92, 127–30

imaging technology in clinical practice, 95, 101, 201–2

imitation of superiors: and authority of instructor, 165; as endpoint of surgical education, 166; and the hidden curriculum, 107; of professional qualities, 29, 109, 113, 118–20, 260; of technical skills, 10, 144, 165–66, 260; and trajectory of career, 105

Immersion Corporation, 202

instruments, surgical: and body of the practitioner, 189–93, 244; for surgical simulation, 234, 241–44

intuition, 109, 133–34. *See also* judgment

joking, 161, 162, 259

judgment: attempts to codify, 134; conceptions of, 132–33; development of, 5, 8, 29, 118, 133–35; embodiment of, 109, 131–35; and emotions, 66, 127–29, 131, 133; and residencies, 105, 109, 118; in surgical decisions, 120, 145–46

Kaplan, Jerry,* 48–51, 52–57

Kristeva, Julia, 67

laboratories, 38–44, 215

Laqueur, Thomas, 98

Latour, Bruno, 228–29, 250

Lenoir, Timothy, 201, 207, 212, 215

Lock, Margaret, 9, 15, 37, 47

Lockheed Martin Corporation, 202

Ludmerer, Kenneth, 106–7, 109

Luhrmann, Tanya M., 109, 126, 133–34

Lynch, Michael, 235

Mahmood, Saba, 8, 67, 196

Martinez, Julie,* 104, 145–46, 157–65, 167

Mauss, Marcel, 10, 66–67, 140, 165, 166, 268n1

Meier, Gabriel,* 78–80, 87–89

mental models, 12–15, 72, 82–89, 98

Merleau-Ponty, Maurice: on habit, 196; on judgment, 132; on perception, 18, 132–33, 267n4; on touch, 86; on use of instruments, 189; on wonder, 52

metaphors of surgeons, 11, 122

Miller, Ken,* 152–57

minimally invasive surgery, 29–30, 172–98; anatomy identification in, 179, 182–83, 184; directional orientation in, 181, 186–87; instruments of, 187–93, 258; movement of surgeon in, 160, 272nn18–19; objectification in, 194; and open surgeries, 173–76; positioning patients for, 177–78; sensory aspects of, 189–94, 195; and simulation technologies, 232–33, 266; spatial perception in, 186–87, 189–94, 197–98, 258–59; and surgical embodiment, 157–65, 172, 195–96; and surgical perception, 171–72, 173–76, 176–86; teaching methods for, 157–65; two-dimensional imagery in, 177, 187, 258; verbal navigation of, 158–59, 189, 258–59

Mol, Annemarie, 7, 24, 59, 185, 236

moral formation. *See* ethics and moral formation

muscular gestalt, development of, 227–28, 240, 249

mutual articulation, 16, 228–31, 248–51

Myers, Natasha, 158

Nassif, Amal:* disorientation of, 103–4, 117; emotional reaction of, 131–32, 133; and minimally invasive surgery, 197; and sterility protocols, 142, 167; and surgical perception, 177–86

National Library of Medicine, 202

Nguyen, Cory,* 142, 177–86, 197, 198

nuclear weapons design, 71

nurses, 226

object formation, 18, 19, 24

objectification, 16–19; in cadaver dissection, 28, 33, 34–38, 42, 58–59, 62, 67–68, 84, 256, 257; and detachment, 257; in language, 63; as learned response of practitioners, 38; and minimally invasive surgery, 194; patients-as-products ideal, 205–6, 223; and Satava's technological vision, 206; self-objectification of students, 58–59, 268n2; in surgery, 62–65, 178, 180

objectivity, 36, 37, 66–67, 129–31

ontological choreography, 17, 38, 58, 63, 256

operating room, hierarchies and protocols in, 140–42

organ donation, 46, 47

pathologies, 18, 37, 97, 258

patients: objectification of own bodies, 38; as products, 205–6, 223; and Satava's technological vision, 205–6, 207; standardized patients, 273n8; and surgeons' emotional management, 127–31; and trends in medicine, 4. *See also* body of the patient; objectification

perception in biomedicine, 18–19; and action, 171–72, 177, 178, 183–84, 186, 188, 190, 195; in cadaver dissection, 180–81; development of, 195; and lack of visibility, 173–75; and the medical "gaze," 175–76, 193; and minimally invasive surgery, 171–72, 173–76, 176–86; and role of touch, 173–76; and surgical embodiment, 198; technology's effect on, 172, 258

Perrotta, Nick:* affective scaffolding of, 122; bedside manner of, 121–22; embodied knowing of, 173–75, 197; on "good hands," 110–11; on stakes of surgical practice, 1, 259–60; surgical restraint of, 145–46, 167

Phillips, Fred,* 243, 245–46, 247, 250

Polanyi, Michael, 147

Pollock, Donald, 36–37

Porter, Stephanie,* 82–84

Porter, Ted, 251

problem-based learning, 83

Rabinow, Paul, 223

Rapp, Rayna, 26

rationalized medical practice: arguments for, 224–25; aspects of medicine lost to, 225, 226; and caring work of medicine, 226; limitations of, 12; and training technologies, 20–21, 27, 224. *See also* reforms

reforms: of residency education, 106, 123, 274n3; standardization emphasis in, 30, 117, 123, 200, 205, 232, 253, 274n3; and training technologies, 2–3, 19–21, 232, 253, 274n3

residencies, 29, 103–35; and anatomical knowledge, 90; and clinical perception, 95; clinical rotations, 115–16; competencies developed in, 122–23; confidence of residents, 197; demands of, 105–6; disorienting quality of, 103, 113, 116, 117; doubts of residents, 103–4; duration of, 269n3; "good hands" in, 110–11; hidden curriculum in, 104–10, 123, 127, 135, 265, 269n5; learning process in, 111–23; nature of, 3–4; preparations of, 115, 271n12; professionalism expected in, 113; reforms advocated in, 106, 123, 274n3; sacrifices expected of, 124–25, 127; transition to, 106, 135; trends affecting, 4; work hours of residents, 105, 123–27

Rosaldo, Michelle, 61

rules-based decision making, 12

Sacks, Oliver, 14–15

Satava, Richard, 99, 202–8, 225, 226, 273n3

scaffolding learning experiences, 120, 122

Scheper-Hughes, Nancy, 37

Sennett, Richard, 112

sensory aspects of biomedicine: auditory cues, 14; in cadaver dissection, 23, 55–57; embodiment of, 257–58; importance of,

sensory aspects of biomedicine (*cont.*)
25; in minimally invasive surgery, 189–
94, 195; overlap of the senses, 172; and
pathology identification, 18; sight, 13–15,
172, 173–76, 190, 197–98. *See also* perception in biomedicine
Sharp, Lesley, 46
sight, 13–15, 172, 173–76, 190, 197–98. *See
also* perception in biomedicine
simulation technologies: advantages of, 6;
and affective abilities, 225; and body
objects (informatic models), 20, 201,
220–23, 225, 238; and body of the practitioner, 194, 197, 198, 218, 227–28, 241–48,
248–49; and errors in clinical practice,
232, 274n4; ethics of, 2, 262–66; and
flight simulation, 202, 273n2; haptic
technologies in, 25, 228, 231, 233–34, 239–
40, 241, 242, 244–48, 249–51; and muscular gestalt, 227–28, 240; and rationalized
medical practice, 224; skill-building
potential of, 259, 263–64, 265–66; and
standardization of medical education,
30, 253; surgical rehearsal, 199. *See also*
surgical simulation
Smith, Allan,* 82–83
Srivastava, Sakti, 107–8
Star, Susan Leigh, 222
sterility rules, 141–42
Stevens, Rosemary, 226
Strathern, Marilyn, 34, 64, 200
Suchman, Lucy, 72
surgeons: anatomical knowledge of, 229–31,
236; authority of, 165 (*see also* imitation of
superiors); as automaton, 129, 223, 226;
autonomy of, 207; competencies embodied by, 11, 111–13, 118–23, 126, 165–66, 168,
197; "good hands" of, 110–11; and "handiness," 148; nondominant-hand proficiency of, 148–52; perceptual capacities
of, 18–19 (*see also* perception in biomedicine); performance evaluations by,
206, 266; and physicians, 126; qualities of,
139, 272n24; Satava's vision for, 226; teaching time of, 144; technological approach
contrasted with, 221–22; in technology
design research, 212–14, 242–43; training
required for, 6, 119

surgery: activation of the person by, 63–65;
emotional toll on, 25–26; fellowships for,
119–21; metaphors for, 11; objectification
by, 62–65, 178, 180; open surgeries, 173–
75, 233; preparations and protocols for,
141–42, 271n3; risks associated with, 145–
46; robotic surgery, 223, 272n19; spatial
awareness in, 120. *See also* control; minimally invasive surgery; surgical simulation
surgical simulation, 30, 227–52; advantages
of, 232, 250–51, 252; collision detection
in, 241–42; and embodied knowledge,
244–48; feedback loops in, 233–34, 242–
43; future of, 233; and haptic technologies, 25, 228, 233–34, 241, 242, 244–
48, 249–51; instruments of, 234, 241–44;
modeling process in, 234–41, 248–49,
274n9; and mutual articulation, 228–31,
248–51; research areas of, 228; surgical
rehearsal, 199; and the user's body, 241–
48, 248–49; and virtual patients, 232–34
Sutherland, Ivan, 201

tacit knowledge, 112, 269n5
Taylor, Frederick W., 205
teaching methods, 29; comparing anatomical differences, 272n22; correcting errors,
259–60; drawing procedures, 153, 154–55;
framing practice, 149–52, 158, 161, 164,
166; guiding, 153–54, 156–57; joking, 161,
162, 259; quizzing students, 153, 154; storytelling, 154, 155–56; and teaching time
of surgeons, 144
technical skills: and affective skills, 11, 226;
as care of self, 218, 226; disassembly/ex-
traction of, for digital technologies, 20,
200, 208, 225, 227; ethical imperative
associated with, 8, 11, 138, 140, 166–68,
226, 260; habituation of, 107, 140, 195–
96; imitation of, 10, 144, 165–66, 260;
and simulation technologies, 252, 265–
66; and virtues of medical morality, 224
techniques of the body: and cadaver dissection, 258; and emotion, 66; ethical practice as, 8, 138; and the hidden curriculum, 110; incorporation of, in medical
learning, 9; intuition as, 109; "prestigious

imitation" in, 165; scholarship on, 10; and technologies for medical training, 12; unquantifiable skills of, 10, 105
technologies for medical training, 30, 199–226; advantages of, 19, 91; and affects, 20; and anticipation of technical requirements, 19; aspects of medicine lost to, 225, 226, 252, 253–54; autonomy-diminishing potential of, 207; body objects (informatic models), 20, 201, 220–23, 225, 238; cadaver-dissection alternatives, 6, 22, 71–73, 91–93 (*see also* anatomy, computational); changes effected by, 4, 19–21; and cognitive model of medical knowing, 13; computer modeling, 237–41; and decision making, 72, 205; and design laboratories, 30, 215; development of, 215–20; and disassembly/extraction of surgeons' skills, 20, 200, 208, 225, 227; electronic medical records, 204, 225; and embodiment in surgical learning, 10, 160; haptic technologies, 25, 228, 231, 233–34, 239–40, 241, 242, 244–48, 249–51; and material practices, 72–73; medical technologies laboratories, 208–12, 215; and military research, 201, 202; motives for moving to, 71–72; multidisciplinary aspects of, 212–14; open-ended exploration in, 81; pace of incorporation of, 27; patient-on-demand concept, 227, 253; and perception, 172, 258; practices developed from, 72–73; and rationalized medical practice, 20–21, 27, 224; and reduction of bodies to parts, 24; and reforms advocated in medical education, 2–3, 19–21, 232, 253, 274n3; robotics, 176, 203, 205, 223, 251, 272n19; and rules-based medicine, 12; Satava's vision for, 202–8, 226; surgeons' competencies contrasted with, 221–22; and variations in anatomy, 96, 100, 204;

virtual reality, 201–8, 232. *See also* simulation technologies; surgical simulation; virtual patients
telemedicine system, 203
Terminologia Anatomica, 73, 76
Thompson, Charis, 17, 38, 268n1
Tomaso, Ernan,* 77, 95–96, 261
touch, role of: in cadaver dissection, 85–86, 87, 89, 93, 100; and sight, 172, 173–76; and surgical simulations, 249–50

Van Gennep, Arnold, 84
Varela, Francisco, 81
Vesalius, Andreas, 41, 73, 76
Vidal, Sonja,* 210–11, 218–23, 240, 243
violence vs. harm, 60, 137
virtual patients: advantages of, 232; killing, ethics of, 2, 262–63; and minimally invasive surgery, 233–34; and reforms advocated in medical education, 2–3; as surrogates for living patients, 2, 262–65. *See also* simulation technologies
virtual reality, 201–8, 232. *See also* surgical simulation
virtues of medical morality, 224
Visible Human Project, 21–22, 76, 91, 98, 267n5, 269n6, 269n8
visual bias in medical training, 13–15

wax models of cadavers, 41
Weber, Max, 224
Wilson, Anna:* anatomical knowledge of, 79–80; on anatomy's future, 78; on "good hands," 110; on killing virtual patients, 2, 262–64; and minimally invasive surgery, 188–94, 198; and object/person duality in surgery, 62–64, 66; on patient relations, 127–29; on readiness of trainees, 147; on surgical instruments, 147; teaching methods of, 148–52, 152–57
wonder, sense of, 51–57, 64, 89

Rachel Prentice is Associate Professor of Science & Technology
Studies at Cornell University.

Library of Congress Cataloging-in-Publication Data
Prentice, Rachel.
Bodies in formation : an ethnography of anatomy and surgery
education / Rachel Prentice.
p. cm. — (Experimental futures)
Includes bibliographical references and index.
ISBN 978-0-8223-5143-6 (cloth : alk. paper)
ISBN 978-0-8223-5157-3 (pbk. : alk. paper)
1. Medical students—Effect of technological innovations on.
2. Residents (Medicine)—Effect of technological innovations
on. 3. Medicine—Study and teaching (Graduate)—Social
aspects. 4. Physician and patient. I. Title. II. Series: Experimental futures.
R840.P74 2012
610.76—dc23   2012011637